Photoreceptors

NATO ASI Series

Advanced Science Institutes Series

A series presenting the results of activities sponsored by the NATO Science Committee, which aims at the dissemination of advanced scientific and technological knowledge, with a view to strengthening links between scientific communities.

The series is published by an international board of publishers in conjunction with the NATO Scientific Affairs Division

A	Life Sciences	Plenum Publishing Corporation
B	Physics	New York and London
C	Mathematical and Physical Sciences	D. Reidel Publishing Company Dordrecht, Boston, and Lancaster
D	Behavioral and Social Sciences	Martinus Nijhoff Publishers
E	Engineering and Materials Sciences	The Hague, Boston, and Lancaster
F	Computer and Systems Sciences	Springer-Verlag
G	Ecological Sciences	Berlin, Heidelberg, New York, and Tokyo

Recent Volumes in this Series

Series A: Life Sciences

Photoreceptors

Edited by

A. Borsellino

University of Genova
Genova, Italy

and

L. Cervetto

Institute of Neurophysiology of the CNR
Pisa, Italy

Plenum Press
New York and London
Published in cooperation with NATO Scientific Affairs Division

Proceedings of a NATO Advanced Study Institute on
Photoreceptors,
held July 1–12, 1981,
in Erice, Sicily, Italy

QP
481
,N345
1981

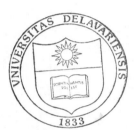

Library of Congress Cataloging in Publication Data

NATO Advanced Study Institute on Photoreceptors (1981: Erice, Italy)
    Photoreceptors.

    (NATO ASI series. Series A, Life sciences; v. 75)
    "Proceedings of a NATO Advanced Study Institute on Photoreceptors, held
July 1–12, 1981, in Erice, Sicily, Italy"—T.p. verso.
    "Published in cooperation with NATO Scientific Affairs Division."
    Bibliography: p.
    Includes index.
    1. Photoreceptors—Congresses. I. Borsellino, Antonio. II. Cervetto, L. III. North
Atlantic Treaty Organization. Scientific Affairs Division. IV. Title. V. Series: NATO
ASI series. Series A, Life sciences; v. 75 [DNLM: 1. Photoreceptors—Congresses.
WL 102.9 N279p 1981]
QP481.N345   1981   591.1'823   84-2131
ISBN 0-306-41629-8

©1984 Plenum Press, New York
A Division of Plenum Publishing Corporation
233 Spring Street, New York, N.Y. 10013

Printed in the United States of America

PREFACE

This volume originates from a NATO Advanced Study Institute on "Photoreceptors" dedicated to M.G.F. Fuortes, held in Erice 1-12 July 1981. The lectures given at the course provided a general review of the photoreceptors functions in both vertebrate and invertebrate eyes. Elaborating on the most recent hypotheses the lectures also added new and interesting details. In order to preserve the novelty and freshness of the subject matter and thus ensure the usefulness of the volume, the authors in their written contributions emphasize more specific findings of their current research rather than the tutorial nature of the lectures actually presented.

The contributors of this volume wish to dedicate their papers to the memory of Mike Fuortes, who has been for many of them an inspiring collegue and friend.

Five papers that do not strictly pertain to the topics of the course are also included in the volume, the authors could not attend the meeting, but wanted to contribute an article to this memorial volume.

A. Borsellino
L. Cervetto

CONTENTS

INTERACTION BETWEEN LIGHT AND MATTER

A. Borsellino

Istituto di Scienze Fisiche, Università di Genova
Italy

In this chapter I will sketch briefly some general idea that can be useful in looking to photoreceptors as devices for detecting light and as informational tools used by the various organisms.

The present volume for many of the contributors -including myself- is thought to be a memorial document for the late M.G.F. Fuortes. Since all who knew him will remember the care and the efforts he was always willing to spend for a better understanding in the field in which he gave such important contributions, the present discussion can find its justification.

1. Photoreceptors

Photoreceptors are cells specialized to detect light, coming mainly from the Sun, in the 240-700 nm wavelength range. Particular structures, developed in order to capture the light photons, contain an absorbing pigment, the retinal or vitamin A, made up, as some other organic pigments (carotene, xanthophyll, lycopene) of combinations of isoprene units. Such molecules can have different isometric states and they can pass from one to the other after absorbing a photon (Fig. 1).

The absorbing molecule is functionally associated to an intrinsic membrane protein, an opsin. By such association, the isometric transition of the retinal triggers a chain of molecular events, changing at the end the ionic permeability of the cell membrane and resulting in this way in the generation of an electric signal.

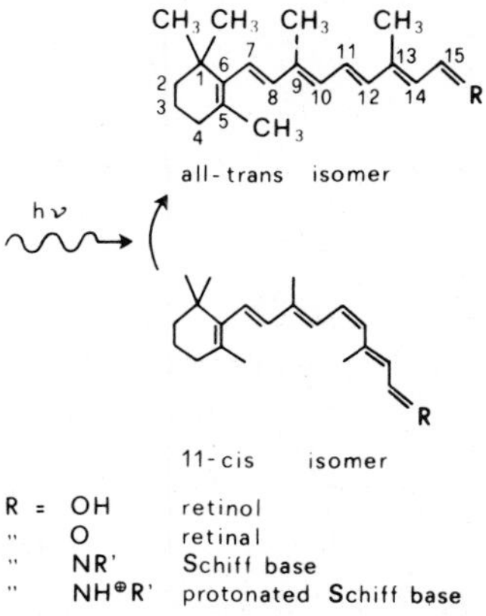

CH₃ CH₃ CH₃   CH₃

all-trans isomer

11-cis   isomer

R = OH   retinol
   "   O   retinal
   "   NR'   Schiff base
   "   NH⊕R'   protonated Schiff base

Fig. 1.   Isometric transition of the visual pigment due the absorp-
          tion of a photon.

To capture light efficiently the pigment-protein complexes
(rhodopsin) must be densely packed and two main evolutionary lines
can be traced (Vinnikov, 1982):

i) the microvillous type, in which the plasma membrane enlarges
and develops folds

ii) the ciliated type, in which the folds develop in the membrane of a modified cilium (cones) and can be pinched off to become
disks (rods).

The first type is found typically in arthropods, molluscs,
flatworms; the second one in the vertebrates, cephalochordata,
echinoderms.

Light, sound and odors are used by animals to obtain information from a distance, to regulate their behavior in the evironment
in which they live. In what follows we will examine briefly how
well photoreceptors operate as informational devices. Furthermore
we will present a short review of the physical interaction between
the light and the receptor structures.

Some aspects of the complicated sequences of events that follow
the initial step of the light absorption are presented in the other
chapters of the book.

2. Photoreceptors as informational devices

It is well recognized that living organisms are open dissipative systems, not in thermodynamical equilibrium with their environment. In a isothermal cavity the electromagnetic radiation has the same density everywhere and in all directions. Such a radiation would not be of any use for informational purposes and in fact animals ended in an ecological niche resembling such a situation (caverns) evolve toward the reabsorption of their photoreceptors.

The solar light, coming from a quite hot source, modulated by reflection or absorption from the cold bodies of the environment, can be informative, when detected with appropriate devices.

We can think of an "ideal" light detector as a device which, without adding noise or distortion, produce a signal when it absorbs energy from the optical field. For very low light intensity, the quantal structure of light shows itself clearly and makes the absorption of photons a discontinuous process, that must be described and analysed by statistical methods. We can make only statements about the probability of arrival of photons, the probability that a photon will be absorbed and revealed by our device, with some efficiency lower than 1.

When the light beam power P is incident on the detector and N is the noise power level, the maximum rate of information is limited by the channel capacity C. The energy spent per bit is given by the ratio $E_o = P/C$. The channel capacity is proportional to the passing bandwidth B of the measuring instrument and depends on the noise to signal power ratio: $C = B \log_2 (1+P/N)$.

Photon beams can be prepared and modulated very finely, becoming a powerful tool in the design of experiments. Some warnings seem appropriate, to keep in mind the quantal structure of light, because the statistical properties of a photon beam often enter the discussion of the results. For example, when the average beam intensity is fixed, giving the number N of photon/cm^2. s, then we must take in account that the number will in fact fluctuate around N, the type of fluctuation depending on the source characteristics. Such fluctuations give rise to an "external" noise for the photoreceptors under study, distinct from the "internal" one, due to the structural properties of the receptor itself. The light noise ΔE can be split in two terms: one due properly to the quantal property of light, the other due to the thermal properties of the source. For each quantum state one has:

$$\Delta E_\nu = h\nu \ \sqrt{(1+a_\nu N) \cdot N}$$

where a_ν is the frequency density per quantum state. In the optical range and for a source in equilibrium at temperature T, one obtains $a_\nu.N \sim \exp(-h\nu/kT) = .001-.1$, therefore only the quantal term dominates the external noise.

$$\Delta E_\nu = h\nu \ \sqrt{N}$$

When one is using a light beam not in thermal equilibrium, the product $a_\nu \cdot N$ can be larger than 1; for a laser beam it can reach values as high as $10^6 - 10^{12}$ and it will become the largely dominant term of the noise energy power (Tarassov, 1981).

It can be of interest to see the limits at which the information can be processed and transmitted, comparing biological and present technical devices. While the minimum energy/bit is few kT, one can see that, technically, the limit is approached by using very sophisticated devices, like the Josephson junction; for biological devices, including photoreceptors, they can normally operate by using 10-20 kT per bit (Wyner, 1981).

Another way to see the sophistication reached by the biological devices and organs is to compare them to the today technically advanced systems dealing with information processing. For such systems a relationship (known as Rent's rule) has been extablished between the number of off-chip signal connections and the number of logic gates. Fig. 2 shows this relation (Keyes, 1981). One can see that the technical rule can be extrapolated to include the eye, represented in terms of number of photoreceptors versus the number of optic nerve fibers. The extrapolation can be extended to the cerebral emispheres. The sophistication of the nervous system can appear by far more advanced if one is not counting a neuron simply as a logic gate.

3. Light and molecular structures

The interaction between light and the electric charges of matter is one of the best known property of Nature. The agreement between theory and experiments can reach the precision of 10 significant figures.

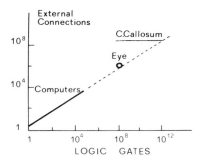

Fig. 2. Rent's rule showing a relationship between number of ex-
         ternal connections and number of logic gates (from Keyes,
         1981).

The optical field in its propagation in space interacts with
the electric charges of matter, organized in atoms, molecules,
bodies, etc., giving rise to a large variety of processes, all of
which can be reduced in principle to the absorption or to the
emission of a photon by an electric charge.

Such a simple picture starts its way to complication because
energy and momentum cannot be conserved simultaneously in the simple
exchange pictured above and something else must happen. For example
electrons must transfer momentum to another particle or structure.
In ordinary matter the electrons are bound, it means that they are
confined by electrostatic attraction in a small volume, around a
nucleous in an atom or molecule. All our difficulties arise not
in the validity of the "a priory" principles, but in our limited
ability to describe and make accurate calculations about the material
structures with which light interacts, together with modifications
in them due to the same light interaction.

Molecules can absorb a photon by making a transition to an
electronic excited state or to a vibrational or rotational state
of higher energy. While the last two types of transitions require
photons in the infrared range, for many molecules the first empty
energy state, able to accept the electron, is too high ($\sim$6eV) and
the transition cannot be induced by a photon in the visual range
(about 2 eV for the average wavelength λ = 600 nm). This is a
consequence of the fact that the electrons in a molecule are in
general too strongly localized, each in the proximity of one or a
few of the constituent atoms of the molecule. This is true also
in general for the most external electrons, shared by adjacent atoms

to form a covalent chemical bond. The situation is different for
molecules presenting an alternate sequence of simple and double
bonds. In a series of conjugated double bonds, the electrons involved in this type of chemical bonds fill π-orbitals and are distributed or delocalized over all the sequence of conjugated bonds.
As a consequence, the separation of the excited electronic energy
states from the resting state is smaller, the excitation energy
falling in the range of the optical photons.

The importance of conjugated double bonds for pigment molecules,
which absorb light in the visual range, was already recognized by
Graebe and Liebermann in 1968. A class of such molecules can be
described as made by isoprene units (see fig. 1). The most important
parameter is the length L in which the π-electrons are delocalized.
Assuming l = 1.4 Å as the length of a single bond, we have in the
case of retinal L = 10xl = 14 Å.

The localized atomic p-orbitals, of two adjacent atoms fuse
together to form a π-orbital. If they fuse together without nodal
planes the π-orbital is bonding, otherwise is antibonding.

One very simple picture useful to understand the behavior of
such molecules is obtained if we consider the electrons as free
inside a one-dimensional box of length L (see Karplus & Porter,
1970; Salem, 1966). To confine the electrons inside the box, their
accompanying wave function must be zero at the boundary and outside
the box. This wave function must have therefore two nodes at the
extremes of the length L. It can have no other nodes inside the
box, or it can have 1, 2, 3,... other nodes. Fig. 3 shows how the
electronic wave function looks like when there is only one node
inside or only two. When there are only the nodes at the extremes
(and an antinode in the middle) the electronic wavelength will be

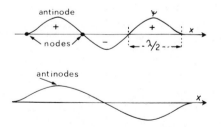

Fig. 3. Examples of electronic wave function for "a particle in a
         box".

2 L, while when there are 1, 2, 3,... interior nodes the wavelength
will be shorter, being 2 L divided by 2, 3, 4,....

Electronic states associated with shorter wavelength have a
higher level of energy. One must remember that the momentum of an
electron is inversely proportional to the wavelength of its associated wave, therefore its kinetic energy is inversely proportional
to the square of the wavelength. In the simplified discussion of
the electronic states of our molecule, we can conclude that the
excited electronic states will have energy higher than the resting
state by a factor 4, 9, 16,.... Remembering that in each electronic
state we can accomodate at most 2 electrons with opposite spin, we
must fill in succession the electronic states with electron pairs,
starting from the orbital with the lowest energy (as sketched in
Fig. 4). In this way the fundamental energy state of the molecule
will have a zero total spin and it is therefore a singlet state. In
the case of retinal we must accomodate 12 electrons in 6 electronic
orbitals.

By absorbing one photon, one of electrons of the highest filled
electronic state will be raised to the next excited empty orbital,
as indicated in the same Fig. 4. The resulting excited state of
the molecule can be still a singlet state or can be a triplet state,
if the total final spin is 1.

It is interesting to consider that in the resulting excited
state, the atoms in the molecule are less strongly bound togegher,
as a consequence of the extra nodal plane of the newly occupied
electronic state. In an intuitive picture, one can think of the
molecule as a compressed spring, for which the internal tension is

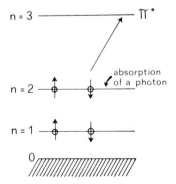

Fig. 4.   Excitation of an electron from the highest filled π-orbital
          to the next empty π^*-orbital.

in part suddenly released. Thereafter the molecule will start to
elongate, with the possibility to dispose of the excitation energy
through vibrational or rotational modes. The transition to an
isometric rotated state, like that indicated in Fig. 1, can be
accomplished in this way, if this transition is favored by other
factors, like steric repulsion due to side groups, possible distor-
tions from the planar structure of the molecule, etc.. The possibility of vibration and rotational modes for the excited molecular
state explains also the fact that the absorption spectrum of the
molecule is not a single line, but a broad band, centered in the
case of the all trans retinal around 360 nm (Birge, 1981).

4. Essentials of photochemistry

We mentioned already that the isomerization of retinal due to
the absorption of a photon is only the first step of a chain of
events, that in some part or at the end must include a modification
of the electric conductance of the photoreceptor membrane. One
part or the essential parts of this chain of events can be a cascade
of chemical reactions (Borsellino A. & Fuortes M.G.F., 1968) and
we are still in difficulty to make explicit the real nature of the
reactions and the molecular species involved. Since photochemistry
studies the chemical reactions initiated or modified by light, it
can be appropriate to revise briefly here the basic laws of photochemistry.

It was first extablished by Grotthus (1818) and later by Draper
(1839) that only that part of light that is absorbed is chemically
active. When associated with the Bunsen-Roscoe law of reciprocity
- we are allowed to trade intensity I with duration Δt - we conclude
that only the absorbed part of the energy $I \cdot \Delta t$ is the important
factor determining the chemical effects. We are in this way led
to the formulation of the Stark-Einstein law (1908), saying that
to each absorbed photon will correspond a chemically active molecule.
In symbols $A + h\nu \longrightarrow A^*$. The activated molecule A^* can give rise
to various processes and can modify the state of other molecules
or structures. So if we call Z^* the modified structures to which we
are looking, we can have that the quantum efficiency or quantum
yield, as valued looking only to the number of Z^* for each of the
absorbed photons:

$$\Phi_{Z^*} = \frac{N_{Z^*}}{N_{abs}}$$

can be different from 1 (100 percent) in many ways. For example it
can be lowered by quenching agents or be increased to values larger
than 1 if some multiplicative chain reaction is intervening, producing many Z^* particles for each molecule A^* that was directly activated by the light.

The absorption of light is measured by sending a beam of light
of intensity I_o through a slab of the material and observing the
emerging intensity I. The ratio I/I_o defines the transmission factor
τ; its complement to 1 defines the absorption factor $a = 1 - \tau$.
Care must be taken to correct for the laterally scattered light, as
well as for other factors, due to reflection, fluorescence, etc..

For a homogeneous slab of finite thickness, the beam is gradually extinguished, the intensity decreasing with an exponential law
(Lambert-Beer law) and one can express this law writing, for a slab
of thickness l and absorption factor a:

$$a = 1 - e^{-\alpha\, C \cdot l}$$

where C is the concentration of the absorbing molecules and α is
defined as the absorption coefficient. By the practical use of
decimal logarithms one is led to define the so called optical density
D (or OD) of the slab:

$$D = \log_{10} I_o/I = 0.43\, \alpha\, C \cdot l$$

the factor 0.43 intervening to convert natural to decimal logarithms.
We can recall now the definition of the extinction coefficient ε as:

$$\varepsilon = 0.43\, \alpha = \frac{D}{C \cdot l}$$

There is sometime a degree of ambiguity and confusion about
the units in which ε can be expressed, ranging from a pure number
(that is not) to a more or less satisfying choice. If C is measured
in mol. L^{-1}, (moles/liter), ε is referred also as molar absorptivity
(another name!), its values usually given in the unit L. mol^{-1}.
cm^{-1}.

In photobiology one has frequently quite small OD and one can
then substitute the previously given relation for a by the simpler
relation $a = \alpha\, C \cdot l$, taking the linear approximation for the exponential in the previous equation. In this way the absorption factor
results simply proportional to the absorption coefficient.

The dependence of a or α or ε on the wavelength of light defines the absorption spectrum of the material. For a pigment molecule the spectrum has a broad maximum, with a dominant peak for a given wavelength λ_{max}. Because the plot of a_λ has the ordinate proportional to the concentration C, sometimes it is indicated as a density spectrum.

Values of ε_{max}, for intense absorption, are in the range $10^4 \div 10^5$ L/mol/cm. Changes in ε_λ can be estimated with a sensitivity of the order 10^{-8} to 10^{-10}. Being difficult to make absolute measures, it is usual to report relative values, by fixing $\alpha_{max} = 1$.

For complex systems, as said before, the primary absorption of light can be followed by a rather involved chain of events. As we specified in defining the quantum yield Φ, we can decide to study a supposed well defined effect. Then we can rightly assume that the looked for response R will be a function of the fraction $\Phi \cdot a \cdot I$ of the light intensity I that has been absorbed with absorption coefficient a and quantum yield Φ:

$$R = f(\Phi \cdot \alpha \cdot I)$$

As a first step toward the analysis of the functional dependence of the response R, we can establish the dependence on the light wavelength λ, by controlling the intensity of the light in such a way that the value of the response R can be kept the same for two different wavelength λ and λ'. From the assumed functional relationship we can write:

$$\Phi \cdot a \cdot I = \Phi' \cdot a' \cdot I'$$

Now we can define what is called the spectral sensitivity: $s = \Phi \cdot a$ of the response R and one can write:

$$\frac{S'}{S} = \frac{\Phi' \cdot a'}{\Phi \cdot a} = \frac{I}{I'}$$

A plot of s or $1/I$ versus λ is called the action spectrum, as defined by the chosen standard response R.

REFERENCES

Birge, R.R. (1981). Photophysics of light transduction in rhodopsin
    and bacteriorhodopsin, Ann. Rev. Biophys. Bioeng., 10, 315-354.
Borsellino, A., Fuortes, M.G.F. (1968). Responses to single photons
    in visual cells of Limulus, J. Physiol., 196, 507-539.
Karplus, R.W., Porter, R.N. (1970). Atoms and Molecules. New York,
    W.A. Benjamin, pag. 77 and 536.
Keyes, R.W. (1981). Fundamental limits in digital information
    processing, Proc. IEEE, 69, 267-279.
Salem, L. (1966). The molecular orbital theory of conjugated systems.
    New York, Benjamin.
Tarassov, L. (1979). Bases physiques de l'électronique quantique
    (domain optique). Moscow, Edition Mir.
Vinnikov, Y.A. (1982). Evolution of receptor cells. Berlin,
    Springer.
Wyner, A.D. (1981). Fundamental limits in information theory,
    Proc. IEEE, 69, 239-251.

RECEPTOR PIGMENTS IN LIGHT-INDUCED BEHAVIOR OF MICROORGANISMS

G. Colombetti

Istituto di Biofisica, C.N.R., Via S. Lorenzo, 26

56100 - Pisa (Italy)

One of the most interesting phenomena that have fascinated scientists of many different cultural backgrounds, from biologists to physicists, is the alteration by light of the motile character-istics of many unicellular organisms (Lenci & Colombetti, 1978), known as photomovement or photobehavior. Many different types of photobehaviors are known, and without going into too many details, we will briefly describe some of them, using a terminology accepted by most of the groups working in the field (Diehn et al., 1977).

When the motile response, commonly a more or less tumbling swimming in flagellates or a reversal of ciliary beating in ciliates, is caused by a sudden alteration in the homogeneous illumination of a specimen, we speak of a phobic reaction. The response is referred to as a step-up photophobic response if the light intensity increases, and a step-down photophobic response if it decreases. Usually, after a certain time that depends on the organism, the stimulus and the environmental conditions, the cell resumes its previous swimming pattern.

The orientation of cell motion with respect to light direction is referred to as phototaxis. Some authors (Doughty & Diehn, 1980) believe that phototaxis is not a response per se, but rather the result of a series of phobic responses. More recently, however, many different research groups have reported convincing evidence that this is not always true (Nultsch et al. 1979; Song et al. 1980; Häder et al. 1981) and that phototaxis may be a response strictu sensu.

13

Finally, there are responses in which the swimming speed of the moving organism is controlled by the light intensity: these are the so called photokinetic responses or photokinesis, defined as positive when the speed during illumination is higher than in the dark and as negative when the speed decreases upon illumination.

Photokinetic responses are usually considered a particular case among photoresponses, since the response remains as long as the stimulus is present and no adaptation occurs. Moreover, photokinesis has been shown to be brought about via a photocoupling process (one in which the energy of the impinging photon is directly used to drive the metabolic process, for instance an increased supply of ATP to the motor apparatus), whereas the other photomotile responses are believed to be photosensory processes (in which the light energy serves as a trigger for the motile reaction that is driven through previously stored metabolic energy).

Different experimental techniques can be used to study these motile behaviors in a quantitative manner. Presently, the most widely adopted set-up is of the type shown in Fig. 1. It consists mainly of a microscope coupled to an infrared sensitive TV-camera, which allows the experimenter to use a non perturbing infrared observation light, a video recorder and a video monitor. The trajectories of single cells can thus be analyzed and all the necessary information on their parameters collected, such as speed, number of directional changes per unit time, and average direction.

The fact that many unicellular organism are able to react to variations in the parameters of external illumination raises the interesting question of how these supposedly simple systems can perceive the light stimulus, transform it into a signal understandable by the cell metabolism and finally transfer this information to the motor apparatus. In other words, one has to face the problem of finding the single pieces that when put together form the so-called photosensory transduction chain in these cells. Until now, only a few cases seem to have come close to a solution, even if not complete.

In many other instances, unfortunately, only some parts of the transduction chain have been more or less clarified, and much work is required in order to have more definite ideas on this question.

Naturally, one of the first goals of research on sensory transduction is the identification and characterization of the photoreceptor pigments, those molecules which upon photon absorption

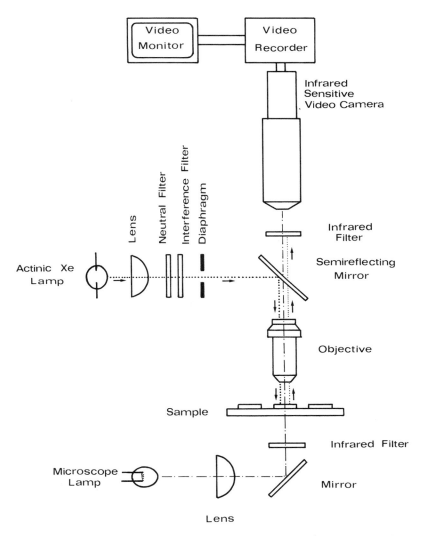

Fig. 1. Experimental set-up used in the analysis of the photomotile
         reactions of single cells.

undergo the physico-chemical change that initiates the chain of
events leading eventually to the motor response.

This short contribution will be mainly devoted to the problem
of the identification and characterization of the photoreceptor
pigments, with a general look at the possible different techniques
that can be used. Particular attention will be given to the case
of Euglena, in which the application of these techniques has allowed

reasonable conclusions to be drawn about the nature of the photoreceptor pigments out knowledge of the photoreceptor pigments involved in the photomotile reaction of microorganisms is not yet
satisfactory; in fact, there are many organisms in which only a few
experiments have been performed to identify these molecules. This
is true even in systems such as the flagellated green alga Chlamydomonas reinhardtii, which are being extensively investigated with
respect to other aspects of the photosensory transduction chain.
However, some progress has been achieved recently, and at present
there are a number of systems in which the photoreceptor pigments
have been identified with a reasonable reliability.

One of the main reasons for this difficulty in identifying the
receptor molecules lies in the fact that in many cases the photoreceptor structures, i.e. the subcellular organelle(s) where the
pigments are localized, are not known. This is a consequence of
the fact that the photoreceptor pigment concentration in several
systems is so low as to prevent a direct (and easy) optical identification of the pigment localization, and even electron microscopy
is not very helpful if one does not know where to look. Following
an idea by Walne & Arnott (1967), (Melkonian and Robenek, 1980;
Ristori, et al. 1981), it has recently been suggested, both in
Chlamydomonas and Haematococcus pluvialis, that the photoreceptor
could lie in a thickening of the plasma membrane in a region facing
the stigma area. In Haematococcus this finding has been substantiated with the help of electrophysiological measurements which have
shown that only that portion of the plasmalemma generates an electrical signal when the cell is illuminated (Ristori et al. 1981).

However, in the cases of Gyrodinium dorsum, Gymnodium splendens
Volvox, Ochromonas, and others, this problem is quite unsolved.
(Lenci & Colombetti, 1978). This fact makes it very difficult both
to try and isolate the photoreceptor structures and to measure in
vivo absorption or fluorescence spectra.

One of the most widely used techniques in the study of the
receptor pigments is still the determination of action spectra
(Colombetti & Lenci, 1980). As it is well known, this kind of
approach does not allow in general a positive identification of the
pigments involved. This is due to several reasons: action spectra
are poorly resolved, many pigments have similar absorption spectra
in the visible range, and the absorption properties of a pigment
in vivo can be deeply modified by the environmental conditions, so
that shoulders or even absorption bands may be present or absent.
However, the measurement of action spectra is often the only

technique available that can give an idea, even if only a rough one, of the pigments involved.

An action spectrum is usually determined by measuring the response at different wavelengths of light. Certain requirements have to be fulfilled in order to have meaningful measurements, and usually the action spectra reported in the modern literature can be considered reliable. If the action spectrum is measured properly, it ought to be proportional to the absorption spectrum of the pigment involved in the light reaction, with the limitation described above.

One of the problems of major concern is the way in which the response is measured. In some cases, for example in photochemistry or electrophysiology, the measured response is a well defined chemical or physical quantity, so no problem should arise. In the case of photomovements, however, the response is defined in a more or less arbitrary way, and sometimes different authors measure different parameters (see, e.g. Colombetti & Lenci, 1980). For example, a step-down reaction could be characterized by the average number of directional changes that take place in unit time (Doughty & Diehn, 1980), or by the average time it takes for the cells to resume normal swimming, or, as we do in our group, by the percentage of cells that show the tumbling reaction upon stimulation (Colombetti & Lenci, 1980). More and more groups are presently accepting the percentage of responding cells as a good operational parameter to measure, since it is clearly defined and certainly related to the photoresponsiveness of the cells, whereas other quantities might be related to adaptation phenomena.

We will now turn our attention to results obtained in the special case of a Euglena gracilis, a green flagellated alga, that can survive either using photosynthesis or an external carbon source. A schematic representation of this organism is shown in Fig. 2. The photoreactivity of Euglena has been known for over a century, and it has been the main organism of choice in studies of photo-movements in unicells.

Euglena shows both step-up and step-down photophobic reactions (Colombetti et al. 1982). It is also able to orient its motion toward or away from the light source, in other words it is both positively and negatively phototactic. Phobic reactions can be easily observed in this alga under a variety of experimental conditions, whereas phototaxis is more difficult to observe. Very recently we have been able to show (Häder et al. 1981), that only a statistical analysis of the orientation of cell trajectories under

a light stimulus can reveal phototactic movements in Euglena, with
a clear indication that the mechanism of orientation of the cell is
not very efficient. The step-up (Diehn et al. 1975), and the step-
down responses (Combetti & Lenci, unpublished) that result in a
tumbling swimming are caused by a sudden flagellar reorientation
with respect to the cell body (Fig. 2 B). In summary, we may say
that at present the photomotile behaviors of Euglena are reasonably
well known.

However, until a few years ago, no real progress had been
achieved in understanding the nature of the photopigments involved
in the photoresponses of this alga. The situation was better as far
as the photoreceptor structure(s) was concerned. In fact, even
the oldest authors reported that the light sensitivity of the cells
of Euglena resided in the anterior part of the cell, i.e. the part
bearing the emerging flagellum (see Fig. 2). The two subcellular
organells that were suggested as photoreceptors are the stigma and
the paraflagellar swelling (PFB) (see Fig. 2). This hypothesis is
mainly based on the fact that a natural colorless form of Euglena,
Astasia longa, which does not posses either a stigma or a PFB, does
not show any light-induced motor response (Pringshein, 1948, Gössel,
1957).

The stigma in Euglena, unlike in other green algae, is an ex-
trachloroplastic organelle located at the base of the reservoir.
It consists of a cup-shaped group of orange-red pigmented granules.
It has been shown (Benedetti et al., 1976), by in vivo microspectro-
spectrophotometry, that the stigma contains carotenoids, in agreement
with the findings of other authors on isolated stigma granules
(Batra & Tollin, 1964; Bartlett, et al., 1972).

The PFB in Euglena is formed from a quasi-crystalline body
located near the base of the emerging flagellum. The ordered structure of the PFB has been studied by Piccinni & Mammi (1978) by
diphractometric analysis. The PFB has been described by these
authors as a crystal with a monoclinic or slightly distorted hexag-
onal unit cell, the dimensions of which are a = 8.9 nm, b = 7.7 nm,
c = 8.3 nm, β = 110°.

It is presently accepted by the majority of the researchers
working in this field that the PFB is the true photoreceptor of
Euglena. Streptomycin bleached mutants of this alga, which do not
possess any stigma-like organelle, do respond to light stimuli
(Ferrara & Banchetti, 1976). Moreover, a direct stimulation of the

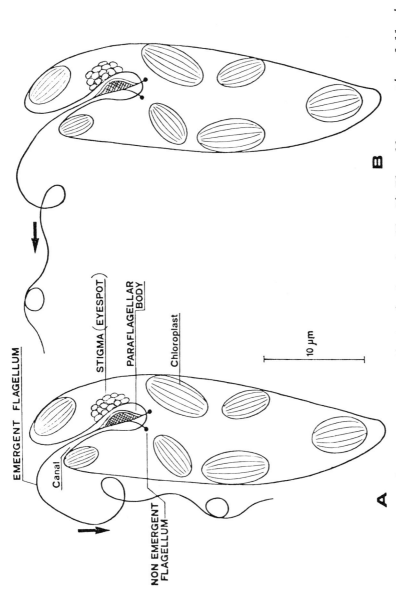

Fig. 2. Schematic drawing of Euglena. A) Unstimulated cell; B) Flagellar erection following a light stimulus.

PFB with a laser beam of about 0.8 μm in diameter causes a flagellar
reorientation, whereas no response is evoked when the beam strikes
the stigma or any other region of the cell. (Colombetti & Lenci,
unpublished). However, we cannot really exclude any role of the
stigma in the process of light detection by the cell. In fact, it
has been suggested (Lenci & Colombetti, 1978), that the stigma could
at least play an indirect role in positive phototaxis, as a shading
device. Without going into unnecessary details, this "passive" role
of the stigma has been invoked by many authors (Lenci & Colombetti,
1978; Foster & Smyth, 1980), to explain how these cells are able
to detect the anisotropy in the external light field when tracking
the light source.

Moreover, according to some of our recent results (Colombetti
& Lenci, unpublished), it looks as if the light sensitivity in
Euglena decreases with the age of the culture examined. We have
also observed that during the aging process the stigma grows larger.
Even if we have established no positive relation between these two
facts, it is interesting to observe that streptomycin-bleached
Euglena (no stigma present) are very sensitive to light stimulation
(Colombetti et al., 1982).

As already mentioned, the first and easier approach to the
identification of photoreceptor pigments is the determination of the
action spectra of the light response. We will not review the old
literature in the field; the interested reader may consult recent
papers (Colombetti e Lenci, 1980; Douthty & Diehn, 1980). In the
last few years, our group has been devoted to a thorough determination of the action spectra of the photoresponse of Euglena.

In earlier work we have determined (Checcucci et al., 1977)
the action spectrum of the red-light response (shown in Fig. 3),
which is pratically identical to the absorption spectrum of chloro-
phyll. This red-light induced accumulation, described by other
authors and misinterpreted by them as a true photoresponse (Wolken
& Shin, 1958) has been shown by us to be in fact caused by a chemo-
response toward the O_2 evolved by the illuminated cells, the photo-
synthetic activity of which is stimulated by the red light. It is
of interest to note that an investigation of the behavior of single
cells has demonstrated that Euglena does indeed show motile reactions
induced by oxygen (Colombetti & Diehn, 1978).

More recently, we have evaluated the action spectra for photoresponses in the range 330 nm 550 nm, both in populations of cells
and on single cells of the wild type, dark-bleached strain and the

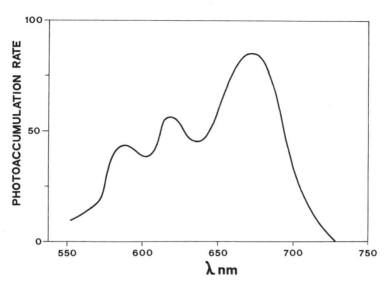

Fig. 3. Action spectrum of photoaccumulation of Euglena cells in the red portion of the spectrum.

streptomycin mutant (Checcucci et al., 1976; Barghigiani et al., 1979). It should be mentioned that the streptomycin bleached cells show a dispersal for the illuminated region. They also do not have any step-down, but only step-up responses. These two facts could be related, but the problem requires further investigation.

In all cases the action spectra show a strict resemblance to that of a typical flavoprotein, as shown in Fig. 4, with two major peaks at 370 nm and 450 nm. The latter shows a good degree of fine resolution, very likely due to flavin embedded in a hydrophobic environment or strongly immobilized. This hypothesis might be in good agreement with the quasi-crystalline structure of the photo-receptors organelle.

It should be noted that the threshold for the step-down reaction at 450 nm has been determined to be of the order of 6.10^{11} photons cm^{-2} sec^{-1} (Barghigiani et al., 1979), which is quite high compared to higher organisms. This threshold value is, however, quite close to the threshold for positive phototaxis, as determined both theo-retically and experimentally, as we will see later on. No photo-taxis action spectra are presently available and work is in progress in our group in this direction. In summary, the action spectra of Euglena point to the presence of flavin-containing photoreceptors.

As already mentioned, action spectra cannot give a definite identification of the pigments involved. However, the fact that flavins might be involved suggested the investigation of the fluorescent properties of the photoreceptor region. Fluorescence microscopy (Benedetti & Checcucci, 1975) showed indeed fluorescence from the PFB region. Then, emission microspectrofluorometry (Benedetti & Lenci, 1977) confirmed that the emitted light was compatible with a flavinic fluorophore. More recently, using a tunable dye laser coupled to an optical microscope (Colombetti et al., 1981), we have been able to determine fluorescence excitation spectra from the PFB. The results, shown in Fig. 6, strongly indicate the presence of flavin pigments in the PFB, thus confirming the previous investigation. From these measurements it has also been possible to obtain an estimate of the fluorescence quantum yield in vivo, which is on the order of 10^{-2}.

Now, if flavins are indeed the photoreceptor pigments, what do we know about the steps that follow photon absorption? In other words, what are the molecular events that lead to the transduction of the luminous information into a biophysical or biochemical message that the organism is able to understand? Unfortunately, not much is really known in the case of Euglena. Experiments have been carried out (Diehn & Kint, 1970; Mikolajczyk & Diehn, 1975) using quenchers of the triplet excited states of flavins, mainly potassium iodide (KI). These studies seem to indicate a quite specific effect of KI on both the step-down response and photoaccumulation of Euglena, but the concentrations used (up to 100 mM) were so high that non spefific effects of both K^+ and I^- were very likely involved, and no definite conclusion can therefore be drawn. Given the role played by flavins in the electron transport chains, one could suggest that photoredox reactions might have a direct role in producing, for instance, light induced membrane potential changes (Colombetti et al., 1982). However, much more work is necessary to clarify this important point.

Before concluding, we would like to show how, using behavioral measurements and a suitable model, it is possible to extract information about the number of photoreceptor molecules contained in the PFB of Euglena. The main idea of the model is that phototatic orientation in this alga is brought about via a modulation of the light falling on the PFB, the modulation being caused by the screening effect of the stigma.

What is the minimum light that can orient the movement of Euglena? The answer depends on many variables (for example the ability of the cell processor to extract the signal from the noise) but the lower limit is certainly set by the amount of the photo-receptor pigment available for light absorption and by the efficiency of the screen. Let N_L be the photon count rate of the photoreceptor during direct illumination and N_D represent the photon count rate during the screening phase. Also let t_L and t_D represent the re-spective count durations. $N_L \, t_L$ and $N_D \, t_D$ are the total counts under full and screened light, respectively. Assuming Poisson statistics, the variances in each of these counts are $N_L \, t_L$ and $N_D \, t_D$. The signal is determined by the difference in the count rates:

$$N_L - N_D \tag{1}$$

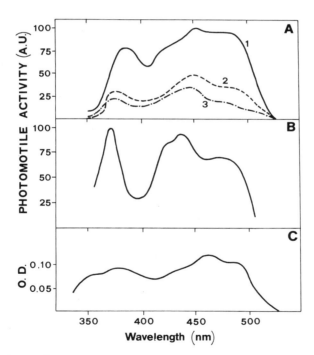

Fig. 4. (A–B) Action spectra of the photoresponses of <u>Euglena</u> cells in the region between 330–550 nm. A1) Green cells A2) Dark-bleached cells A3) Streptomycin bleached mutant cells (see text) B) step-down in single cells C) Absorption spectrum of a flavoprotein, D-amino acid oxidase.

The variance for this quantity is given by:

$$\frac{N_L}{t_L} + \frac{N_D}{t_D} \tag{2}$$

Accordingly, this counting process has a signal to noise ratio given by

$$\frac{S}{N} = \frac{N_L - N_D}{\sqrt{\dfrac{N_L}{t_L} + \dfrac{N_D}{t_D}}} \tag{3}$$

The lowest detectable signal has S/N = 1, therefore

$$N_L - N_D = \sqrt{\frac{N_L}{t_L} + \frac{N_D}{t_D}} \tag{4}$$

Now, let M be the number of receptor molecules in the photoreceptor, let $\emptyset$ be the quantum yield of the process, σ the photon absorption cross section and I the number of quanta cm^{-2} s^{-1}. Let us, moreover, assume that the screen has a transmittance T, so that the screened number of quanta cm^{-2} s^{-1} is $I_D = T I$.

Hence

$$N_L = M \emptyset \sigma I \tag{5}$$

and

$$N_D = M T \emptyset \sigma I \tag{6}$$

Substituting (5) and (6) in (4) and rearranging, we obtain

$$M \sigma \emptyset I = \frac{t_D + T t_L}{t_L t_D} \frac{1}{(1 - T^2)} \tag{7}$$

from which

$$M = \frac{1}{\sigma \emptyset I} \frac{t_D + T t_L}{t_L t_D} \frac{1}{(1 - T^2)} \tag{8}$$

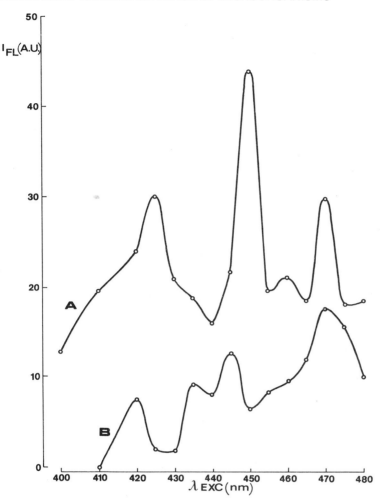

Fig. 5.   Fluorescence excitation spectrum determined by means of the
microspectrofluorometer, as discussed in the text. A) PFB,
spectrum corrected for cytoplasm emission B) Riboflavintet-
rabutyrate (RFTB) in ethanol, corrected for ethanol emission.

Let us now see what this means in the case of _Euglena_.   In this
alga, t_L = 0.3 s and t_D = 0.2 s.   T, the transmittance of the screening organelle (the stigma) has been determined to be about 0.46
(Benedetti et al., 1976).   The photoreceptor of _Euglena_ is probably
a flavin, as discussed previously, the absorption cross section of
which, σ, is about 3.8 10^{-17} cm^2, and we may assume for $\emptyset$ a value
of about.5.

With these values (8) becomes

$$M = \frac{1.016}{I} \; 10^{18}$$ (9)

We have recently determined from behavioral measurements (Häder et al., 1981), that the threshold for positive phototaxis is about 9.5 10^{11} quanta cm^{-2} s^{-1} at 450 nm. Substituting this value in (9) we obtain that the number of receptor molecules is of the order of 10^6. This value is in pretty good agreement with other independent estimates based on microspetroscopical techniques (Colombetti & Lenci, 1980) or on crystallographic considerations (Creutz, personal communication).

REFERENCES

Barghigiani, C., Colombetti, G., Franchini, B. and Lenci, F. (1979). Photobehavior of Euglena gracilis: Action spectrum for the step-down photophobic response of individual cells. Photochem. Photobiol. 29, 1015-1019.

Bartlett, C.M., Walne, P.L., Schwarz, O.J. and Brown, D.H. (1972). Large scale isolation and purification of eyespot granules from Euglena gracilis. Plant Physiol. 49, 881-885.

Batra; P.P. and Tollin, G. (1964). Phototaxis in Euglena. I. Isolation of the eyespot granules and identification of the eyespot pigment. Biochim. Biophys. Acta, 79, 371-378.

Benedetti, P.A., Bianchini, G., Checcucci, A., Ferrara, R., Grassi, S. and Percyval, D. (1976). Spectroscopic properties and related functions of the stigma measured in living cells of Euglena gracilis. Arch. Microbiol. 111, 73-76.

Benedetti, P.A. and Checcucci, A. (1975). Paraflagellar body (PFB) pigments studied by fluorescence microscopy in Euglena gracilis Plant Sci. Lett., 4, 47-51.

Benedetti, P.A. and Lenci, F. (1977). "In vivo" microspectrofluorometry of photoreceptor pigments in Euglena gracilis. Photochem. Photobiol. 26, 315-318.

Checcucci, A., Colombetti, G., Del Carratore, G., Ferrara, R. and Lenci, F. (1974). Red-light induced accumulation of Euglena gracilis. Photochem. Photobiol. 19, 223-226.

Checcucci, A., Colombetti, G., Ferrara, R. and Lenci, F. (1976). Action spectra for photoaccumulation of green and colorless Euglena: Evidence for identification of receptor pigments. Photochem. Photobiol. 23, 51-54.

Colombetti, G. and Dehn, B. (1978). Chemosensory responses toward
oxygen in Euglena gracilis. J. Protozool. 25, 211-217.

Colombetti, G., Ghetti, F., Lenci, F., Polacco, E. and Quaglia, M.
(1981). "In vivo" microspectrofluorimetry of photoreceptor
pigments. Journal of Photochemistry 17, 36.

Colombetti, G. and Lenci, F. (1980). Identification and spectroscopic characterization of photoreceptor pigments. In: Photo-
reception and Sensory Transduction in Aneural Organisms (F.
Lenci, G. Colombetti, eds.). Plenum Press, New York, London
pp. 173-188.

Colombetti, G., Lenci, F. and Diehn, B. (1982). Response to photic
chemical and mechanical stimuli. In: The Biology of Euglena,
Vol. 3 (D.E. Buetow, ed.) Academic Press, 169-195.

Diehn, B., Feinleib, M., Haupt, W., Hildebrand, E., Lenci, F. and
Nultsch, W. (1977). Terminology of behavioral responses of
motile microorganisms Photochem. Photobiol. 26, 559-560.

Diehn, B., Fonseca, J.R. and Jahn, T.L. (1975). High speed cinemi-
crography of the direct photophobic response of Euglena and the
mechanism of negative phototaxis. J. Protozool., 22, 492-494.

Diehn, B. and Kint, B. (1970). The flavin nature of the photoreceptor pigments for phototaxis in Euglena. Physiol. Chem.
Phys. 2, 483-488.

Doughty, M.J. and Diehn, B. (1980). Flavins as photoreceptor pigments for behavioral responses in motile microorganisms,
especially in the flagellated alga, Euglena sp., in: Structure
and Bonding, Vol. 41, Molecular Structure and Sensory Physiology
(P. Hemmerich, ed.) Springer, Berlin, pp. 45-70.

Ferrara, R. and Banchetti, R. (1976). Effect of streptomycin on the
structure and function of the photoreceptor apparatus of
Euglena gracilis. J. Exp. Zool. 198, 393-402.

Foster, K.W. and Smyth, R.D. (1980). Light antennas in phototactic
algae. Microbiol. Reviews 44, 572-630.

Gössel, I. (1957). Über das Aktionsspektrum der Phototaxis chloro-
phyllfreier Euglenen und über die Absorption des Augenflecks.
Arch. Mikrobiol. 27, 288-305.

Häder Donat-P., Colombetti, G., Lenci, F. and Quaglia, M. (1981).
Phototaxis in the Flagellates, Euglena gracilis and Ochromonas
danica. Arch. Mikrobiol. 130, 78-82.

Lenci, F. and Colombetti, G. (1978). Photobehavior of microorganisms: a biophysical approach, Ann. Rev. Biophys. Bioeng.
7, 341-361.

Melkonian, M. and Robenek, H. (1980). Eyespot membranes of Chlamydomonas reinhardii: a freeze-fracture study. J. Ultrastruc.
Res. 72, 90-102.

Mikolajczyk, E. and Diehn, B. (1975). The effect of potassium iodide
on photophobic responses in Euglena: Evidence for two photoreceptor pigments. Photochem. Photobiol. 22, 268-271.

Nultsch, W., Schuchart, H. and Höhl, M. (1979). Investigations the
phototatic orientation of Anabaena variabilis. Arch. Microbiol., 122, 85-91.

Piccinni, F. and Mammi, M. (1978). Motor apparatus of Euglena
gracilis: ultrastructures of the basal portion of the flagellum
and the paraflagellar body, Boll. Zool. 45, 405-414.

Pringsheim, E.G. (1948). The loss of chromatophores in Euglena
gracilis New Phytol. 47, 52-87.

Ristori, T., Ascoli, C., Banchetti, R., Parrini, P. and Petracchi,
D. (1981). VI International Congress of Protozoology, Warszawa,
Book of Abstracts, A 314.

Song, P.S., Häder, D.P., Poff, K.L. (1980). Phototactic orientation
by the ciliate Stentor coeruleus Photochem. Photobiol. 32,
781-786.

Walne, P.L. and Arnott, H.J. (1967). The comparative ultrastructure
and possible function of eyespots: Euglena granulata and
Chlamydomonas eugametos Planta (Berl), 77, 325-353.

Wolken, J.J. and Shin, E. (1958). Photomotion in Euglena gracilis.
J. Protozool. 5, 39-46.

SENSITIZATION OF THE VISUAL PIGMENT IN A PHOTORECEPTOR

K. Kirschfeld

Max-Planck-Institut für biologische Kybernetik
Spemannstrasse 38, D-7400 Tübingen, W.-Germany

INTRODUCTION

Detection of light in a photoreceptor begins with the absorption of quanta of light. Highly evolved photoreceptors should absorb light with a high probability. This can be important for an animal for several reasons, for instance in order to allow vision at low ambient intensities where only few quanta are available, or, when the animal has to detect small optical signals (small modulation of intensity) in a short time. The detection of such signals can be a problem even in bright light because the light quantum noise must be smaller than the signal, and the only way to achieve a low light quantum noise is to absorb many quanta per unit time.

The Absorption Probability of Light in Photoreceptors

Highly evolved photoreceptors or, more exactly their light absorbing organelles (outer segments, rhabdomeres), are dieletric lightguides: light imaged by a dioptric system onto the distal ending of such a lightguide travels, due to total internal reflection, along the length of it whereby it is absorbed by the visual pigment. According to basic laws of physics high absorption probability needs high visual pigment concentrations and an extended length of the structure.

In vertebrates as well as in invertebrates high visual pigment concentrations are achieved by maximizing the membrane density in the receptors (disc in outer segments, microvilli in rhabdomeres),

29

by packing the visual pigment molecules (membrane bound proteins) as close together in the membranes as possible and using as the visual pigment a molecule with the highest extinction coefficient possible.

The molecular weight of rhodopsin is on the order of 40 000, which means that a rhodopsin molecule, if spherical, should have a diameter of some 5 nm. Freeze-etching techniques in membrane of outer segments and rhabdomeres show a very high density of particles which most likely represent rhodopsin molecules. Data from rhodopsin extraction experiments are also consistent with the view that visual pigment molecules are incorporated into the receptor membranes in the highest possible concentration.

For the extinction coefficient of a molecule there is an upper limit since the area under the absorption band of a single electronic transition is limited. For the usual halfwidth of electronic transitions in organic molecules there is a peak extinction coefficient of some 5000 m^2/mole, which is rarely exceeded (Hagins 1972). Experimental values for rhodopsin are on the order of 4000 m^2/mole, which is close to the theoretical maximum (see review in Handbook of Sensory Physiology VII/1, 1972, ed. H. J. A. Dartnall).

If the retinal pigment concentration and the extinction coefficient are maximal, a further increase in absorption probability in a receptor requires an increase in the length of the absorbing organelles. One can easily see that in real eyes in which either absolute or contrast sensitivity must be high the length of the receptors is also considerable.

If concentration, extinction coefficient and length are maximised in a receptor we might think that this is all that can be done to optimize absorption. How could absorption probability be further improved? If rhodopsin molecules could be made smaller this would allow their concentration in the receptors membrane, and hence absorption, to be increased. But it might well be that the process of transduction needs a protein of sufficient complexity, and therefore size, which means that the molecular weight of rhodopsin perhaps cannot be further reduced. That there is nevertheless a realistic possibility of increasing the number of absorbed quanta per length of receptor emerges from the analysis of the properties of photoreceptors in the housefly and some related diptera.

UV-sensitivity in Fly Photoreceptors

The measurement of the spectral sensitivity of photoreceptors

in the fly (more precisely: that of the most common fly receptors,
called no. 1-6) led to an unexpected result: there are two maxima
rather than one. One is in the green spectral range, close to 500
nm, the other in the ultraviolet at 365 nm (Burkhardt 1962). Dual-
peak sensitivity of this type cannot be explained on the basis of
extinction spectra of known rhodopsins: these pigments have only a
small peak at shorter wavelengths, of less than 25% of the maximum
(β -peak).

Possible explanations for this finding have been , among others:
two different visual pigments in one and the same photoreceptor
(Horridge and Mimura, 1975; Rosner, 1975), or waveguide effects that
can selectively enhance short wavelength extinction of light (Snyder
and Pask, 1973). The waveguide concept as an explanation (together
witha selfscreening effect as it was originally proposed) has in
fact already been eliminated by older experiments, in which spectral
sensitivity of white eye mutants has been determined by means of
the ERG (e.g. Goldsmith and Fernandez, 1968; Minke et al. 1975;
Stark, 1975; Harris et al., 1976). These spectral sensitivities
also exhibit a pronounced UV-peak. Since in these mutants, with
the kind of illumination chosen, rhabdomeres were stimulated primarily by stray light crossing the rhabdomeres obliquely, waveguide
effects and selfscreening were considerably reduced and hence cannot explain the high UV-sensitivity.

It can be shown microspectrophotometrically that UV light
creates the same metarhodopsin as blue light. There is, however,
no decrease in extinction in the UV at the same time (Kirschfeld
et al., 1977). Furthermore, whatever pair of wavelengths of light
is used to shift the visual pigment(s) to a different state - rhodopsin or metarhodopsin - the isosbestic point always remains at
the same wavelength, and the shape of the difference spectrum remains unaltered. This is true as long as the pH is sufficiently
low to prevent the formation of alkaline metarhodopsin. These results strongly indicate that there should be only one visual pigment
present in the rhabdomeres of these photoreceptors.

The difficulty in interpreting the UV-sensitivity in these
flies in a classical way led to the hypothesis that there might be
in these rhabdomeres, in addition to the visual pigment, another
(photostable) pigment absorbing in the ultraviolet. This pigment
should be able to transfer energy of absorbed quanta to the visual
pigment which then could behave as it had absorbed a light quantum

itself. That is, according to this concept rhodopsin is sensitized
by a UV-absorbing pigment, thus accounting for the high UV sensitivity. The sensitizing pigment hypothesis can be formulated as follows

$$X + h\nu \rightarrow X^*, \tag{1}$$

$$X^* + R \rightarrow R^* + X \;\;, \tag{2}$$

$$R^* \rightarrow M. \tag{3}$$

Or, in other words, due to the the absorption of a light quantum, the
unspecified, photostable molecule X^+ is converted into the excited
state X^* (Eq. 1). In a secondary process it then may interact with
a rhodopsin molecule R, converting it into an excited state R (Eq. 2)
which finally leads to metarrhodopsin M (Eq. 3). Alternatively, the
molecule X^* may loose the extra energy by fluorescing

$$X^* \quad X + h\nu', \tag{4}$$

or by suffering deactivating collisions with other molecules. In the
later case the energy is dissipated as heat. There is a growing body
of evidence that unanimously supports this hypothesis and, furthermore, the evidence favours the view that the transfer follows the
rules of Försters (1951) type of dipole – dipole energy transfer.

If the energy transfer occurs by this mechanism several conditions must be fulfilled.
    1. The donor (= sensitizing) molecule should be close to the ac-
    ceptor (sensitized) molecule. Estimates show that distances
    should be not much larger than 5 nm.
    2. The absorption spectrum of the acceptor molecule should over-
    lap sufficiently with the fluorescence spectrum of the donor
    molecule.
    3. The dipoles of both molecules should be parallel (the effi-
    ciency is proportional to the cosine of the angle between the
    dipoles).

The conditions for the efficiency of energy transfer as formulated above can be used for predictions that can be checked experimentally.

Evidence for the sensitizing concept includes the following:
A) in the rhabdomeres type 1-6 there is a strong extinction in the
UV, which is not significantly altered by light (small changes can
be interpreted as due to contribution of the short wavelength shoul-
ders of rhodopsin and metarhodopsin) (Kirschfeld et al., 1977).
More recent microspectrophotometrical results show furthermore

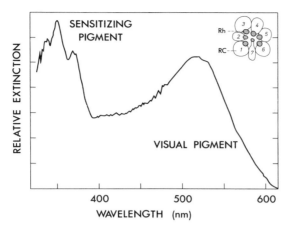

Fig. 1.   Extinction spectrum of rhabdomeres type 1-6 of a male
           Musca (wild type).   The spectrum was measured in "pho-
           toequilibrium" with the measuring light, which means
           that in the range from 400 to 600 nm there is a mixture
           of the two states of the visual pigment present, rhodopsin
           and metarhodopsin, respectively.
           Inset: cross section through ommatidium indicating recep-
           tor cells (RC) no. 1-7 and rhabdomeres (RH).
           Modified from Kirschfeld et al., 1983.

that there is a typical vibrational substructure in the UV-extinc-
tions, not known from visual pigments (Fig. 1). This fine structure
agrees with electrophysiological results in which the UV-sensitivity
has been determined with high resolution, (Gemperlein et al., 1980;
Kirschfeld et al., 1983).
B) According to condition 2 (see above) the photosensitivity not
only of rhodopsin, but also that of metarhodopsin should be high.
This conclusion follows from the fact that the absorption spectra
of rhodopsin and metarhodopsin overlap considerably (Fig. 2).
Hence the fluorescence spectrum of the sensitizing pigment should
overlap not only with the absorption spectrum of rhodopsin but also
with that of metarhodopsin.   We found that the photosentivity of
metarhodopsin in th UV is very high indeed, and furthermore that
the maxima and halfwidth of the UV photosensitivity spectra of rhodopsin and metarhodopsin are practically identical, as is to be
expected if both spectra are created by the same sensitizing pigment (Fig. 2) (Minke and Kirschfeld, 1979).
C) Flies grown on a carotene free diet have a reduced rhodopsin
concentration in their microvilli (Boschek and Hamdorf, 1976;

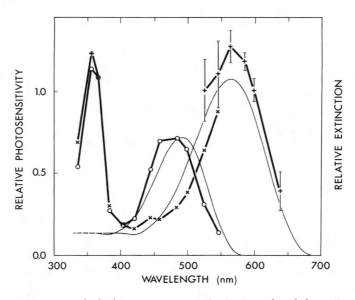

Fig. 2.   Photosensitivity spectra of rhodopsin (o) and metarho-
           dopsin (x, +) in the fly (Calliphora).   The methods
           used to derive the spectra measure the efficiency with
           which rhodopsin and metarhodopsin are converted into
           each other, depending upon wavelength and intensity of
           light.   Therefore instead of absorption spectra, photo-
           sensitivity spectra are derived, which include the ef-
           fects of sensitizing pigments.   For the spectrum of me-
           tarhodopsin two different methods had to be applied for
           shorter and longer wavelengths.   This explains the
           somewhat different results at wavelengths from 520 to
           540 nm.   Thin lines: extinction spectra of rhodopsin
           (Hamdorf, Schlecht, Täuber, pers. comm.) as derived
           from a difference spectrum of Calliphora.   Note the
           lack of pronounced UV-extinction in these spectra.
           Modified from Minke and Kirschfeld (1979).

Harris et al., 1977; Razmjoo and Hamdorf, 1976).   Their content of
sensitizing pigment is also significantly reduced (Kirschfeld et
al., 1983), and their receptors no longer exhibit the high UV-sensitivity (Goldsmith et al., 1964; Stark and Zitzmann, 1976; Kuo,
1980).   More detailed analysis has shown, in addition, that the
vibrational structure of the UV sensitivity is lost together with
the selective loss in UV sensitivity (Kirschfelf et al., 1983).

These results are easily interpreted as being due to a loss of
sensitizing pigment in these receptors, the remaining UV sensiv-
ity then being due to β - peak absorption of the rhodopsin
itself.

D)   As far as polarization sensitivity is concerned, we could find
no dichroic absorption in the UV using microspectrophotometry
(Kirschfeld, unpublished). Polarization sensitivity of receptors
1-6, measured electrophysiologically, is also confined to the visible part of the spectrum (Hardie, 1978, Kuo, 1980).   The absence
of dichroic absorption in the UV could, in principle, be explained
by a specific dipole alignment of the β - peak of the visual pigment.
However, if one measures polarization sensitivity in vitamin A de-
prived flies in the UV it turns out that photoreceptors type 1-6
are sensitive to polarised light, and that the polarization sensitivity is similar in size and of the same phase as that in the
visible (at 500 nm). This shows that the dipoles of the sensitizing
pigment are aligned in a different way to those of the visual pigment
(Vogt and Kirschfeld, 1983).   These observations again are strong
evidence for the sensitizing pigment hypothesis.

The Chemical Identity of the Sensitizing Pigment

     The biosynthesis of the sensitizing pigment molecules, or at
least their incorporation into the microvillar membrane, obviously
depends on the presence of carotenoids in the diet: not only is
the visual pigment concentration reduced in flies grown on a carotenoid deficient diet, but also the typical UV-extinction (Fig. 1)
is lost (Kirschfeld et al., 1983).   Therefore one candidate for
the sensitizing pigment could be retinal or a compound related to
retinal, because these molecules depend biosynthetically on the
presence of carotenoids and they absorb in the spectral range of
325 to 380 nm.

     The microspectrophotometrical as well as the electrophysiologi-
cal data in the ultra violet show a clear cut vibrational fine
structure which is not usually found in retinal or retinal derivates.
Under special circumstances such a fine structure can nevertheless
be expected also in this kind of molecules. The lack of a fine
structure is considered as being due primarily to the fact that
there are a large number of conformers differing in the torsional
angle about the single bond connecting the β -ionylidene ring and
the sidechain of retinal or related compounds, that is the carbon
atoms called C6 and C7. The absorptions of the various conformers
are all shifted with respect to one another with the consequence

that when they are superimposed the spectrum is broad and unresolved
(Hemley and Kohler, 1977).

If now the C6 - C7 bond is stabilised not only is a vibrational
fine structure in the extinction spectrum to be expected but also a
redshift of some 30 nm if the -ionylidene ring becomes coplanar
with the side chain (Reppe, 1970).   There are several possibilities
for such a stabilization.   Either by a sterical hindrance, e.g. if
retinol is incorporated into a membrane, or if a protein - retinol
complex is formed, or, if the conjugated chain of C = C double bonds
is shifted by one C.   In the latter case the C6 - C7 bond now is a
double bond and therefore no longer torsional. The extinction spectra of such retinol derivates are all quite similar to the spectrum
of the sensitizing pigment as discussed in detail elsewhere (Kirschfeld et al., 1983; Franceschini, 1983), and they are therefore candidates for the sensitizing pigment.

However, the distance of some 20 nm between the UV-peaks
of the sensitizing pigment only indicates that the extinction
should be due to a conjugated system as has already been suggested
by Gemperlein et al., 1980; it needs not be due to a retinol deriv-
ative.   Since the presence of the sensitizing pigment depends upon
the presence of carotenoid in the diet, it might be that the sensitizing molecule is a C40-carotenoid.   However, carotenoids like
 -carotene with a system of 11 conjugated double bonds absorb in
the range of 400 to 500 nm, that is at much longer wavelength than
the sensitizing pigment.   If, however, some of the double bonds
in the carotene are hydrated, as e.g. in the phytofluene molecule
the extinction would be shifted to shorter wavelengths (Zechmeister,
1962).

Recently a class of rather exotic naturally occuring substances
has been described that cannot yet be completely excluded as a candidate for the sensitizing pigment: polyene fatty acids, or lipids
containing these acids.   These subsatnces, like parinaric acid
from the plant Parinarium laurium, exhibit the typical vibrational
structure in their extinction spectrum.   Actually, it has already
been shown that parinaric acid, artificially incorporated into rod
outer segment membranes is able to transfer energy to rhodopsin
(Sklar et al., 1979).   Of course, the sensitizing pigment needs
not be a fatty acid by itself; the fatty acid could be incorporated

into a lipid, similar to the parinaric acid-labeled lecithins that are used as membrane probes.

We are still unable to precisely specify chemically the sensitizing pigment molecule. But several naturally occuring candidates with properties similar to those of sensitizing pigment do exist, and model systems have been shown to behave in just the same way that we suggest for the fly photoreceptors with high UV and green sensitivity.

CONCLUSION

If there is the possibility of incorporating a sensitizing pigment into the membranes of photoreceptors, then there is the possibility of overcoming the limitation, as far as absorption probability is concerned, given by membrane density, rhodopsin concentration and length of the absorbing photoreceptor organelle. The advantage of such a sensitizing pigment is obvious: these molecules, since they do not directly mediate transduction, need not be large and hence can be incorporated into the membranes in addition to the visual pigment without demanding much space. Most likely candidates for the sensitizing pigment in fly rhabdomeres have a molecular weight of 600 or less, which is about 1,5% of that of rhodopsin. Such a sensitizing pigment in principle can be used to extend the spectral range over which the receptor is sensitive, and by this means photoreceptors can be made more efficient light quantum collectors. Or, for a given total absorption, the receptors can be made shorter.

It is surprising that this kind of sensitization has up to now been demonstrated only in insects. In vertebrates, the similarity between spectral sensitivities as determined electrophysiologically and the absorption spectra of the rhodopsin indicates that there are no sensitizing pigments present, at least in receptors analysed up to now in sufficient detail. This means that with respect to their absorption properties vertebrate photoreceptors could in principle still be further improved.

ACKNOWLEDGEMENT

I thank Drs. N. Franceschini, R. Hardie and K. Vogt for discussion and for reading the manuscript.

REFERENCES

Boschek, C. B. and Hamdorf, K. (1976). Rhodopsin Particles in the
    Photoreceptors Membrane of an Insect, Z. Naturforsch., 31c,
    763.
Burkhardt, D. (1962). Spectral sensitivity and other response
    characteristics of single visual cells in the arthropod eye,
    Symp. Soc. Exp. Biol., 16, 86 - 109.
Dartnall, H.J.A. (1972). Handbook of Sensory Physiology. Vol. VII/1,
    Photochemistry of Vision, Dartnall H. J. A. ed., Springer,
    Berlin - Heidelberg - New York.
Förster, T. (1951). Fluoreszenz organischer Verbindungen.
    Göttingen: Vandenhoek und Ruprecht.
Franceschini, N. (1983). In Vivo Microspectrofluorimetry of visual
    pigments, Symp. Soc. Exp. Biol. (in press).
Gemperlein, R., Paul, R., Lindauer, E. and Steiner, A. (1980).
    UV fine structure of the spectral sensitivity of flies visual
    cells. Revealed by FIS (Fourier Interferometric Stimulation),
    Naturwissenschaften, 67, 565 - 566.
Goldsmith, T. H., Barker, R. J., Cohen, C. F. (1964). Sensitivity
    of visual receptors of carotenoid-depleted flies: A vitamin A
    deficiency in an invertebrate, Science,146, 65 - 67.
Goldsmith, T. H. and Fernandez, H. R. (1968). The sensitivity of
    house fly photoreceptors in the mid-ultraviolet and the limits
    of the visible spectrum, J. Exp. Biol., 49, 669 - 677.
Hagins, W. A. (1972). The visual process: excitatory mechanisms
    in the primary receptor cells, Ann. Rev. Biophysics and
    Bioengineering, 1, 131 - 158.
Hardie, R. (1978). Peripheral visual function in the fly. Thesis,
    University of Canberra, Australia.
Harris, W. A., Stark, W. S., Walker, J. A. (1976). Genetic dissec-
    tion of the photoreceptor system in the compound eye of
    Drosophila melanogaster, J. Physiol. (Lond.), 256, 415 - 439.
Harris, W. A., Ready, D. F., Lipson, E. D., Hudspeth, A. J., Stark,
    W. S. (1977). Vitamin A deprivation and Drosophila photopig-
    ments, Nature, 266, 648 - 650.
Hemley, R. and Kohler, B. E. (1977). Electronic structure of
    polyenes related to the visual chromophore. A simple model
    for the observed band shapes, Biophys. J., 20, 377 - 382.
Horridge, G. A. and Mimura, K. (1975). Fly photoreceptors. I.
    Physical separation of two visual pigments in Calliphora
    retinula cells 1-6, Proc. R. Soc. Lond. (Biol.), 190, 211-224.
Kirschfeld, K., Minke, B. and Franceschini, N. (1977). Evidence

for a sensitizing pigment in fly photoreceptors, Nature, 269, 386 - 390.

Kirschfeld, K., Feiler, R., Hardie, R., Vogt, K. and Franceschini, N. (1983). The sensitizing pigment in fly photoreceptors: properties and candidates, Biophs. Struct. Mech., 9 (in press).

Kuo, A. (1980). Elektrophysiologische Untersuchungen zur Spektral und Polarisationsempfindlichkeit der Sehzellen von Calliphora Erythrocephala, I. Scientia Sinica Vol. XXIII, no. 9, 1182 - 1196.

Minke, B. Wu, C. F., Pak, W. L. (1975). Isolation of the light induced response from the electroretinogram of Drosophila, J. Comp. Physiol., 98, 345 - 355.

Minke, B. and Kirschfeld, K. (1979). The contribution of a sensitizing pigment to the photosensitivity spectra of fly rhodopsin and metarhodopsin, J. Gen. Physiol., 73, 517 - 540.

Razmjoo, S. and Hamdorf, K. (1976). Visual sensitivity and the variation of total photopigment content in the blowfly photoreceptor membrane, J. Comp. Physiol., 105, 279 - 286.

Reppe, K. (1970). In Houben-Weyl, Methoden der Organischen Chemie, Müller, E., ed., Vol. V/1 d, 7 - 31. Stuttgart: Thieme Verlag.

Rosner, G.(1975). Adaptation und Photoregeneration im Fliegen-auge, J. Comp. Physiol., 102, 269 - 295.

Sklar, L. A., Hudson, B. S. and Simoni, R. D. (1975). Conjugated polyene fatty acids as membrane probes: preliminary characterization, Proc. Nat. Acad. Sci. USA, 72, 1649 - 1653.

Sklar, L. A., Miljanich, G. P. Bursten, S. L. and Dratz, E. A.(1979). Thermal lateral phase separations in bovine retinal rod outer segment membranes and phospholipids as evidenced by parinaric acid fluorescence polarization and energy transfer, J. Biol. Chemistry, 254, 9583 - 9591.

Snyder, A. W. and Pask, C. (1973). Spectral sensitivity of dipteran retinula cells, J. Comp. Physiol., 84, 59 - 76.

Stark, W. S. (1975). Spectral selectivity of visual response alterations mediated by interconversions of native and intermediate photopigments in Drosophila, J. Comp. Physiol., 96, 343 - 356.

Stark, W. S. and Zitzmann, W. G. (1976). Isolation of adaptation mechanisms and photopigment spectra by vitamin A deprivation in Drosophila, J. Comp. Physiol., 105, 15 - 27.

Vogt, K. and Kirschfeld, K. (1983). Sensitizing pigment in the fly. Biophys. Struct. Mech. (in press).

Zechmeister, L. (1962). CIS-TRANS Isomeric Carotenoids Vitamins A and Arylpolyenes. Wien: Springer - Verlag.

IN VITRO REGENERATION OF VISUAL PIGMENT IN ISOLATED VERTEBRATE
PHOTORECEPTORS[*]

Ferenc I. Harosi

Marine Biological Laboratory
Woods Hole, MA 02543 U.S.A.

ABSTRACT

By the addition of exosenous 11-cis retinal to bleached retina
fragments in vitro, homolog pigments have been obtained in carp
(Cyprinus carpio), clawed frog (Xenopus laevis) and mudpuppy (Necturus maculosus) rods and cones. In each case the 11-cis retinal
spontaneously condensed with the available opsin in situ and thus
produced rhodopsin-type homologs instead of the original por-
phyropsin-type chromo-proteins. Visual pigments were identified
by microspectrophotometry in side-on oriented and optically isolated
cells. It was found that rod and cone outer segments can soak up
large quantities of 11-cis retinal. From these stores visual pigments are spontaneously generated even after repeated bleaches.
Cones under identical conditions regenerate their homologous visual
pigments 2.5 to 3-fold faster than rods.

INTRODUCTION

The use of exogenous 11-cis retinal to regenerate rhodopsin
in aqueous digitonin solutions was pioneered by Wald and Brown
(1950) and Hubbard and Wald (1952). Several aspects of visual pigment regeneration have been investigated (for a review see Baumann,

---

[*] Dedicated to the memory of Mike Fuortes, who not only was an out-
standing scientist, but also a fair-minded and concerned individual.

1972). Well established, for instance, is that the pigment epithelium normally plays a decisive role in the regeneration process
(Dowling, 1960; Bridges and Yoshikami, 1970; Reuter et al., 1971;
Bridges, 1973). Conditions for pigment regenerability have also
been studied, such as those concerning the phospholipid requirement
(Zorn and Futterman, 1971; Shichi, 1971), and the effect of digitonin
concentration on the regeneration of cattle rhodopsin (Matsumoto et
al., 1978). Visual pigment regeneration in isolated retinas has
also been investigated in the frog (Reuter, 1966; Baumann, 1970;
Azuma et al., 1977) and in the rat (Cone and Brown, 1969). More
recently Pepperberg et al., (1976, 1978) applied 11-cis and 9-cis
retinals externally to the isolated skate retina, whereas Witkovsky
et al. (1978, 1981) injected exogenous chromophores into Xenopus
and attained in vivo synthesis of artificial pigments. Although
Bridges (1977) investigated the utilization of 11-cis retinol, and
their 9-cis isomers in fragmented and intact frog rod outer segments in suspension, visual pigment regeneration in isolated photoreceptors received very little attention. Except for brief references by Liebman (1972, 1973) and Tsin et al. (1981) to successful
regeneration of visual pigments and their detection in isolated
rods and cones of goldfish and mudpuppy, no experimental details
have been pubblished on either the procedures involved or the absorption spectra obtained from regenerated visual pigments in isolated receptors.

    This microspectrophotometric study was undertaken to investi-
gate the necessary conditions for in vitro regeneration of rod and
cone pigments and to establish the extent to which the obtained
spectra can be useful in the spectroscopic characterization of the
artificial chromo-proteins. Important motivation for this work was
provided by the recent successes on the synthesis of organic molecules analogous to the natural chromophores of 11-cis retinal (and
3-dehydroretinal) that spontaneously condense with various opsins
in forming pigments (Arnaboldi et al., 1979; Honig et al., 1979;
Balogh-Nair and Nakanishi, 1982 a,b). The hope is that by virtue
of the single-cell technique, it will be possible to combine a
variety of opsins with analogs of known structure. The pigments
thus obtained are expected to yield a series of spectral shifts
which, in turn, would add new dimensions to our understanding of
opsin-chromophore interactions.

    Carp, Necturus and Xenopus, were chosen for this study for
several reasons. First, the natural prosthetic group for the visual
pigments in these animals is 3,4-dehydroretinal. Therefore, when

their opsins condense with 11-cis retinal, the resulting pigments
are blue-shifted with respect to the natural ones, making them easily
distinguishable. Second, the rod and cone outer segments are of
relatively large size so that they are readily accessible to single-
cell measurements. Third, due to the fact that their visual pigments cover the entire visible spectrum, they are attractive for
spectroscopic studies. Included in this report is the initial phase
of the work. Although the results are still preliminary, they are
interesting enough to warrant continued, more detailed investigations.

METHODS

    Animals. Carps (Cyprinus carpio) of 15 cm body length were
purchased from Sea Plantations, Inc., Salem, Mass. They were kept
in an aerated aquarium at room temperature (20-24°C) and under
natural light conditions (daylight and dark cycles of roughly equal
duration). Their diet consisted of daily portions of dried fish
food. Before use each fish was dark-adapted for at least three
hours in an aereated dark container and in the final minutes anes-
thetized with Tricaine (Crescent Research Chemicals, Scottsdale,
Arizona) at a concentration of 0.5 g/1 of water. Adult specimens
of frogs (Xenopus laevis) and mudpuppy (Necturus maculosus) were
purchased from Nasco, Fort Atkinson, Wisc., and were kept under
normal laboratory conditions. While the Xenopus were fed live
crickets, the Necturus remained unfed in the laboratory. These
animals were also dark adapted before use in the same manner as the
carp, but then quickly decapitated under dim red light.

Solutions. For all experiments in this series the same saline
solution was used for both dissection and suspension. It contained
105 mM NaCl, 2 mM KCl, 3 mM $CaCl_2$, 1 mM $MgSO_4$, 0.5 mM $NaHCO_3$, 0.5
mM NaH_2PO_4 and 10 mM Hepes buffer adjustated with NaOH to pH 7.3
at 22°C. The measured osmolality (mean value of three determina-
tions) was 257 mOs/Kg.

    The retinal stock solution was prepared by Ms. Bridgette
Barry. 2 mg of 11-cis retinal (a gift from Dr. Richard Mathies,
University of California at Berkeley) was dissolved in 2 ml of
hexane under dim red light. The solution was stored air-tight,
light-tight, in a freezer. At the time of each experiment, the
desired volume of hexane-retinal was pipetted into an empty vial
again under dim red light. The hexane was evaporated by blowing

high purity, dry N_2 gas over it for a few minutes. The 11-<u>cis</u> retinal was redissolved in absolute pure ethyl alcohol (0.1 ml) and
pipetted into a small volume (5 ml) of saline previously saturated
with N_2 gas. This served as incubation as well as suspension medium
for bleached pieces of retinas.

<u>Experimental Procedures</u>. Eyes were removed under a deep red photo-
graphic safety lamp (carp) or under a low power dissecting microscope
equipped for infrared work (frog and mudpuppy). The retinas were
peeled out of the eye cup in a small dish of saline solution, and
cut into four quarters or even smaller pieces, while always kept
submerged.

The experimental protocol consisted of three types of preparations: two controls and one test. The first control was a piece
of dark-adapted tissue. Recordings from this were intended to establish the native pigment properties. The second control was an
externally bleached retina preparation. The aim was to test the
effectiveness of the bleach and to record the long-term optical
properties (photoproduct content) of the outer segments. The test
preparation was an externally bleached tissue transferred to the
incubation medium containing 11-cis retinal. This was to test for
visual pigment regeneration in isolated rods and cones.

The external bleaching device consisted of a metal housing
equipped with a 60 W bulb, a 6mm thick heat-absorbing glass, a ≠ 2E
Wratten (Kodak) gelatin filter, and a 2mm thick glass diffuser.
Below these was the tissue to be bleached in a small Stender dish
placed atop a flat mirror. The distance between bulb and tissue
was ca. 13 cm. Routine exposure time was 5 minutes.

Specimens for microspectrophotometry were prepared each time
in an identical manner. Small pieces (1-2 mm^2) of retina were
minced on a No. 1.5 microscopic cover glass in a drop of saline (or
ethanolic saline), carefully covered with a second cover glass, and
sealed (Harosi and MacNichol, 1974 b).

The dichroic microspectrophotometer (DMSP) was used for spectral recordings. With recent modifications of the earlier version
(Harosi and MacNichol, 1974 a), the DMSP now is more sensitive and
has an improved signal-to-noise ratio (Harosi, 1982). It simultaneously records the average and modulated light fluxes. When a
recording is taken through a sample and one through a reference
area, a dedicated digital computer calculates the average density

(OD) and the linear dichroism (LD) of the sample. If a prebleach
and a postbleach recording of the same sample is available, the
bleaching optical density difference (BD) spectrum can be obtained.
These three spectra proved to be useful in distinguishing visual
pigment absorption from those of the late photoproducts. The cross
section of the light beam used in these measurements was adjusted
to be ca. 1.5 x 8 μm in the plane of the specimen.

RESULTS

        Fragments of retina, whether derived from carp, Necturus or
Xenopus, bleached nearly equally well in the external bleaching
device. With a 5-min exposure, 90-100% of the native visual pigment was photolized in all rod and cone outer segments. Mounted in
saline, no spontaneous, dark-regeneration was detected in any of
the cells. The small amounts of porphyropsin encountered occasionally in large rods (Necturus) were believed to indicate incomplete
bleaching rather than regeneration. In small cells, such as carp
rods or Xenopus cones, no light absorption (≥ 0.001 O.D.) could be
detected postbleach between 325 and 695 nm. This is to be contrasted with bleached cells of larger size, such as carp and Necturus
cones or Xenopus and Necturus rods, in which considerable amounts
of shortwave absorption persisted for as long as they were tested
(up to 6 hours).

The dark-adapted preparations yielded single-cell records
indicating the presence of previously identified visual pigments.
Significant LD was found in every outer segment. When bleached in
the DMSP, some of the later photoproducts could be observed as
changes in both OD and LD.

When bleached tissues were placed in ethanolic saline containing 11-cis retinal, regenerated pigments were found in every preparation. When the final concentration of 11-cis retinal was 10 μs/ml
and a large piece of carp retina (ca. 10 mm^2) was incubated, few
cells showed significant regeneration. However at 30 μg/ml, small
pieces of Necturus retina yielded rods and cones with an overabun-
dance of new prostetic groups. Although the best result was obtained
at 20 μg/ml of 11-cis retinal with a 2% ethanol-to-saline volume
ratio, no sharp optimum was noted (cf. Bridges, 1977; Pepperberg
et al., 1978; Pepperberg, 1982).

One of the interesting findings in this work was that, given
the change, rod and cone outer segments gorge themselves with 11-cis
retinal. To be sure, other lipophilic structures also load up

significant amounts of this prosthetic group, such as the Xenopus
cone oil droplets. However, while the oil droplets concentrate
these molecules randomly, outer segments exhibit a strong axial
anisotopy at wavelengths where 11-cis retinal absorbs light. The
implication therefore is that the excess chromophores line up with
the phospholipid hydrocarbon chains throughout the transverse membranes; the cone outer segment infoldings as well as the rod discs.

Even more interesting, perhaps, is the finding that when these
11-cis retinal- loaded rods and cones are exposed to light at the
λ_{max} of their regenerated visual pigments, there is a loss of density
at wavelengths corresponding to the main absorption bands. Thus,
the newly formed pigments bleach in analogous manner to the natural
pigments. However, in these cells, there is spontaneous regeneration following the bleach. Moreover, the rate of recovery in all
cones (carp, Necturus and Xenopus) is quite rapid (a few minutes)
whereas much slower (2.5 to 3 fold) in rods. These cells were also
capable of repeated spontaneous regenerations following repeated
bleaches. They appeared, in fact, as if they had an inexhaustible
capacity to regenerate visual pigments incorporating the exogenous
11-cis retinal.

Figure 1 shows spectral records obtained from the outer segment of an apparently complete carp rod (about 2 μm in diameter)
that had been incubated with 11-cis retinal. Although the average
optical density spectrum (OD) is distorted due to noise and light
scattering, the LD and BD spectra indicate the presence of a light-
sensitive, transversely dichroic peak near 500 nm (rhodopsin), and
some axially dichroic shortwave-absorbing substance (various forms
of retinal). OD has its usual meaning: the negative logarithm
(base 10) of the average transmittance (the ratio of average fluxes
transmitted by sample and reference). LD is defined as a fraction
formed by the difference of polarized transmittances divided by the
sum of the polarized transmittances (thus a perfect linear polarized
would yield +1 if crossed and −1 if aligned parallel with the reference direction; the axes of cells are brought to coincide with this
direction). BD is defined as the difference in average optical
density between a prebleach and a postbleach recording. Although
not shown here, it is an easy matter to prove that several parameters are obtainable from these spectra. From Fig. 1, for instance,
the dichroic ratio ($R = D_{\perp}/D_{\parallel}$) of the α-band is computed to be
2.5. Also, the transverse specific density (at λ_{max}) is determined
to be 0.01/μm which implies that this carp rod regenerated only 64%

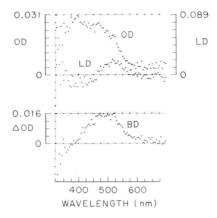

Fig. 1. Spectral records from a single carp rod previously bleached
in vitro and then incubated and mounted in ethanolic saline
solution containing 10 μs/ml of 11-cis retinal. Averages
of 8 spectral scans taken from 325 to 695 nm. Upper trace,
optical density (OD) of the outer segment compared with a
cell-free area in the preparation. Middle trace, linear
dichroism (LD), defined ad $(T_{||} - T_{\perp})/(T_{||} + T_{\perp})$, where the
symbols are polarized transmittances referred to the long
axis of the cell. Lower trace, bleaching difference (BD)
spectrum, showing changes in optical density of the outer
segment between a prebleach and a postbleach recording.
The bleach was a 2-min. steady exposure to the measuring
light at 505 nm.

of its pigment when compared with a rhodopsin-containing rod of
Bufo marinus (cf. Harosi, 1975). However, the comparison is probably unfair, because small cells are notorious for yielding "diluted"
OD spectra. Combined with an additional observation, namely, that
regenerated carp rods were unsusually denser (optically) than native
carp rods, it is estimated that the regeneration in this cell was
ca. 75% complete (Note that equal OD and LD would imply 71% regeneration, since the molar extinction coefficient of rhordopsin is 1.4-
fold greater than that of porphyropsin).

    The regeneration of rhodopsin for the second time in the same
carp rod was tested subsequently. As shown in Fig. 2, the optical
density at 505 nm recovers spontaneously and at a rapid rate. The
theoretical curves drawn to the experimental points were fitted by
eye and constitute no proof that they are indeed simple exponential
functions. Nevertheless, the exponential nature of regeneration

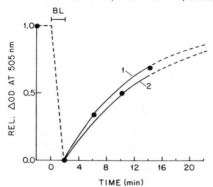

CARP ROD, T=22.5°C

curves: $(1-e^{-1/\tau})$

$\tau_1 = 10$ min

$\tau_2 = 12$ min

Rel. $\triangle OD$ of 1.0 corresponds to 0.016 opt. dens. unit

Fig. 2.   Regeneration of rhodopsin in a carp rod outer segment
           (same one as in Fig. 1). Following the recording of the
           BD spectrum depicted in Fig. 1, the cell was left in the
           dark and remeasured periodically. BD spectra (consisting
           of averages of 8 spectral scans) were obtained and the
           changes in optical density determined at 505 nm as a
           function of time. The values were normalized to the peak
           (0.016). It was found that the experimental points fall
           between two exponential curves, differring only in their
           time constant (τ_1=10 min., τ_2=12 min.).

is indicated by previous investigations (es. Rushton, 1961, 1963;
Matsumoto, et al., 1978). Incidentally, in this process the α-band
linear dichroism recovers as well as the optical density so that
the amplitude change in LD could also be plotted. One complication
in the LD spectrum, however, is that it is a composite response of
at least two anisotropically absorbing species of molecules: rhodopsin and "free" prosthetic group. Whereas the former has a
positive LD-band near 505 nm, the latter exhibits a negative LD peak
around 370 nm (e.g. Fig. 5). In the overlapping spectral regions
these two peaks counteract one another. At the crossover point
they cancel each other exactly. Moreover, the mutual cancellation
brings about a shifting of the peaks from their true values outward,
away from the main overlap region. The relative amplitudes of the
peaks will determine the apparent shifts. Additional complications

arise from transient photoproducts (meta II and meta III) as well
as from the non-specifically bound native and artificial chromophores. No attempt is made here to quantitatively account for all
these phenomena.

Carp photoreceptors have a strong resenblance to those of
goldfish, both spectrally and morphologically. For the latter the
nomenclature used for goldfish (Stell and Harosi, 1976) was borrowed.
A carp double cone (unequal) was measured extensively. The short
member, having an outer segment of 3.6 μm diameter at its base,
tapering to 1.8 μm at the apex in its 17 μm length was recorded first
(not illustrated). The computed dichroic ratio was 2.3. The peak
transversely polarized optical density at 510 nm divided by the
average outer diameter (i.e. transverse specific density) was 0.0123/
μm. Upon completion of the prebleach recording, the cell was exposed
to the measuring light at 510 nm for 2 min., and then remeasured
several times. Ten min. later the bleaching exposure was repeated.
Following both bleaches, the cell recovered its α-band extinction
rapidly. The long member of the double cone was measured next. Its
outer segment was about 5 μm at its base and tapered to 2 μm along
the length of 22 μm. The recorded spectra are shown in Fig. 3.

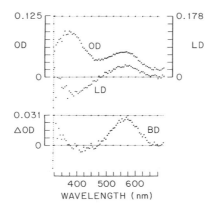

Fig. 3. Spectral records from a carp cone (long member of double)
         previously bleached in vitro, and then incubated and
         mounted in ethanolic saline solution containing 20 μs/ml
         of 11-cis retinal. The details given in the legend of Fig.
         1 for explanation of the traces are also valid here. The
         only exception being the wavelength of the bleaching ex-
         posure which, in this case, was 570 nm.

Based on the α-bands, the dichroic ratio was computed to be 2.7 and the transverse specific density (at 565-570 nm) to be 0.0120/μm. When compared with the rods of <u>Bufo marinus</u>, as was done with the carp rod earlier, the conclusion is that regeneration in this cell is 78% complete.

The regeneration of visual pigment in this cone after several bleaches was recorded for more than an hour. The time-course of optical density changes is plotted in Fig. 4. The exponential functions are identical. Curve-fitting was done be eye to the experimental points in the first period. Subsequent periods were not fitted separately even though scaling would have improved the fit. The rapid recovery is plainly visible, just as it was in the case of the short member of this double cone. The cell was photographed after the last recording. Cellular dimensions were obtained from enlarged prints with an estimated accuracy of ± 10%.

Representative results from Xenopus receptors are shown in Figures 5-8. Spectral record obtained from a rod fragment is presented in Fig. 5. Although it was not photographed so that its exact dimensions are unavailable, a diameter of 9 μm was assumed. This is about the average size for principal rod outer segments (7-12 μm), accordings to Witkovsky et al. (1981). In the course of evaluating the records, the question arose whether the OD or the BD spectrum (at 500 nm) would better represent the rhodopsin content of the cell. When using OD and LD, the dichroic ratio was 2.7, whereas from BD and LD a dichroic ratio of 10 was calculated. Since the last figure was extraordinarily high, it was decided that neither OD nor BD be used, but instead, their average. With that, the dichroic ratio was 3.8. For the transverse specific density, 0.008/μm was calculated. When compared with <u>Bufo</u> rods (Harosi, 1975), this <u>Xenopus</u> rod contained only about 50% as much rhodopsin as it could. In estimating the 11-<u>cis</u> retinal content of the cell, the OD at 365 nm was determined from Fig. 5. The obtained value was reduced by the sum of the β-band OD and the OD of the original amount of 3,4-dehydroretinal (since all of that could still be present). An additional assumption was that the molar extinction coefficient of rhodopsin is 1.5-fold greater than that of 11-<u>cis</u> retinal (cf. Wald and Brown, 1953). The result of the calculation showed that the outer segment has an 11-<u>cis</u> retinal concentration of 8-10 mM, representing a roughly 5-fold molar excess to the observed rhodopsin. The dichroic ratio at 365 nm was 0.54, meaning that the axial density is nearly twice the magnitude of the transverse

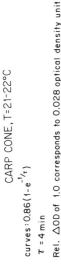
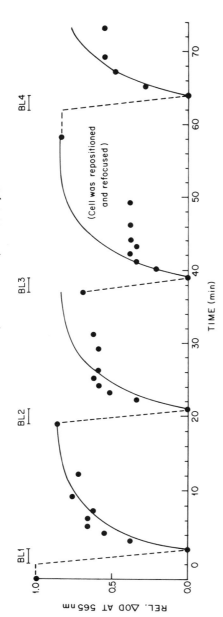

Fig. 4. Repetitive dark regenerations of visual pigment in a carp cone (long member of double) imbibed with 11-cis retinal (see Fig. 3 for details). Each regeneration period was preceeded by a 2-minute steady exposure to 570 nm light derived from the measuring beam of the DMSP. The change in optical density at 565 nm following the first bleach (0.028) was used to normalize all subsequent BD values. The plot depicts relative bleaching difference densities vs. time, beginning with a prebleach recording taken 2 min. prior to the onset of the first bleach. Each point was derived from the average of 8 consecutive spectral scans, the first of which was started at the marked time. An 8-scan recording takes about 20 sec. to complete. The BD spectrum shown in Fig. 3 is one such 8-scan average.

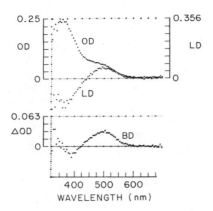

Fig. 5.   Spectral records from a broken rod outer segment of <u>Xenopus</u>.
The tissue was externally bleached (5-min exposure to white
light) and then incubated (6 hrs) and mounted in saline
(pH 7.3) containing 22 µs/ml of 11-<u>cis</u> retinal (2.2% ethanol to saline volume ratio).   Sample traces are 8-scan
averages (combined with a 16-scan reference).   For further
details see the legend of Fig. 1.

optical density at this wavelenght. Rhodopsin regeneration in the
same rod was briefly tested; the result is depicted in Fig. 6. The
theoretical curve was neither scaled nor fitted to the experimental
points.

     Spectral records obtained from a <u>Xenopus</u> cone are presented
in Fig. 7. The preparation from which this cell originated was
exceptional. Instead of freshly injecting saline with the ethanol
solution of 11-<u>cis</u> retinal as described in the Methods, a solution
prepared the day before was used. Most of the cells incubated in
this medium did not regenerate visual pigments. However, one of
the cones found in this preparation not only had acceptable regenerated density and dichroism, but also was able to regenerate after
two subsequent bleaches (Fig. 8). The dichroic ratio at 570 nm
was calculated from Fig. 7; it was 3.1. The transverse specific
optical density could only be obtained approximately since cellular
dimensions were not established by photography. By assuming an
average cell diameter of 3 µm, it was 0.008/µm (cf. Witkovsky et
al. 1981). When compared with <u>Bufo</u> rods, this cone was estimated
to have about 50% of its pigment in the regenerated form. Again,
this is probably an underestimation of the true concentration, as

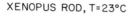

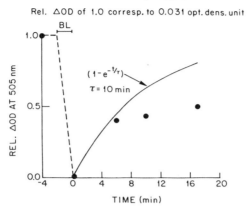

XENOPUS ROD, T=23°C

Rel. ΔOD of 1.0 corresp. to 0.031 opt. dens. unit

Fig. 6.   Time course of rhodopsin formation in the Xenopus rod of
Fig. 5.   Bleaching exposure (BL) was 2 min.   at 505 nm.

often is the case with small cells (cf. carp rods in connection
with Fig. 1).   Repeated pigment regeneration was observed in the
same cone outer segment. This is demonstrated in Fig. 8.

    The final set of records (Figures 9-12) concern Necturus rods
and cones.   Spectra obtained from a rod outer segment is shown in
Fig. 9.   From calculations, similar to those described above, the
dichroic ratio at 505 nm was either 3.4 (using OD and LD) or 17.6
(for BD and LD); it was 5.2 when the average of OD and BD was combined with LD. The transverse specific density, by assuming 10 μm
for the pathlength (cf. Harosi, 1975), resulted in 0.011/μm.
Again, comparing this to the parameter already used (Bufo rods)
indicated that this Necturus rod had 66% of its opsin bound as rhodopsin. The in situ concentration of 11-cis retinal could also be
estimated from the spectral traces (at 375 nm) and from additional
measurements of bleached but non-regenerating rods. Control measurements established that Necturus rods, under the stated experimental conditions, retained essentially 100% of their native prosthetic
groups, detectable as a broad axially dichroic absorption band that
peaked near 390 nm. It was therefore assumed that the bleached
native chromophores contributed to the uv-absorption of rods. Thus,
the OD at 375 nm was reduced by the expected photoproduct absorption.
Accounting for the molecular anisotropies as well, the calculated
11-cis retinal concentration was 3.5 mM. At that, it enjoyed nearly
a 2-fold molar excess to rhodopsin that regenerated in 4 hrs of

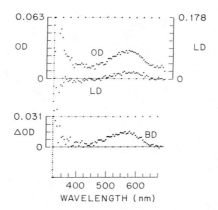

Fig. 7. Spectra from a Xenopus cone outer segment. The externally
         bleached tissue was incubated (2 hrs) and mounted in saline
         solution prepared 21 hrs earlier and contained 30 μs/ml
         of 11-cis retinal (at 1% ethanol). Each record is based
         on 8 spectral scans (and a 16-scan reference). The bleach-
         ing difference (BD) spectrum was recorded immediately
         following a 2-min, 575-nm exposure.

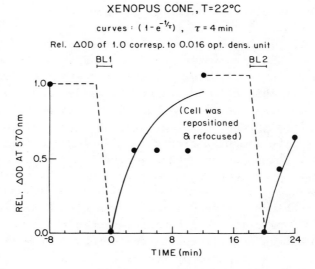

Fig. 8. Time course of pigment regeneration is the Xenopus cone
         of Fig. 7. Bleaching exposures (Bl 1 and BL 2) were 2
         min. each at 575 nm.

incubation. This rod was bleached with a 3-min exposure to monochromatic light (505 nm). Its recovery of pigment at 505 nm is
illustrated in Fig. 10, as is evident in the plot, it regenerated
rhodopsin to only 37% of its prebleach concentration in 50 min.
Although this is relatively poor recovery, it occurred nearly in an
exponential fashion with a 10 min time constant.

   Spectra obtained from <u>Necturus</u> cone outer segment (fractured)
are shown in Fig. 11. The computed dichroic ratio at 540 nm was
3.0 and the transverse specific density 0.009/μm. For the calculation of the latter, 5 μm pathlengh was assumed (cf. Brown et al.
1963). Based on comparison with Bufo rods, the estimated visual
pigment formation was 57% complete. From a calculation similar to
those already used above, the in situ concentration of 11-<u>cis</u> retinal was determined 8.3 nM and the retinal to visual pigment ratio
was about 5. The same cone was repeatedly bleached and remeasured.
The recovery of the α-band OD was plotted in Fig. 12. Again, without
elaborate curve-fitting, the data points appear to fall near the
exponential of τ = 4 min.

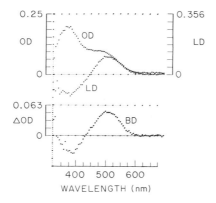

Fig. 9.   Spectra from a smaller than average <u>Necturus</u> rod outer
          segment. The retina was externally bleached and incubated
          (4 hrs) at room temperature in 1% ethanolic saline contain-
          ing 30 μs/ml of 11-cis retinal. Sample recordings are 8-
          scan averages (the reference is 16). The BD spectrum was
          recorded following a 3-min. 505-nm bleach.

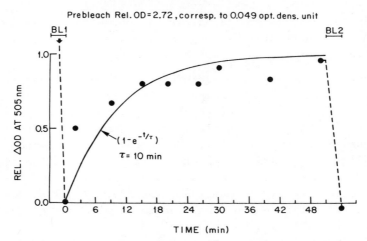

Fig. 10. Time course of rhodopsin recovery in the Necturus rod
          of Fig. 9. BL 1 and BL 2 designate two 3-min bleached at
          505 nm.

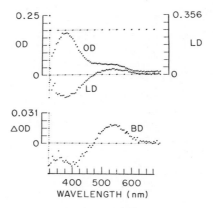

Fig. 11. Spectra recorded from a broken-off outer segment of
          Necturus cone. The externally bleached tissue was incu-
          bated (2 hrs) and mounted in 1% ethanolic saline contain-
          ing 30 μs/ml of 11-cis retinal. OD and LD are averaged
          from 16 scans. The BD spectrum (based on 8 scans) was
          recorded following a 3-min. 540-nm bleach.

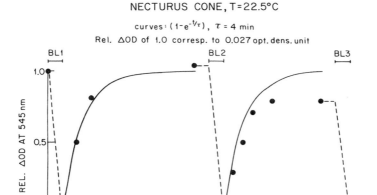

Fig. 12. Time course of pigment recovery in the Necturus cone of
          Fig. 11. BL 1, BL 2 and BL 3-min exposure at 540 nm.

DISCUSSION

    With regards to the λ_{max}, the native and artificial visual
pigments measured in this work agreed well with the previously
published values. Although elaborate curve-fitting to the α-bands
were not carried out here, the estimated λ_{max} in each case was close
(within 5-10 nm) to what was expected. These expectations were
based on former studies, e.g. by Crescitelli and Dartnall (1954),
Marks (1963, 1965), Liebman and Entine (1964); Harosi and MacNichol
(1974 b); Harosi (1976); Tsin et al. (1981) on carp and goldfish;
by Witkovsky et al. (1978, 1981) on Xenopus; by Crescitelli (1958);
Brown et al. (1963); Liebman (1972, 1973); Harosi (1975) on Necturus.

    Success in generating visual pigments in freshly removed and
bleached pieces of retinas with externally applied chromophores
came as no surprise. In the present study ethanolic 11-cis retinal
was used in 35-105 nmol/ml (10-30 µs/ml) final concentration. This
range is somewhat higher than that applied by Bridges (1977) to
fragmented frog rod outer segments (6-20 nmol/ml), but much lower
than the suspension that Pepperberg et al. (1976, 1978) delivered
to the skate retina (1.5-4.5 µmol/ml) (see also Pepperberg, 1982).

    Following light exposure and long incubation periods (usually
hours) in the dark, rods and cones still attached to small patches
of retina generated visual pigments with exogenous 11-cis retinal.

The amount of pigment formed was spectroscopically determined in optically isolated photoreceptors and found to be 50-78% of what an equivalent "standard" cell could maximally have. The standard was based on measured properties of rhodopsin-containing Bufo rods (Harosi, 1975). This estimate compared favorably with the result of Pepperberg et al. (1978) who found that in the skate retina rhodopsin regenerated to 56% of the amount initially present.

A significant result of this study is the finding of large intracellular quantities of externally applied retinal. It appears that the only manner in which the observed high optical densities can be produced is by having the retinals partitioned into all the transverse membranes (i.e. filling only the plasma membrane would be insufficient). The large OD and axial LD imply that the newly acquired 11-cis retinal molecules (in addition to any retinals and retinols already there) intercalated with the hydrocarbon chains of membrane lipids throughout the outer segments. This arrangement not only places the fat-soluble retinal in its preferred medium, but also ensures the closeness of available opsins with which it can react to form visual pigments.

In the course of the present experiments the total quantity of opsin remained unknown. However, the overall concentration of opsin and of 11-cis retinal may not be the relevant parameters for regeneration. A more relevant parameter appears to be the relative concentration of 11-cis retinal to free opsin in the outer segment membranes. Microspectrophotometric measurements can furnish the needed information, as demonstrated in the Results section.

Based on the present investigation, the emerging view is that retinals can readily penetrate the plasma membrane from ethanolic suspension; rod and cone outer segments may accumulate them to high concentrations (e.g. 10 mM). However, in the presence of whole retina, other lipoid structures compete with photoreceptors for the suspended chromophores, thereby reducing their effective concentration. Such a "sponge-effect" by other than the receptor membranes may prevent outer segments from accruing lavish amounts of 11-cis retinal. Nevertheless, the utilization of 11-cis retinal by rods and cones may still be relatively inefficient, as was suggested by Bridges (1977) and by Pepperberg et al. (1978).

Figure 7 poignantly demonstrated that large stores of 11-cis retinal may not be necessary for rapid visual pigment generation. The spectral records reveal little, if any, accumulated retinal (the uv absorption is indicative of the presence of retinol). The preparation contained many cells. Testing several rod and cone outer segments showed that they supported no pigment regeneration at all. Thus, 11-cis retinal was scarce. And yet, the recorded cone was capable of repeated regenerations. Another curious observation concerns the time-course of rhodopsin formation in the skate retina (Pepperberg et al., 1978). It appears that their result was quite similar to that of the rods found in the present study (cf. Figs. 2, 6 and 10). However, it is less than clear why that should be so, when the experimental conditions were quite different.

The most significant finding in this work is that a difference in the rate of pigment regeneration between rods and cones exists at the cellular level; it seems that this property is already programmed into the outer segments (cf. Figs. 5 and 6 with Figs. 11 and 12). This suggests the possibility that rod pigments are different from cone pigments on a fundamental level. The illucidation of this difference in the rate of visual pigment regeneration remains a challenge for future endeavors.

As a final point, an interesting comparison can be made between the time-courses of pigment regeneration in vitro with those of the human visual pigments determined in vivo by Rushton (1961, 1963). He found that rhodopsin in the living human eye after strong light exposures regenerates with an exponential time-course, having a time constant of $\tau = 6$ min. The green-absorbing cone system (chlorolabe) in the living human eye also recovers exponentially, but at a faster rate having $\tau = 120-140$ sec (2-2.23 min). The ratio of these time constants is 2.6-3. Thus, the relative rate of pigment regeneration between the human rods and cones (6 min and 2 min) is similar to that found in this work for carp, Xenopus and Necturus (10 min and 4 min). The absolute rates appear more difficult to compare. Based on the temperature-dependence of cattle rhodopsin regeneration found by Matsumoto et al. (1978), a more than 2-fold increase in the rate constants would be expected to occur for a 15° temperature increase (viz. from 22 to 37°C). Thus, in view of cattle and human rhodopsins, the absolute rates of regeneration encountered at 22-23°C in this work appear to be too high. This implies that factors other than temperature are also involved. Although the high 11-cis retinal concentrations found to occur in situ under the chosen experimental conditions were probably crucial for the fast kinetics, a satisfactory interpretation of the disparity must await the outcome of further experiments.

REFERENCES

Arnaboldi, M., M.G. Motto, K. Tsujimoto, V. Balosh-Nair, K. Nakanishi
    (1979). Hydroretinals and Hydrorhodopsins, J. Am. Chem. Soc.,
    101, 7082-7084.
Azuma, K., M. Azuma and W. Sickel (1977). Regeneration of rhodopsin
    in frog rod outer segments, J. Physiol. 271, 747-759.
Balogh-Nair, V. and K. Nakanishi (1982 a). Synthetic analogs of
    retinal, bacteriorhodopsin, and bovine rhodopsin, in: "Methods
    in Enzymology". Vol. 88, Biomembranes, Part I, V.P. and P.M.
    II, L. Packer, ed., pp. 496-506, Academic Press, New
    York.
Balogh-Nair, V., and K. Nakanishi (1982 b). The stereochemistry of
    vision, in: "New Comprehensive Biochemistry", chap. 7, Ch.
    Tammed, ed., pp. 283-334, Elsevier Biomedical Press, Amsterdam.
Baumann, C. (1970). Regeneration of rhodopsin in the isolated
    retina of the frog Rana esculenta, Vision Res., 10, 627-637.
Baumann, C. (1972). The regeneration and renewal of visual pigment
    in vertebrates, in: "Handbook of Sensory Physiology", Vol.
    VII/1, Photochemistry of Vision H.J.A. Dartnall ed., pp. 395-
    416, Springer-Verlag, Berlin, Heidelberg; New York.
Bridges, C.D.B. (1973). Interrelations of visual pigments and
    "Vitamins A" in fish and amphibia, in: "Biochemistry and
    Physiology of Visual Pigments", H. Langer ed., pp. 115-121,
    Springer-Verlag, New York, Heidelberg, Berlin.
Bridges, C.D.B. (1977). Rhodopsin regeneration in rod outer seg-
    ments: Utilization of 11-cis retinal and retinol, Exp. Eye
    Res., 24, 571-580.
Bridges, C.D.B. and S. Yoshikami (1970). The rhodopsin-porphyropsin
    system in freshwater fishes. 2. Turnover and interconversion
    of visual pigment prosthetic groups in light and darkness-
    role of the pigment epithelium, Vision Res., 10, 1333-1345.
Brown, P.K., I.R. Gibbon and G. Wald(1963). The visual cells and
    visual pigment of mudpuppy, Necturus, J. Cell Biol., 19, 79-
    106.
Cone, R.A. and P.K. Brown (1969). Spontaneous regeneration of rho-
    dopsin in the isolated rat retina, Nature 221, 818-820.
Crescitelli, F. (1958). The natural hystory of visual pigments.
    Ann. N.Y. Acad. Sci., 74, 230-255.
Crescitelli, F. and H.J.A. Dartnall (1954). A photosensitive pig-
    ment of the carp retina, J. Physiol., 125, 607-627.

Dowling, J.E. (1960). Chemistry of visual adaptation in the rat, Nature, 188, 114-118.

Harosi, F.I. (1975). Absorption spectra and linear dichroism of some amphibian photoreceptors. J. Gen. Physiol., 66, 357-382.

Harosi, F.I. (1976). Spectral relations of cone pigments in goldfish, J. Gen. Physiol., 68, 65-80.

Harosi, F.I. (1982). Recent results from single-cell microspectrophotometry: Cone pigments in frog, fish and monkey, Color Res. Applic., Vol. 7, n. 2, Part 2, pp. 135-141.

Harosi, F.I. and E.F. MacNichol, Jr. (1974 a). Dichroic microspectrophotometer: A computer-assisted, rapid, wavelength-scanning photometer for measuring linear dichroism in single cells, J. Opt. Soc. Amer., 64, 903-918.

Harosi, F.I. and E.F. MacNichol, Jr. (1974 b). Visual pigments of goldfish cones. Spectral properties and dichroism, J. Gen. Physiol., 63, 279-304.

Honig, B., U. Dinur, K. Nakanishi, V., Balogh-Nair, M.A. Gawinowicz, M. Arnaboldi, M.G. Motto (1979). An external point-charge model for wavelength regulation in visual pigments, J. Am. Chem. Soc., 101, 7084-7086.

Hubbard, R. and G. Wald (1952). Cis-trans isomers of vitamin A and retinene in the rhodopsin system, J. Gen. Physiol., 36, 269-315.

Liebman, P.A. (1972). Microspectrophotometry of photoreceptors, in: "Handbook of Sensory Physiology", Vol. VII/1, Photochemistry of Vision, H.J.A. Dartnall ed., pp. 481-528, Springer-Verlag, Berlin, Heidelberg, New York.

Liebman, P.A. (1973). Microspectrophotometry of visual receptors, in: "Biochemistry and Physiology of Visual Pigments", H. Langer ed., pp. 299-305, Springer-Verlag, Berlin, Heidelberg, New York.

Liebman, P.A. and G. Entine (1964). Sensitive low light level microspectrophotometer: detection of photosensitive pigments of retinal cones, J. Opt. Soc. Amer., 54, 1451-1459.

Marks, W.B. (1963). Difference spectra of the visual pigments in single goldfish cones, Ph.D. Thesis. The Johns Hopkins University, Baltimore, MD.

Marks, W.B. (1965). Visual pigments of single goldfish cones, J. Physiol., 178, 14-32.

Matsumoto, H., K. Horiuchi and T. Yoshizawa (1978). Effect of digitonin concentration on regeneration of cattle rhodopsin, Biochem. Biophys. Acta, 501, 257-268.

Pepperberg, D.R. (1982). Generation of rhodopsin and "artificial" visual pigments in electrophysiologically active photoreceptors in: "Biomembranes, Part H, Visual Pigments and Purple Membranes", I. (L. Packer, ed.) Methods in Enzymology, Vol. 81, pp. 452-459. Academic Press, New York.

Pepperberg, D.R.; M. Lurie, P.K. Brown and J.E. Dowling (1976). Visual adaptation: Effects of externally applied retinal on the light-adapted isolated skate retina, Science, 191, 394-396.

Pepperberg, D.R., P.K. Brown, M. Lurie and J.E. Dowling (1978). Visual pigment and photoreceptor sensitivity in the isolated skate retina, J. Gen. Physiol., 71, 369-396.

Reuter, T. (1966). The synthesis of photosensitive pigments in the rods of the frog's retina, Vision Res., 6, 15-38.

Reuter, T., R.H. White and G. Wald (1971). Rhodopsin and porphyropsin fields in the adult bullfrog retina, J. Gen. Physiol., 58, 351-371.

Rushton, W.A.H. (1961). Dark-adaptation and the regeneration of rhodopsin, J. Physiol., 156, 166-178.

Rushton, W.A.H. (1963). Cone pigment kinetics in the protanope. J. Physiol., 168, 374-388.

Shichi, H. (1971). Biochemistry of visual pigments. II. Phospholipid requirement and opsin conformation for regeneration of bovine rhodopsin, J. Biol. Chem., 246, 6178-6182.

Stell, W.K. and F.I. Harosi (1976). Cone structure and visual pigment content in the retina of the goldfish, Vision Res., 16, 647-657.

Tsin, A.T.C., P.A. Liebman, D.D. Beatty and R. Drzymala (1980). Rod and cone visual pigments in the goldfish, Vision Res., 21, 943-946.

Wald, G. and P.K. Brown (1950). The synthesis of rhodopsin from retinene, Proc. Nat. Acad. Sci. (U.S.A.), 36, 84-92.

Wald, G. and P.K. Brown (1953). The molar extinction of rhodopsin, J. Gen. Physiol., 37, 189-200.

Witkovsky, P., G.A. Engbretson and H. Ripps (1978). Formation, Conversion and utilization of isorhodopsin, rhodopsin and porphyropsin by rod photoreceptors in the Xenopus retina, J. Gen. Physiol., 72, 821-836.

Witkovsky, P., J.S. Levine, G.A. Engbretson, G. Hassin and E.F. MacNichol, Jr. (1981). A microspectrophotometric study of normal and artificial visual pigments in the photoreceptors of Xenopus laevis, Vision Res., 21, 867-873.

Zorn, M. and S. Futterman (1971). Properties of rhodopsin dependent
    on associated phospholipid, J. Biol. Chem., 246, 881-886.

RETINAL-BINDING PROTEIN IN THE HONEYBEE RETINA

I.M. Pepe[*], J. Schwemer[+], R. Paulsen[+] and C. Cugnoli[*]

[*]Institue of Cybernetics and Biophysics of CNR
Camogli, Italy
[+]Institut fur Tierphysiologie, Ruhr-Universitat
Bochum, West Germany

INTRODUCTION

The morphology and physiology of the honeybee visual system have accumulated enough data to formulate general ideas on the structure and function of the compound eye. In contrast, the study of its chemistry has encountered unusual difficulties. For example important problems as the isolation and identification of the visual pigments as well as that of their turnover, have not ben solved so far.

It has been known for a long time that bees are able to discriminate colours (von Frisch, 1914) and are also capable of orientation to the plane of polarized light (von Frisch, 1949). Behavioural observations had led to the hypothesis that colour vision in bees is based on a trichmatic system. Daumer (1956) postulated the existence in the bee retina of a yellow, a blue-violet and an ultra-violet receptor. By extracellular recordings of the spectral sensitivity after selective adaption. Goldsmith (1960) found two maxima, one at about 345 nm, the other at about 535 nm. Finally spectral sensitivity measurements on single photoreceptor cell with intracellular microelectrodes showed in honeybee workers maxima at 340, 430, 460 and 530 nm and in honeybee drones at 340, 450 and 530 nm (Autrum and von Zwehl, 1964; Autrum, 1965). The dominant receptor, found throughout the entire compound eye, has sensitivity maximum at 530 nm for the workers and at 450 nm for the drones.

The structure of the honeybee compound eye has been revealed in details by a number of electron microscopic studies (Goldsmith, 1962; Varela and Porter, 1969; Perrelet, 1970). The single unit, the ommatidium contains nine retinula cells. Each cell forms a rhabdomere which contribute to a central rhabdom. The microvillar membranes of the rhabdomeres, which correspond to the disk membranes of the vertebrate rods, are thought to contain the visual pigments. The observation that the rhabdomeres undergo structural changes upon irradiation (Gribakin, 1969) revealed three photoreceptor cells with different spectral sensitivities in a single ommatidium (Gribakin, 1972). Freeze-etching of the rhabdomeric microvilli demonstrated membrane particles with a diameter of 70-90 Å which seem to be related to visual pigment molecules (Perrelet, Bauer and Fryder, 1972).

The only direct information on visual pigments of the honeybee come from microspectrophotometry. Bertrand, Fuortes and Muri (1979) were able to find one visual pigment in drone eye with λ_{max} 445 nm which is converted by light to metarhodopsin with λ_{max} 505 nm. All attempts to bring visual pigments from honeybee compound eyes into detergent solution have failed so far. Fernandez and Bishop (1973) isolated a photosensitive pigment from honeybee heads, but the authors assume that this pigment originated from ocelli and not from compound eyes.

In 1958, Goldsmith already extracted a light sensitive pigment from honeybee heads. On exposure to light, the pigment bleached leading to a maximal absorbance decrease at about 450 nm and an increase in the near ultraviolet which was attributed to retinaldehyde, the chromophore of visual pigments. Yet, in contrast to all visual pigments which had been isolated so far, this retinalprotein complex was water-soluble. Goldsmith first suggested that this pigment could be the visual pigment of the drone because of the agreement between the absorbance maximum and the sensitivity maximum of the most common photoreceptor in the drone retina. Later on, however, the unusual property of being water-soluble as well as the fact that most of the animals used for preparing this extract were worker bees (dominant receptor at 535 nm) led to some doubt about the nature of this pigment (Goldsmith, 1972).

However vitamin A was demonstrated to be involved in the visual cycle of the bees. Dark-adapted bees contain more retinaldehyde than light-adapted animals which contain correspondingly more retinal.

Moreover, a NADH-dependent enzyme capable of reducing retinal retinol was found in bee heads (Goldsmith and Warner, 1964).

Starting from these data, Pepe, Perrelet and Bauman (1976) injected tritiated retinol into the hemolymph of live drones and analysed the labeled proteins in the retina 6 hours after the inijection by gel electrophoresis. They found that the radioactivity was only bound to a water-soluble, light-sensitive protein. The label, introduced as retinol, seemed to be converted to retinal, associated with the protein via a Schiff base linkage.

A similar retinal-protein complex could be isolated from heads of worker bees, which were homogenized and then incubated with tritiated retinol (Pepe and Cugnoli, 1980). Material from some hundres of bee heads was purified by preparative electrophoresis on polyacrylamide gel, the radioactive band was eluted and analysed.

Molecular weight and structure of the protein

Protein isolated by preparative electrophoresis behaved as a single band on standard polyacrylamide gel. However, analysis of the sample by SDS-gel electrophoresis showed that the extracted protein was not homogeneous. When samples were first irradiated in presence of sodium borohydride and then subjected to SDS-gel electrophoresis, two protein bands were found with apparent molecular weights of 27.000 and 24.000 Daltons (Pepe and Cugnoli, 1980). Both proteins bind retinaldehyde. The pigment having a molecular weight of 27.000 was further purified by means of ion-exchange chromatography on a DEAE-Sephacel column. The molecular weight was estimated by gel filtration chromatography, yielding a value of about 50.000 Daltons. This result suggests that the native protein has a quaternary structure of a dimer (Schwemer, Pepe, Paulsen and Cugnoli, in preparation). The number of retinaldehyde molecules bound to one protein molecule has not yet been determined.

Spectrophotometry

The absorbance properties of the bee-pigment (MW 27.000) are shown in Fig. 1. Besides a protein peak at 280 nm, an absorbance maximum at about 440 nm can be observed. Upon irradiation with light of the wavelength 493 nm the pigment bleaches. The absorbance in the blue spectral range is decreased (maximally at about 445 nm), whereas an increase in absorbance is found in the ultra-violet (maximally at about 370 nm) which is due to the formation of a photoproduct (Fig. 2).

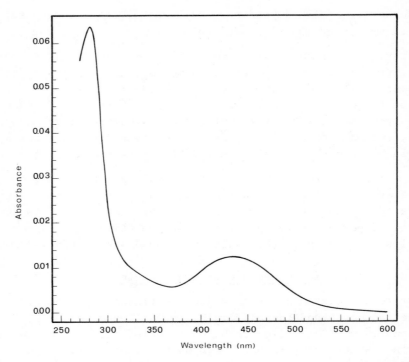

Fig. 1. Absorbance spectrum of the bee-pigment in 0.1 M phosphate
         buffer (pH 7.0); room temperature).

If 0.1 M hydroxylamine is added to an unbleached sample in the
dark, the absorbance at 440 nm decreases with a concomitant increase
at approximately 360 nm (Pepe, Schwemer and Paulsen, 1982) characteristic of the formation of retinal oxime. The molar extinction
coefficient (ε) of the 440-pigment was estimated to be approximately
47.000 M^{-1} cm^{-1}. Based on this value, estimation of the molar absorbance coefficient of the photoproduct (Fig. 2) leads to approximately 24.000 M^{-1} cm^{-1} which is very close to values for cis-
isomers of retinal. From this it is suggested that all-trans
retinal which is bound to the protein is transformed by light into
a cis isomer. Moreover, when the chromophore of the photoproduct
is extracted and then incubated with freshly prepared frog opsin
the formation of frog rhodopsin (λ_{max} 502 nm) can be observed
indicating that at least some of the retinal had been converted to
the 11-cis conformation.

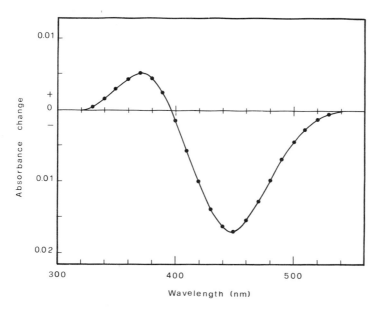

Fig. 2.   Absorbance change after irradiating the bee-pigment for
          10 min with light of λ 493 nm (pH 6.9; room temperature).

Binding between retinal and protein

When the pH of a solution of the bee-pigment is changed from
6.5 to 9.5 in the dark, a decrease in absorbance at 440 nm and an
increase with maximum at about 365 nm is found. Changing the pH
of the solution subsequently from 9.5 to 7.0, the absorbance changes
are reversed, i.e., the alkaline product with λ_{max} 365 nm is recon-
verted to the 440-form. The titration curve shows a pK of 8.4
(Pepe, Schwemer and Paulsen, 1982). These results suggest that
retinal is bound to the protein via a Schiff base linkage which can
exist in a protonated (λ_{max} 440 nm) and an unprotonated form (λ_{max}
at about 365 nm).

Irradiation of the pigment in the presence of 1% sodium cyanoborohydride leads to the formation of a photoproduct with absorbance
maximum at about 330 nm (Pepe, Schwemer and Paulsen, 1982). This
photoproduct is most likely a retinyl-protein in agreement with the
observation that the radioactive chromophore remains covalently
attached to the protein after reduction (Pepe and Cugnoli, 1980).
Since the reaction with cyanoborohydride does not occur in the dark,
it is assumed that light causes an isomerization of the chromophore
which is followed by some conformational change of the tertiary

structure of the protein as well as a deprotonation of the binding
site which then becomes accessible to the reducing agent.

Isomeric form of the chromophore

When the chromophore of the protein band was extracted from
dark-adapted bees (1 hour) and then analyzed by thin layer chromatography on silica gel, a mixture of all-trans retinal and 11-cis
retinal was found with a ratio trans/cis of about 3/1. After
irradiation of an identical sample with light (30 min), the analysis
of the chromophore gave a ratio trans/cis of about 1/1 showing that
part of all-trans retinal was transformed by light into 11-cis
retinal (Pepe and Cugnoli, 1980).

Recently, the chromophore of the purified pigment (MW 27.000)
was analyzed by high pressure liquid chromatography (HPLC). A
protein extract was divided into two samples, one of which was kept
in the dark and the other one was irradiated for 20 min with light
of the wavelength 530 nm. Subsequently, retinal was extracted from
the two samples with methylene-chloride (Pilkiewicz et al., 1972),
evaporated under nitrogen, dissolved in 20 μl hexane and run on a
5 μm Ultrasphere-Si column (Altex).

Table 1. Isomeric composition of the bee-pigment chromophore before
and after irradiation with λ 530 nm. The values are given
as percentage of the total concentration of retinal.

	dark sample	irradiated sample
all-trans retinal	62%	16%
ii-cis retinal	38%	84%
ʽ-cis retinal	0%	8%

The chromatogram from HPLC showed mainly the presence of all-
trans and 11-cis retinal with the exception of a small peak of
13-cis retinal which was formed during irradiation. Table 1 which
gives the results as percentage of the total retinal concentration
shows that after 20 min of irradiation with a wavelength primarily
absorbed by the protonated Schiff-base, 40% of all-trans retinal
are converted to the 11-cis isomer.

Discussion

The results summarized in Table I clearly show that the chromophore of the bee-pigment, all-trans retinaldehyde, is isomerized
by light almost exclusively to the 11-cis isomer. This latter

isomer was shown to be the prerequisite to rhodopsin synthesis in flies (Schwemer, in press). Since this isomerization process requires light, earlier results can now be explained in which, after injection of tritiated retinol into live drones, no radioactivity was found to be associated with membrane proteins (Pepe, Perrelet and Baumann, 1976). After injection, the animals had been kept in the dark and thus, radioactive all-trans retinal was not isomerized. Consequently, the labeled chromophore remained bound to the water-soluble protein, and rhodopsin synthesis did not occur.

In flies, a renewal of visual pigment has been demonstrated which includes also a light-dependent isomerization of all-trans retinal with a peak of the efficiency spectrum in the blu-violet spectral range (Schwemer, 1979; 1982 a; 1982 b). On the basis of his experiments, Schwemer postulated that the isomerization of all-trans retinal requires a protein which shifts the absorbance maximum of retinaldehyde from the near ultraviolet into the visible spectral range. The protein extracted from honeybee heads could provide such an enzymatic function in the compound eye. Further support of this hypothesis come from the fact that the bee-protein shares some remarkable similarities with the well characterized retinochrome of cephalopods (Hara and Hara, 1972), e.g. photoconversion of all-trans retinal to 11-cis retinal, pH-dependent absorbance properties, as well as a smaller molecular weight than that of the visual pigment. Despite the fact that the bee-protein differs from retinochrome with respect to its solubility, it nevertheless may have the same function as is suggested for retinochrome, i.e. the isomerization of all-trans retinal into 11-cis retinal.

REFERENCES

Autrum, H. (1965). The physiological basis of colour vision in honeybees, in: "Ciba Foundation Symposium on Physiology and Experimental Psychology of Colour Vision", Little, Brown and Co, Boston.

Autrum, H. and von Zwehl, V. (1964). Die spektrale Empfindlichkeit einzelner Sehzellen des Bienenauges, Z. vergl. Physiol., 48, 357-384.

Bertrand, D., Fuortes, G. and Muri, R. (1979). Pigment trasformation and electrical responses in retinula cells of drone, Apis mellifera, J. Physiol., 296, 431-441.

Daumer, K. (1956). Reizmetrische Untersuchung des Farbensehens der Bienen, Z. vergl. Physiol., 38, 413-478.

Fernandez, H.R. and Bishop, L.G. (1973). Photosensitive pigment from the worker honeybee, Apis Mellifera, Vision Res., 13, 1379-1381.

von Frisch, K. (1914). Der Farbisnn und Formensinn der Biene, Zool. Zoll. Jb., Abt. Zool. u. Physiol., 35, 1-182.

von Frisch, K. (1949). Die Polarization des Himmelslichtes als orientierender Faktor bei den Tanzen der Bienen, Experientia, 5, 142-148.

Goldsmith, T.H. (1958). The visual system of the honeybee, Proc. Natl. Acad. Sci. USA, 44, 123-126.

Goldsmith, T.H. (1960). The nature of the retinal action potential and the spectral sensitivities of ultraviolet and green receptor systems in the compound eye of the worker honeybee, J. gen. Physiol., 43, 775-799.

Goldsmith, T.H. (1962). Fine structure of the retinulae in the compound eye of the honeybee, J. Cell. Biol., 14, 489-494.

Goldsmith, T.H. (1972). The natural history of invertebrate visual pigments, in: "Handbook of Sensory Physiology, vol. 7, Photochemistry of Vision. Dartnall, H.J.A., ed., pp. 684-719, Springer-Verlag, New York.

Goldsmith, T.H. and Warner, L.T. (1964). Vitamin A in the vision of insects, J. gen. Physiol., 47, 433-441.

Gribakin, F.G. (1969). Cellular basis of colour vision in the honeybee, Nature, 223, 639-641.

Gribakin, F.G. (1972). The distribution of long wave photoreceptors in the compound eye of the honeybee as revealed by selective osmic staining. Vision Res., 12, 1225-1230.

Hara, T. and Hara, R. (1972). Cephalopod retinochrome, in: Hanbook of Sensory Physiology. vol. 7, part 1, Photochemistry of Vision, Dartnall, H.J.A. ed., pp. 720-766. Springer-Verlag, New York.

Pepe, I.M. and Cugnoli, C. (1980). Isolation and characterization of a water-soluble photopigment from honeybee compound eye. Vision Res., 20, 97-102.

Pepe, I.M. Perrelet, A. and Baumann, F. (1976). Isolation by polyacrylamide gel electrophoresis of a light-sensitive vitamin A-protein complex from the retina of the honeybee drone, Vision Res., 16, 905-908.

Pepe, I.M. Schwemer, J. and Paulsen, R. (1982). Characteristics of retinal-binding proteins from the honeybee retina, Vision Res., 22, 775-781.

Perrelet, A. (1970). The fine structure of the retina of the honeybee drone, Z. Zellforsch, 108, 530-562.

Perrelet, A. Bauer, H. and Fryder, V. (1972). Fracture faces of
an insect rhabdome, J. de Microscopie, 13, 97–106.
Pilkiewicz, F.G. Pettei, M.J. Yudd, A.P. and Nakanishi, K. (1977).
A simple and non-isomerizing procedure for the identification
of protein-linked retinals, Expl. Eye Res., 24, 421–423.
Schwemer, J. (1979). Molekulare Grundlagen der Photorezeption bei
der Schmeissfliege Calliphora erythrocephala Meig. Habilitations-
schrift Abt. Biologie, Ruhr-Universitat, Bochum (W. Germany).
Schwemer, J. (1982 a). Visual pigment turnover in fly photoreceptors. Abstract book of the Fifth International Congress of
Eye Research, October 3–8. Eindhoven. The Netherlands p. 9.
Schwemer, J. (1982 b). Pathways of rhodopsin regeneration in fly
photoreceptors, Biophys. Struct. Mech., in the press.
Varela, F.G. and Porter, K. (1969). Fine structure of visual
system of the honeybee (Apis mellifera). The retina, J. Ultrastruct. Res., 29. 236–259.

EARLY STEPS IN THE ACTIVATION OF PHOTORECEPTOR ENZYMES BY LIGHT: INTERACTIONS BETWEEN DISK MEMBRANE PROTEINS TRIGGERED BY LIGHT AND REGULATED BY GTP

Hermann Kühn

Institut für Neurobiologie der Kernforschungsanlage Jülich
5170 Jülich, Federal Republic of Germany

1. INTRODUCTION

1.1. Light-activated enzymes in rod outer segments

Absorption of visible light by rhodopsin in vertebrate rod outer segments (ROS) leads to the activation of several enzymes or enzymatic reactions. Light triggers, for instance, the exchange of (guanosin triphosphate) GTP for bound (guanosin diphosphate) GDP on a GTP-binding protein (Godchaux & Zimmerman, 1979). This nucleotide exchange is highly amplified, i.e., up to several hundred exchanges can be triggered for one photon absorbed (Fung & Stryer, 1980). The GTP-binding protein consists of three polypeptides G_α (M$_r$ 37-40 K), G_β (35-37 K), and G_γ (6-10 K) (Kühn, 1980 a,b; Fung, Hurley & Stryer, 1981). It also has GTPase activity (Wheeler & Bitensky, 1977; Godchaux & Zimmerman, 1979; Kühn, 1980 a,b), and has therefore also been termed "GTPase" (Weeler & Bitensky, 1977; Kühn, 1980 a,b), as well as "transducin" (Fung & Stryer, 1980); it will be abbreviated throughout this paper by the term "G-protein".

Following nucleotide exchange (i.e., in the GTP-binding form), the α-subunit of G-protein activates a cyclic GMP-phosphodiesterase (Fung et al., 1981; Uchida, Wheeler, Yamazaki & Bitensky, 1981). Phosphodiesterase (PDE) activation is also highly amplified as has been reported first by Yee & Liebman (1978).

Light absorption furthermore converts rhodopsin into a substrate for phosphorylation by a specific protein kinase and ATP (e.g., Kühn

75

& Dreyer, 1972; Bownds, Dawes, Miller & Stahlman, 1972; Kühn, 1978).
Up to nine phosphate groups can be incorporated per bleached rhodopsin; incorporation is 50-100 times greater into bleached than
into dark-adapted rhodopsin (Wilden & Kühn, 1982). Other light-
stimulated enzyme reactions reported in ROS include a Ca-dependent
GTPase (Biernbaum & Bownds, 1979; Robinson & Hagins, 1979) and one
or several ATPases (Thacher, 1978; Uhl, Borys & Abrahamson, 1979).

1.2. Some facts and speculations about the mechanism of light activation

All these enzymatic reactions are activated by visible light
that is not absorbed by the enzyme proteins themselves but by rhodopsin. Whenever the action spectrum of enzyme activation has been
measured, it has coincided with the absorption spectrum of rhodopsin
(reviewed by Pober & Bitensky, 1979). This implies that photo-
excitation of rhodopsin is the first step in enzyme activation and
that photoexcited rhodopsin must somehow, directly or indirectly,
interact with the enzymes in order to activate them.

One requirement for such interactions is that the enzymes must
recognise photoexcited rhodopsin (R^*) and distinguish it from dark-
adapted rhodopsin; i.e., absorption of light must lead to conformational changes in rhodopsin, not only around the chromophore inside
the hydrophobic core (Chabre & Breton, 1979; Rafferty, 1979), but
also at the cytoplasmic-exposed surface of rhodopsin that is expected to interact with peripheral and soluble proteins. Such
surface-conformational changes have recently been reported. One
SH group becomes more accessible to chemical modification (Chen &
Hubbell, 1978), and the carboxyl terminus becomes more accessible
to proteolytic cleavage by thermolysin (Kühn, Mommertz & Hargrave,
1982). The earliest photoproduct at which increased accessibility
to proteolysis can be observed is metharodopsin II. Further conformational changes are expected to occur and should be detected
by different probes sensitive to other regions of rhodopsin's surface.

Light-induced interactions between peripherally associated or
soluble ROS proteins and the disk membrane have been observed in
binding experiments (Kühn, 1978, 1980 a,b, 1981) and have been
further analyzed by light scattering techniques (Kühn, Bennett,
Michel-Villaz & Chabre, 1981). Guanosine triphosphate (GTP) plays
an important role in these interactions. The experimental results

(all obtained with bovine ROS preparations) will be reviewed here
and will be briefly discussed with regard to hypothetical mechanisms
of enzyme activation.

2. LIGHT-INDUCED BINDING/DISSOCIATION OF PROTEINS

The most simple way of studying interactions between extractable
proteins and the disk membrane is the separation of soluble and
membrane-bound proteins by centrifugation. The supernatants are
then analyzed for enzymatic activities, as well as for their polypeptide composition, using polyacrylamide gel electrophoresis in
the presence of sodium dodecyl sulfate (SDS-PAGE); the pellets may
be subjected to further treatments in order to release bound proteins. This centrifugation technique allows one to detect only
strong, long-lasting interactions ("binding"). The supernatants
from bleached ROS are called "light extracts", and those from unbleached ROS "dark extracts".

The five most prominent light-dependent polypeptides and their
corresponding enzymatic activities are listed in Table I. These
polypeptides are present in dark extracts and are more or less
absent in corresponding light extracts because they sediment with
the bleached membranes. The α and β subunits of G-protein are the
most abundant of these polypeptides; ROS contain about one molecule
of both α and β subunit per 10 rhodopsin molecules (Kühn, 1981).
The 48 K protein is about 5-10 times less abundant; its function
is not yet determined. The kinase is present in very small quantities and yields only a faint band on SDS gels (Kühn, 1978, 1981)
but can be easily followed by its enzymatic activity. Kinase activity in dark extracts is typically about 10 times higher (up to
20 times; see Kühn, 1978) than in corresponding light extracts.
GTPase activity is typically 20-50 times higher in dark extracts
than in light extracts. Since rhodopsin is needed in such enzyme
assays to serve as a substrate for kinase, or to mediate light
activation of the G-protein (GTPase), respectively, washed disk
membranes devoid of intrinsic enzyme activities are added to the
enzyme assays of soluble supernatant (Kühn, 1978, 1980 a, b, 1981).

The light-induced binding is <u>reversible</u>: the bleached membranes
slowly relax in the dark into a form which releases the bound proteins in soluble form. The half-time of this spontaneous relaxation is of the order of 15 min (Kühn, 1978, 1980 a,b, 1981) but
varies among ROS preparations. A rapid and specific dissociation
of the G-protein from the bleached membranes is induced by GTP,

Table I. Polypeptides (enzymes) that undergo light-induced binding
          to the disk membrane

Polypeptide	Solubility at moderate ionic strenght	Enzymatic activity	Typical ratios of activities present in dark vs. light extracts
68 000	mostly soluble	rhodopsin-kinase	ca. 10 : 1
48 000	soluble	?	
37 000 35 000 6 000	membrane associated	G-protein (GTPase)	ca. 30 : 1

independently of the spontaneous release (see later section on
"effect of nucleotides").

Besides the five polypeptides shown in Table I, two additional
polypeptides can be found under certain extraction conditions to
be more concentrated in dark extracts than in light extracts: a
polypeptide of ca. 42 000 dalton, the light dependence of which
is seen if 1 M NH$_4$Cl is the extractant (Kühn, 1980 b), and a faint
polypeptide band above the kinase band (ca. 80 000 dalton). It is
interesting to note that the phosphodiesterase (doublet band at
about 95 K) does not undergo light-induced binding.

Several aspects of the light-induced binding will be discussed
in more detail in the following subsections.

2.1. Influence of ionic strength

Most of the extractable ROS proteins are soluble at any ionic
strength and will therefore be termed "soluble proteins" for con-

venience. The 48 K protein and the major part of rhodopsin-kinase
belong to this category (see Table I). Other proteins, particularly
the G-protein and the phosphodiesterase, are membrane-associated
at moderate ionic strength (100-150 mM salt) and need extremely low
ionic strength (e.g., < 10 mM salt) to be eluted from the membranes.
They are termed "peripheral proteins".

Extraction of ROS in light and darkness at moderate ionic
strength reveals mainly two light-dependent proteins in the supernatants, namely the kinase and the 48 K protein (Kühn, 1978). The
G-protein also undergoes light-induced binding at moderate ionic
strength (Kühn, 1980 a, 1981), but this is not revealed in the
corresponding supernatant since most of the G-protein remains membrane-bound in both light and darkness due to the ionic strength
(Fig. 1, left side). That light-induced binding has occurred can
be demonstrated by a subsequent treatment of the pellet with low
ionic strength-buffer in the dark: the G-protein is then readily
extracted from the unbleached pellet but not from the previously
bleached pellet (Fig. 1, middle). The subsequent treatment thus

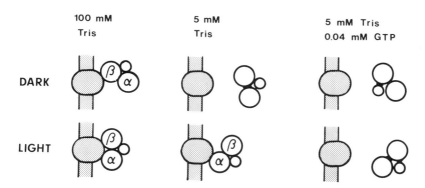

Fig. 1. Schematic presentation of the interactions of G-protein
         (subunit α, β, γ) with the rhodopsin membrane (shaded
         symbols) as a function of ionic strength, light, and GTP.
         The scheme (modified from Kühn, 1981) results from binding
         experiments and analysis of the supernatants by SDS-PAGE
         and GTPase assays (Kühn, 1980). The G-protein is membrane-
         bound at moderate ionic strength (left side); light induces
         and additional binding (α-subunit) which is not broken by
         lowering the ionic strength (middle) but is broken by GTP
         (right side). Both the ionic strength-dependent and the
         light-induced binding (i.e., the condition shown in lower
         left corner) are required for the enzyme to operate.

breaks the ionic strength-dependent but not the light-dependent mode
of binding. GTPase assays have shown (Kühn, 1981) that moderate
ionic strength is as important for optimal enzymatic activity as is
light; i.e., both modes of binding, the ionic strength-dependent
and the light-induced binding, are required for a proper functioning
of the enzyme.

Light-induced binding of the proteins shown in Table I also
takes place when ROS are illuminated at low ionic strength i.e.,
when the G-protein is soluble before illumination (Kühn, 1980 a, b).
In this case, the G-polypeptides are the most prominent light-dependent polypeptides in the corresponding supernatants (i.e., present
in dark extracts and nearly absent in light extracts). The kinase
and the G-protein also undergo light-induced binding when ROS are
illuminated at very high ionic strength (1 M NH$_4$Cl; Kühn, 1980 b).
The light-induced binding thus appears to be independent of the
ionic strength, and vice versa.

The ionic strength-dependent mode of binding is reversible.
If a dark extract, prepared at low ionic strength and therefore
contanining all of the extractable ROS proteins, is added to washed
disk membranes and the ionic strength is then raised by the addition
of 100-150 mM salt, both G-protein and PDE become nearly quantita-
vely membrane-associated whereas most of the other proteins remain
in solution (Kühn & Hargrave, 1981).

2.2. Effect of nucleotides

Guanosine triphosphate reverses the light-induced binding of
the G-protein and strengthens the binding of the 48 K protein (Kühn,
1980 a,b). At low ionic strength, the whole G-protein (α, β, and
γ subunits) is rapidly solubilized from bleached disk membranes
upon addition of GTP. This solubilizing effect is nearly specific
for GTP and its non-hydrolyzable analogs GTP-γ-S (Kühn, unpublished
experiments) and, to a lesser extent, guanylyl imidodiphosphate
(Kühn, 1980 b). The light-induced binding of G-protein, and its
specific elution from the bleached membranes with GTP after the
removal of the other extractable proteins, can be used to purify
the G-protein to homogeneity simply by repeated centrifugation of
the membranes under proper conditions of light, ionic strength and
GTP addition (Kühn, 1982).

Even at moderate ionic strength where the G-protein is normally
membrane-associated, illumination in the presence of GTP leads to

partial solubilization of the G-protein (Figs. 2 and 3). The α-subunit becomes preferentially solubilized whereas most of the β-subunit remains membrane associated due to the ionic strength. Typically, about 3-4 times as much α-subunit as compared to β-subunit is in the supernatant. (The correct results are shown by the gels of Fig. 3; the scheme in Fig. 2 oversimplifies somewhat since it does not show that some of the β-subunit is also solubilized). GTP without illumination has no solubilizing effect (Fig. 3, first gel). The light-induced solubilization of the α-subunit is related to the light-triggered exchange of GTP for bound GDP (Fung & Stryer, 1980; Fung et al., 1981; Uchida et al., 1981). The α-subunit in its GTP-binding form (G_α-GTP) obviously has no affinity for R^* and a relatively low affinity for the β-subunit; this leads to its dissociation from the membrane. The non-hydrolyzable analog GTP-γ-S, in contrast to GTP, is able to fully dissociate the α-subunit from the membranes even without illumination (Emeis, Kühn, Reichert & Hofmann, manuscript submitted), by displacing the bound GDP already in the dark.

2.3. Influence of temperature and pH

The light-induced binding of the G-protein occurs so rapidly even at 0°C that no difference in the extent of binding is seen between 0°C and 29°C (Kühn, 1980 b) (the time resolution of the centrifugation method is about 7 min). The spontaneous release of bound G-protein in the dark after bleaching is, on the other hand, a slow reaction and is highly temperature-dependent. No release

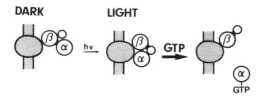

Fig. 2. Effect of light and GTP on the solubility of G-protein at moderate ionic strength. The α-subunit is solubilized following nucleotide exchange (this has been tested using ^{3}H-guanylyl-imidodiphosphate; Kühn, unpublished experiments), whereas most of the β-subunit remains membrane-associated due to the ionic strength (130 mM KCl-Ringer). The scheme is derived from the gels of Fig. 3 which show that in fact some of the β-subunit is also solubilized together with α.

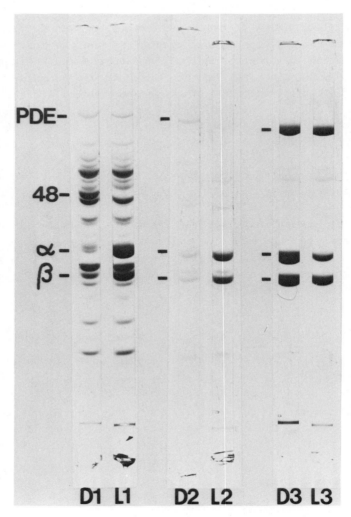

Fig. 3.   Preferential solubilization of the α-subunit of G-protein
          by illumination in the presence of GTP at moderate ionic
          strength. The first two gels show supernatants obtained
          after centrifugation of unbleached (D1) and bleached (L1)
          ROS, suspended in KCl-Ringer's solution containing 1 mM
          GTP and 2 mM ATP (results are similar if only GTP is
          present). Both the unbleached and the bleached pellet were
          reextracted in the dark with 50 mM Tris-HCl/0.5 mM GTP
          (supernatants D2 and L2) and finally with 5 mM Tris-HCl/
          ca. 0.05 mM GTP (supernatants D3 and L3). (Reproduced
          with kind permission from Academic Press; Kühn, 1981).

is observed within 90 min at 0°C, and low release at 11°C and 16°C, whereas the release is completed within 90 min at 29°C (Kühn, 1980 b). The light-induced binding of the 48 K-protein is much slower than that of G-protein and does not take place to an appreciable extent at 0°C (Kühn, unpublished observations).

The pH-dependence of light-induced- binding of G-protein gives some interesting insights about the "active" photoproduct of rhodopsin, R*, that causes the binding. At 0°C, bovine metarhodopsin I (MI) and MII are in a stable, pH-dependent equilibrium; MI predominates at alkaline pH, MII at acid pH, and about equal amounts of MI and MII are present at pH 7.0 in the "classical" equilibrium extensively described in the literature (reviewed in Emeis & Hofmann, 1981). Recent data by Emeis & Hofmann (1981) have shown, however, that this classical equilibrium holds only in the case of washed disc membranes but not in ROS at low bleaching extents. An extractable protein, which has recently been identified to be G-protein (Emeis, Kühn, Reichert & Hofmann; Bennett, Michel-Villaz & Kühn, manuscripts submitted), shifts the equilibrium towards MII (see also next section).

At moderate ionic strength, the G-protein undergoes light-induced binding at all pH conditions tested i.e., between pH 5.8 and 8.4. At pH 8.4/0°C, MI would "normally" be the only photoproduct present in the classical equilibrium; however, the spectra show that MII is nevertheless formed ("extra MII" due to the presence of G-protein), and the binding experiments show that light-induced binding takes place under these conditions of ionic strength. The situation is different at low ionic strength: here, light-induced binding of G-protein at 0°C takes place at pH 5.8 and pH 7 but not at pH 8.4. The spectra show that no MII is formed at low ionic strength, pH 8.4. Moderate ionic strength, that causes the G-protein to be peripherally membrane-associated before illumination, is obviously required to enable the shift of the equilibrium towards MII and also to enable light-induced binding at alkaline pH (Bennett et al., submitted). These results strongly suggest that MII is the active photoproduct that causes the binding.

2.4. Evidence that light-induced binding occurs to photoexcited rhodopsin (R*)

In the case of rhodopsin-kinase, it is plausible that R* is che binding target since it is the substrate for the kinase. In the case of G-protein and 48 K protein, it is at least clear that

the binding occurs to the <u>disk membrane</u>: the bound proteins do not
only sediment with the bleached membranes as they do in the usual
extraction procedure, they also float with purified bleached disks
in a procedure (Smith, Stubbs & Litman, 1975) in which pure, osmotically intact disks are separated from other membraneous material
by flotation in 5% Ficoll/water (Kühn, 1981). The following evidence indicates that G-protein binds in fact to R^* (i.e., more
specifically, to MII).

(i) G-protein shifts the photoproduct equilibrium

As already discussed in the previous section, G-protein shifts
the MI/MII equilibrium towards MII. If washed disk membranes,
suspended in moderate ionic strength buffer at pH 8.3, are bleached
at 0°C, MI (480 nm) is virtually the only photoproduct found, in
agreement with the "classical" MI/MII equilibrium. Addition of
G-protein to the bleached membranes causes a significant loss in
OD_{480} and an increase in OD_{380} indicating that MII is formed at
the cost of MI. If GTP is then added, both OD_{480} and OD_{380} return
to their original values (if correction is made for dilution) i.e.,
the MII formed due to the addition of G-protein reverts to MI as
soon as GTP has reacted with the G-protein (and thereby solubilized
its α-subunit, see Fig. 2). These results are summarized in the
following scheme (Bennett et al., submitted):

$$\text{Rhodopsin} \xrightarrow{\text{hv}} \dots \text{MI} \rightleftharpoons \text{MII} \quad \begin{array}{c} G_{GTP} \\ \\ G_{GDP} \end{array} \quad \begin{array}{c} (MII - G_{GDP}) \\ \\ MII - G_{GDP} \end{array} \quad \begin{array}{c} GDP \\ \\ GTP \end{array}$$

where G_{GDP} and G_{GTP} represent the G-protein with GDP or GTP bound,
respectively. The most simple interpretation of the data is that
G_{GDP} binds to MII that is present (in small quantities at alkaline
pH) in the equilibrium and thereby draws MII from the equilibrium
("extra MII" formation). This view is supported by recent kinetic
data (Emeis et al., submitted). If GTP is present, it displaces
the bound GDP, followed by dissociation of the putative complex
$MII-G_{GTP}$. Since G_{GTP} obviously has no affinity to R^* (see Figs.
2, 3, 7; and Kühn, 1980 a, 1981), the equilibrium turns back to
the "classical" situation, i.e. virtually pure MI, at alkaline pH
after addition of GTP.

This shows that not only R^* influences (i.e., activates) the G-protein but also the G-protein exerts an influence on R^* spectroscopy, strongly suggesting that G-protein directly interacts with R^* (MII).

(ii) <u>Proteolytic modification of rhodopsin abolishes light-induced binding of G-protein</u>

Rhodopsin in washed disk membranes can be modified in several distinct ways using limited proteolysis by thermolysin. Long-term digestion leads to internal cleavage of rhodopsin's polypeptide chain, yielding two large, noncovalently associated, membrane-bound fragments (Pober & Stryer, 1975) without changing the absorption spectrum of rhodopsin. After inactivation and removal of the protease, G-protein containing extract was added to such modified disks and to untreated control disks for binding tests in darkness and light (Kühn & Hargrave, 1981). The light-induced binding (i. e., the light-dark difference in binding) of G-protein was found to be greatly diminished in the modified disks, both at low and at moderate ionic strength. The solubilizing effect of GTP on the G-protein after illumination was similarly diminished. Intactness of the major part of rhodopsin's polypeptide chain is thus required for both the light-induced binding of G-protein and its reversal by GTP to take place. On the other hand, a more gentle proteolytic modification of rhodopsin, removing only 12 amino acids from its carboxyl terminus, has no influence, either on the light-induced binding or its reversal by GTP (Kühn & Hargrave, 1981).

(iii) <u>The stoichiometry of light-induced binding is 1:1 (i.e., one photoexcited rhodopsin per molecule of G-protein present)</u>

This can be approximately shown in binding tests using centrifugation: most of the G-protein in ROS is bound when slightly more than 10% of the total rhodopsin has been bleached (Kühn, unpublished results). (ROS contain about 10 G-proteins per 100 rhodopsins; Kühn, 1981). The same result is obtained in a more precise and more elegant way from the saturation behaviour of the ligh-scattering "binding signal", both in ROS and in a reconstituted system (Kühn, Bennett, Michel-Villaz & Chabre, 1981; see next section).

3. KINETIC AND STOICHIOMETRIC ANALYSIS BY LIGHT SCATTERING

Flash photolysis of rhodopsin in ROS suspensions leads not only to the well-known spectral changes due to rhodopsin's photo-

product decay, but also to dramatic and rapid light-scattering
changes observable in the far red or near infrared. Rapid flash-
induced scattering changes (in the absence of added nucleotides)
have been studied by a number of groups for several years in isolated
bovine ROS (e.g., Hofmann, Uhl, Hoffmann & Kreutz, 1976) and in the
toad retina (Harari, Brown & Pinto, 1978); they have led to various
interpretations such as light-induced disk and ROS shrinkage (Uhl,
Hofmann & Kreutz, 1977; Hofmann, Schleicher, Emeis & Reichert, 1981)
and light-induced "rhodopsin cooperativity" (Wey & Cone, 1978).
Bignetti, Cavaggioni, Fasella, Ottonello & Rossi (1980) were the
first who noticed that the sign of the signal was changed in presence
of GTP and suggested that it may be related to the activation of
phosphodiesterase.

     In a recent study (Kühn et al., 1981) we have shown, by using
a reconstituted system with purified G-protein, that two major
light-induced light-scattering changes in ROS membranes specifically
reflect interactions between G-protein and photoexcited rhodopsin:
the "binding signal" which is observed in the absence of GTP, and
the "dissociation signal" which is of opposite sign and is observed
in presence of GTP. Membranes (ROS fragments or washed disk membranes with various extractable proteins added), suspensed in 100
mM KCl/1 mM $MgCl_2$/10-20 mM Tris-HCl, pH 7.4, and 1 mM dithiothreitol
in a thermostated cuvette (normally 20°C) were flash-illuminated
(500 nm; 0.1-0.5 msec), and the changes in light-scattering were
monitored at 708 nm normally in transmission (occasionally also
at 90° scattering angle resulting in signals of opposite sign).

3.1. Binding signal

     Flash illumination of ROS fragments in the absence of GTP
leads to a rapid increase in turbidity termed "binding signal"
(Fig. 4A). Its total amplitude is roughly proportional to the
amount of rhodopsin bleached by the flash, up to ca. 10% bleaching,
where it saturates. If a suspension is subjected to a series of
consecutive flashes (Fig. 4A, tracings a-d), the binding signal
becomes saturated when a bleaching level of ca. 10% is reached;
further flashes evoke no further binding signals but instead, small
rapid signals of opposite sign, termed "rhodopsin signals", are
produced (Fig. 4, tracing d). The rhodopsin signal does not sat-
urate until all of the rhodopsin is bleached; it has previously
been termed "N-signal" and the binding signal has been termed "P-
signal" by Hofmann et al. (1976).

The kinetics of the binding signal are complex, consisting of
rapid (10-100 msec) and slow phases. The rapid phase is shown with
a better time resolution in Fig. 4, tracing e. Its half-time is
about 25 msec at 10% bleach and 60 msec at 1.3% bleach. The kinetics
are strongly dependent on the physical state of the preparation:
any manipulation that breaks the regular array of the disk stack
in ROS fragments (e.g., transient hypoosmotic shock or sonication)
increases the proportion of the slow kinetic components at the cost
of the rapid component, the total amplitude ($\Delta T/T$) remaining approximately constant. The harsher the treatment, the slower the time
course.

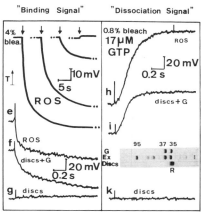

Fig. 4. Light-induced transmittance changes (at 708 nm) in ROS
         membranes (5-7 µM rhodopsin) and in a reconstituted system
         containing purified G-protein. (A) Binding signals in
         absence of GTP. Tracings a-d, ROS membrane suspension
         subjected to four consecutive flashes, each bleaching 4%
         of the rhodopsin. Tracings e and f, rapid recordings after
         bleaching 10% of the rhodopsin in ROS membranes (e) and in
         a reconstituted system of washed discs and purified G-pro-
         tein (f). Tracing g, washed discs alone (8% bleached).
         (B) Dissociation signals in presence of 17 µM GTP, induced
         by a flash bleaching 0,8% of the rhodopsin in ROS membranes
         (tracing h) or in a mixture of washed discs and purified
         G-protein (tracing i). A second flash (tracing h) evoked
         no further dissociation signal. Tracing k, washed discs
         in presence of GTP but absence of G-protein (0,8% bleach).
         (Inset) SDS-PAGE of washed disk membranes (7 µg; bottom
         gel), hypoosmotic dark extract (middle), and purified G-
         protein (upper gel). Reproduced from Kühn et al. (1981),
         slightly modified.

Reconstitution of binding signal. Removal of the extractable proteins by hypoosmotic washing abolishes the binding signal; the washed membranes give only the rhodopsin signal (Fig. 4, tracings g and k). Addition of dark extract, containing all of the extractable proteins, to the washed membranes restores the binding signal (not shown in Fig. 4), though with somewhat slower kinetics depending on the previous washing procedure. (Gentle washing with 10 mM buffer yielded still reasonably rapid reconstituted signals whereas washing with water yielded slow signals).

Addition of purified G-protein (Fig. 4 inset, upper gel) to washed membranes restores the binding signal (Fig. 4 f). The following preparations of extracted proteins were not capable of restoring the binding signal when added to washed membranes: hypoosmotic light extract (containing all of the extractable proteins except G-protein, 48 K-protein, and kinase), isotonic dark extract (containing the soluble proteins but not G-protein nor phosphodiesterase), and purified phosphodiesterase. This clearly demonstrates that the binding signal specifically reflects a light-induced interaction between G-protein and the disk membrane, most probably the binding observed earlier in the centrifugation experiments.

Saturation of the binding signal. We have already mentioned that in ROS, where about 10 molecules of G-protein are present per 100 rhodopsin, the binding signal saturates at about 10% bleaching (Fig. 4, a-d), suggesting a 1:1 stoichiometric binding of G-protein to R*. Saturation has been extensively studied in the reconstituted system of washed membranes and G-protein-containing dark extract, by applying a wide range of mixing ratios of G-protein versus rhodopsin (Kühn et al., 1981; data not shown here). Whatever the amount of G-protein added, from 0.25 to 4 times the native G-protein/rhodopsin ratio, saturation was always reached when the molar amount of rhodopsin bleached was equal to that of G-protein present. The saturation (i.e., the bleaching level, reached by a succession of small flashes, above which a further flash evokes no further binding signal) was independent of the total amount of rhodopsin present but depended only on the amount of G-protein present in the mixture. This further supports the hypothesis of a 1:1 complex formed between G-protein and R*.

3.3. Dissociation signal

Flash illumination of ROS fragments in the presence of GTP (10^{-5} - 10^{-3} M) leads to a rapid decrease in turbidity termed "dissociation signal" (Fig. 4B). The "dissociation signal" differs

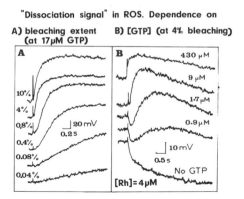

"Dissociation signal" in ROS. Dependence on
A) bleaching extent   B) [GTP] (at 4% bleaching)
   (at 17µM GTP)

Fig. 5.   Dependence of dissociation signal in ROS membranes on
          flash intensity and GTP concentration. Each tracing rep-
          presents one sample. (A) Constant GTP concentration (17
          µM) but varied bleaching extents (% R*) as indicated at
          each tracing. Rhodopsin concentration was 6.6 µM. (B)
          Constant flash intensity (bleaching 4% in each sample) but
          varied GTP concentration as indicated above each tracing.
          Rhodopsin concentration was 3.9 µM. Reproduced from Kühn
          et al. (1981).

from the "rhodopsin signal" by its much greater sensitivity to dim
light flashes, its dependence on GTP, its saturation behaviour (see
later), and its slower time course. The dissociation signal is also,
like the binding signal, a G-protein-specific signal: it is absent
in washed membranes (Fig. 4, tracing K) and is reconstituted upon
addition of purified G-protein to the membranes (Fig. 4, tracing
i). Note that the conditions in which the dissociation signal is
observed (moderate ionic strength, presence of GTP) are the same
as shown in Figs. 2 and 3, where real dissociation of the G_α-sub-
unit takes place upon illumination.

    The kinetics of the dissociation signal are less complex than
those of the binding signal; after a certain delay, the dissociation signal rises with approximately monophasic kinetics. The
kinetics strongly depend on both the flash intensity (Fig. 5A) and
the GTP concentration (Fig. 5B), being more rapid at higher light
intensities and higher GTP concentration. At very low GTP concentration, the dissociation signal is preceded by a transient binding
signal (Fig. 5B). The absence of such transient binding signal at
higher GTP concentration is not due to limited time resolution of

the recording, but is most probably due to the short life time of
the associated complex R^*-G-protein in the presence of GTP such
that too low amounts of the complex accumulate to be visible as a
transient binding signal at normal GTP concentrations (see later,
Fig. 7). The early rise of the dissociation signal is always slower
than that of the binding signal at the same flash intensity.

The saturation of the dissociation signal shows a highly non-
stoichiometric behaviour, in sharp contrast to that of the binding
signal. Flashes between 0.4% and 10% bleaching yield the same,
maximal amplitude (Figs. 5A and 6). Furthermore, a second flash
delivered after a first flash bleaching only 08.% does not evoke
a further signal (except the small rhodopsin signal; see Fig. 4B,
tracing h). This shows that, in the presence of GTP, the system
is saturated at bleaching levels below 0.8%. Note, however, that
about 10 G-proteins are present per 100 rhodopsin. It is important
that the second flash evokes neither a dissociation signal nor a
binding signal, althought the level of bleached rhodopsin (0.8%)
is far below the level of saturation of the binding signal (10%).
This indicates that the first small flash leads to the turnover of
all of the G-protein molecules into a form that is unresponsive to
further flashes, namely the GTP-binding form (abbreviated as G_{GTP})
(see Figs. 2 and 7; see also Fung & Stryer, 1980; Kühn et al.,
1981). G_{GTP} has no affinity to R^*, as is demonstrated by the gels
of Fig. 3 (light-induced dissociation in presence of GTP) as well
as by the MI/MII spectroscopic data (see the reaction scheme in
section 2.4). Because bleaching of only 0.8% of the rhodopsin
obviously transforms all of the G-protein into this unresponsive
form (G_{GTP}), one has to conclude that one R^* can turn over many
G-protein molecules.

Fig. 6 shows responses of submaximal amplitude evoked by non-
saturating dim flashes. If the amplitude evoked by a first flash,
relative to the maximal (saturated) amplitude, is taken as a measure
of the proportion of the total G-protein that has been turned over
by the flash, one arrives at the estimate that 100-130 G-protein
molecules per single R^* have been turned over at each of the three
weakest flash intensities given in Fig. 6. This confirms the biochemical data by Fung & Stryer (1980) indicating amplified nucleotide exchange at low flash intensities.

Requirement of previously bound GDP for the dissociation signal.

ROS membranes containing G-protein depleted of GDP by extensive
isotonic washing do not give dissociation signals. This is ex-

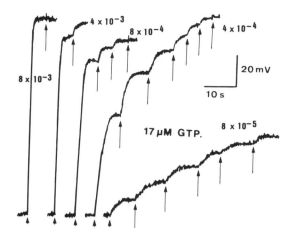

Fig. 6.   Saturation of dissociation signal. Each tracing represents
          a separate sample of ROS membranes (6.6 μM rhodopsin; 17
          μM GTP) subjected to a series of flashes (indicated by
          the arrows). The flash intensity was constant within each
          series. The fraction of rhodopsin bleached per single
          flash is indicated at each tracing. Reproduced from Kühn
          et al. (1981).

plained by the assuption that the nucleotide already binds to the
vacant binding sites on the G-protein before the flash, making it
unresponsive to the flash. Indeed, if GDP (or better, GDP-βS) is
first added, normal dissociation signals are obtained. This demonstrates that nucleotide exchange is an obligatory step needed for
the formation of dissociation signals. (The nucleotide used in such
experiments is guanylyl-imidodiphosphate rather than GTP since GTP
normally contains some GDP).

The conclusions from the light-scattering experiments are
summarized in the following reaction scheme (Fig. 7). Absorption
of light transforms rhodopsin into "photoexcited rhodopsin", R^*,
which is most probably the photoproduct MII (see section 2.4; Emeis
et al.; Bennett et al.; manuscripts submitted). The G-protein,
which in the dark-adapted state contains tightly bound GDP (abbreviated as G_{GDP}; Godchaux & Zimmerman, 1979; Fung and Stryer, 1980),
has a high affinity for R^* and therefore binds to R^* in a 1:1
stoichiometric complex $R^* - G_{GDP}$. The formation of this complex
is revealed by the "binding signal". The complex is stable for
tens of minutes in the absence of GTP. If GTP is present, however,

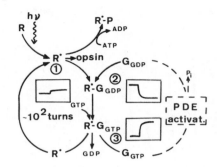

Fig. 7.   Scheme of the reaction cycle of R* leading to amplified
          GDP/GTP exchange. The light-scattering signals that
          accompany the different reaction steps are: 1, rhodopsin
          signal; 2, binding signal; 3, dissociation signal. For
          details see text. PDE, phosphodiesterase; G_{GDP}, G-protein
          in the GDP-binding form, and G_{GTP}, in the GTP-binding form.
          Reproduced from Kühn et al. (1981).

rapid exchange of GTP for bound GDP takes place in the complex.
The resulting GTP-binding form of G-protein (G_{GTP}) has no affinity
for R*; this leads to rapid dissociation of the putative complex
R* - G_{GTP} into R* and G_{GTP}, revealed as the "dissociative signal".
G_{GTP} then activates the phosphodiesterase (Fung et al., 1981; Uchida
et al., 1981) until the GTP is hydrolyzed later on. After dissociation, R* is recycled up to about 100 times, binding further G_{GDP}
molecules and catalyzind the nucleotide exchange on them. This
amplification factor of about 100, estimated from the saturation
behaviour of the dissociation signal compares well with published
biochemical data on amplified GDP/guanylyl-imidodiphosphate exchange
(amplification factor 70-500; Fung & Stryer, 1980; Fung et al.,
1981) and phosphodiesterase activation (factor 500; Yee & Liebman,
1978). The energy required for the multiple interactions of one
R* with many G_{GDP} molecules seems to be provided by the hydrolysis
of GTP in the G-protein (GTPase). The inactivation of the active
photoproduct R* seems to occur via several separate pathways: a
slow spontaneous decay of R* into an inactive photoproduct; and
a much more rapid process utilizing ATP (Liebman & Pugh, 1980) and
a soluble ROS protein (Kühn et al., 1981; Kühn, Bennett & Michel-
Villaz, unpublished experiments).

3.3. <u>Biochemically useful information contained in the light-scattering signals</u>

Light-scattering (or even worse, turbidity) phenomena on biological samples are normally very complex, making it difficult to draw specific information out of the signals. In the case of ROS membranes, however, the system is rather well defined from a biochemical veiwpoint, particularly due to the reconstituted experiments with purified G-protein; this allows one to gain specific information from different parameters of the signals. The parameters that have been used to arrive at the picture of Fig. 7 are briefly summarized below.

(i) <u>The kinetics</u> of the signals have provided insight into the velocity and temporal sequence of the binding and dissociation reactions, showing that these processes are rather rapid. The onset of the dissociation signal is slower than that of the binding signal, indicating that binding takes place before dissociation. (The slow phases of the binding signal are without interest in this context: since only a very small proportion of R^* is needed to turn over all of the G-protein, only the very early time course of the binding signal is important). The absence of an initial binding signal at GTP concentration > 5 μM (Fig. 5B) indicates that the life-time of the complex $R^* - G_{GDP}$ (and also of $R^* - G_{GTP}$, if this complex exists) must be too short at normal GTP concentration to allow for significant accumulation of the complex. The kinetics of the binding signal furthermore provides information about the active photoproduct R^* that triggers the process.

(ii) The <u>saturation</u> behaviour of the signals has provided the stoichiometry of the interactions between R^* and G-protein: a 1:1 stoichiometry of binding, and a highly non-stoichiometric relationship for the dissociation signal, the latter reflecting serial interaction of one R^* with many G-protein molecules, consistent with amplified nucleotide exchange.

(iii) The <u>recovery</u> of the responses <u>after a saturating flash</u> yields information about the life-time of R^* and about mechanisms of deactivation of R^* (not shown in this report).

(iv) Experiments with various nucleotides and analogs can provide biochemical information about <u>nucleotide specificity</u>, affinity constants for the nucleotides, competition, etc. (not shown here).

3.4. Physical origin of the light-scattering changes

The biochemical processes underlying the two signals have been characterized: both signals reflect interactions between R* and G-protein. In the case of the dissociation signal, light in presence of GTP induces a real dissociation of G-protein (mainly its α-subunit) from the membrane (see Figs. 2 and 3). In the case of the binding signal, the centrifugation experiments have shown that under the experimental conditions used (moderate ionic strength) the G-protein is membrane-associated both before and after the flash (see Fig. 1, left side); light changes only the mode of binding. How this can lead to the large scattering changes observed is not yet resolved. Apparently, the binding signal depends not only on the presence of G-protein but also on the physical state of the stack of disk membranes in ROS; this is already indicated by the dependence of its kinetics on mechanical and osmotic manipulations affecting the ROS and disk structure (see section 3.1). The physical events underlying the light-scattering changes are currently being investigated in several laboratories on magnetically oriented ROS; the most rapid components of the signals have thereby been shown to be highly anisotropic (Hofmann et al., 1981; Chabre, Vuong & Stryer, 1982). Such detailed studies of the separate components of the signals will provide further insights into the underlying structural events.

4.   ARE THE OBSERVED LIGHT-INDUCED PROTEIN INTERACTIONS RELATED
     TO ENZYME ACTIVATION?

Several arguments support the idea (but do not strictly prove it) that the observed interactions between certain ROS enzymes and photoexcited rhodopsin mediate activation of the corresponding enzymatic reactions by light. This is most plausible for the kinase since R* is its substrate. It has been shown (Kühn, 1978) that the light-induced capability of rhodopsin to be phosphorylated lasts as long as its capability to bind the kinase; this suggests that the phosphorylating activity is regulated via binding of the kinase.

In the case of the G-protein, the stoichiometry of binding (1:1), and the highly non-stoichiometric dissociation reaction with GTP (Figs. 6 and 7), which is in agreement with reported biochemical amplification data (Yee & Liebman, 1978; Fung & Stryer, 1980), also suggests that these interactions reflect the mechanism by which R* catalyzes the GDP/GTP exchange on the G-protein. Furthermore, the kinetics of the interactions, as revealed by the light-scattering signals, are compatible with the kinetics of phosphodiesterase activation reported by Yee & Liebman (1978). The observation that the binding signal is more rapid than the dissociation signal makes sense in the scheme of reactions leading to GDP/GTP exchange (Fig. 7). The observation that the phosphodiesterase does not undergo light-induced binding (Kühn, 1980 a) is consistent with the recently advanced biochemical knowledge (Fung et al., 1981; Uchida et al., 1981) that the α-subunit of G-protein alone, in the absence of photo-excited rhodopsin, activates the phosphodiesterase. Further experiments, using chemically and enzymatically modified rhodopsins, should further substantiate the relationship between the light-induced interactions and enzyme activation, and should help in localizing the sites of interaction.

REFERENCES

Biernbaum, M.S., and Bownds, M.D. (1979). Influence of light and calcium on guanosine 5'-triphosphate in isolated frog rod outer segments, J. Gen. Physiol., 74 : 649-669.

Bignetti, E., Cavaggioni, A., Fasella, P., Ottonello, S., and Rossi, G.L. (1980). Light and GTP effects on the turbidity of frog visual membrane suspensions. Molecular & Cellular Biochemistry, 30: 93-99.

Bownds, D., Dawes, J., Miller, J., and Stahlman, M. (1972). Phosphorylation of frog photoreceptor membranes induced by light, Nature (London), New Biol., 237: 125-127.

Chabre, M., and Breton, J. (1979). Orientation of aromatic residues in rhodopsin. Rotation of one tryptophan upon the Meta I Meta II transition after illumination, Photochem. Photobiol., 30: 295-299.

Chabre, M., Vuong, M., and Stryer, L. (1982). Anisotropy of the infra-red light-scattering changes induced by illumination of oriented retinal rod outer segments, Biophys. J., 37: 274a.

Chen, Y.S., and Hubbell, W.L. (1978). Reactions of the sulfhydryl groups of membrane-bound bovine rhodopsin, Membrane Biochem., 1: 107-130.

Emeis, D., and Hofmann, K.P. (1981). Shift in the relation between flash-induced metarhodopsin I and metarhodopsin II within the first 10% rhodopsin bleaching in bovine disc membranes, FEBS Letters, 136: 201-207.

Fung, B.K., and Stryer, L. (1980). Photolyzed rhodopsin catalyzes the exchange of GTP for bound GDP in retinal rod outer segments, Proc. Natl. Acad. Sci. U.S.A., 77: 2500-2504.

Fung, B.K., Hurley, J.B., and Stryer, L. (1981). Flow of information in the light-triggered cyclic nucleotide cascade of vision, Proc. Natl. Acad. Sci. U.S.A., 78: 152-156.

Godchaux, W., III, and Zimmerman, W.F. (1979). Membrane-dependent guanine nucleotide binding and GTPase activities of soluble protein from bovine rod cell outer segments, J. Biol. Chem., 254: 7874-7884.

Harari, H.H., Brown, J.E., and Pinto, L.H. (1978). Rapid light-induced changes in near infrared transmission of rods in bufo marinus, Science, 202: 1083-1085.

Hofmann; K.P., Uhl, R. Hoffmann, W., and Kreutz, W. (1976). Measurements of fast light-induced light-scattering and -absorption changes in outer segments of vertebrate light sensitive rod cells, Biophys. Struct. Mechanism, 2: 61-77.

Hofmann, K.L., Schleicher, A., Emeis, D., and Reichert, J. (1981). Light-induced axial and radial shrinkage effects and changes of the refractive index in isolated bovine rod outer segments and disk vesicles, Biophys. Struct. Mechanism, 8: 67-93.

Kühn, H. (1978). Light-regulated binding of rhodopsin kinase and other proteins to cattle photoreceptor membranes, Biochemistry, 17: 4389-4395.

Kühn, H. (1980 a). Light- and GTP-regulated interaction of GTPase and other proteins with bovine photoreceptor membranes, Nature (London), 283: 587-589.

Kühn, H. (1980 b). Light-induced, reversible binding of proteins to bovine photoreceptor membranes: Influence of nucleotides, Neurochem. Int., 1: 269-285.

Kühn, H. (1981). Interactions of rod cell proteins with the disk membrane: Influence of light, ionic strength, and nucleotides, Current Topics in Membrane and Transport, 15: 171-201.

Kühn, H. (1982). Light regulated binding of proteins to photoreceptor membranes, and its use for the purification of several rod cell proteins, in "Methods in Enzymology", Academic Press, New York.

Kühn, H., and Dreyer, W.J. (1972). Light dependent phosphorylation of rhodopsin by ATP, FEBS Lett., 20: 1-6.

Kühn, H, and Hargrave, P.A. (1981). Light-induced binding of GTPase to bovine photoreceptor membranes: Effect of limited proteolysis of the membranes, Biochemistry, 20: 2410-2417.

Kühn, H., Bennett, N., Michel-Villaz, M., and Chabre, M. (1981). Interactions between photoexcited rhodopsin and GTP-binding protein: kinetic and stoichiometric analysis from light-scattering changes, Proc. Natl. Acad. Sci. U.S.A., 18: 6873-6877.

Kühn, H., Mommertz, O., and Hargrave, P.A. (1982). Light-dependent conformational change at rhodopsin's cytoplasmic surface detected by increased susceptibility to proteolysis, Biochim. Biophys. Acta, 679: 95-100.

Pober, J.S., and Stryer, L. (1975). Light dissociates enzymatically cleaved rhodopsin into two different fragments, J. Mol. Biol., 95: 477-481.

Pober, J.S. and Bitensky, M.W. (1979). Light-regulated enzymes of vertebrate retinal rods, Adv. Cyclic Nucleotide Res., 11: 265-301.

Rafferty, C.N. (1979). Light-induced perturbation of aromatic residues in bovine rhodopsin and bacteriorhodopsin, Photochem. Photobiol., 29: 109-120.

Robinson, W.E., and Hagins, W.A. (1979). GTP hydrolysis in intact rod outer segments and the transmitter cycle in visual excitation, Nature (London), 280: 398-400.

Smith, H.G., Stubbs, G.W., and Litman, B.J. (1975). The isolation and purification of osmotically intact discs from retinal rod outer segment, Exp. Eye Res., 20: 211-217.

Thacher, S.M. (1978). Light-stimulated, magnesium-dependent ATPase in toad retinal rod outer segments, Biochemistry, 17: 3005-3011.

Uchida, S., Wheeler, G.L., Yamazaki, A., and Bitensky, M.W. (1981). A GTP-protein activator of phosphodiesterase which forms in response to bleached rhodopsin, J. Cycl. Nucleotide Res., 7: 95-104.

Uhl, R., Hofmann, K.P., and Kreutz, W. (1977). Measurement of fast light-induced disc-shrinkage within bovine rod outer segments by means of a light-scattering transient, Biochim. Biophys. Acta, 469: 113-122.

Uhl, R., Borys, T., and Abrahamson, E.W. (1979). Evidence for structural changes in the photoreceptor disk membrane, enabled by magnesium ATPase activity and triggered by light, FEBS Lett, 107: 317-322.

Wey, C.L., and Cone, R.A. (1978). Light-induced light-scattering changes from rod outer segments, Biophys. J., 21: 135a.

Wheeler, G.L., and Bitensky, M.W. (1977). A light-activated GTPase
    in vertebrate photoreceptors: Regulation of light-activated
    cyclic-GMP phosphodiesterase, Proc. Natl. Acad. Sci. U.S.A.,
    74: 4238-4242.
Wilden, U., and Kühn, H. (1982). Light-dependent phosphorylation
    of rhodopsin: Number of phosphorylation sites, Biochemistry,
    in press.
Yee, R., and Liebman, P.A. (1978). Light-activated phosphodiesterase
    of the rod outer segment. Kinetics and parameters of activation
    and deactivation, J. Biol. Chem., 253: 8902-8909.

INTRACELLULAR CHANGES OF H^+ AND Ca^{2+} IN BALANUS PHOTORECEPTORS

H. Mack Brown

Department of Physiology University of Utah Salt Lake City, Utah U.S.A.

INTRODUCTION

Both H^+ and Ca^{2+} have been under consideration as the intracellular mediator of the receptor potential or light adaptation in both vertebrate and invertebrate photoreceptors. Closer experimental scrutiny has qualified neither of them for an exclusive role in this regard. However, it remains that changes in these ions might represent important sequelae to certain events, such as biochemical changes, that are involved in important functional processes. Intracellular pH changes have been shown to occur with pH electrodes in an invertebrate photoreceptor (Brown and Meech, 1976; 1979). In vertebrate preparations, a suspension of rod disk membranes have been shown to acidify with illumination. This acidification has been shown to be caused by hydrolysis of cyclic GMP (Libman and Pugh, 1981).

Electrophysiologically, intracellular acidification reduces the resting dark conductance of an invertebrate photoreceptor (Brown and Meech, 1975; 1979) and the resting dark conductance of rod outer segments (Pinto and Ostroy, 1978). Both changes are associated with reduced potassium conductance (g_K). Intracellular acidification also reduces the light-induced increase in g_{Na} in Balanus photoreceptors (Brown and Meech, 1979) but the effect of intracellular pH changes are not so clear in rod outer segments since the inferred intracellular acidification (with CO_2) or alkalinization (with NH_4Cl) both augment the receptor potential (Pinto and Ostroy, 1978).

Increasing extracellular Ca^{2+} in invertebrate preparations reduces the light-induced g_{Na} increase (Brown, Hagiwara, Koike, Meech, 1970; Millecchia and Mauro, 1969) and decreases the resting g_{Na} of vertebrate rod outer segments (Yoshikami and Hagins, 1971). An intracellular Ca^{2+} increase has been shown to occur with light in invertebrate photoreceptors (Brown, Brown and Pinto, 1977; Brown and Rydqvist, 1980); this change has been associated with a reduction of the receptor potential at a fixed light intensity (Brown and Lisman, 1975). A light-induced extracellular increase in calcium in rod outer segments (Gold and Korenbrot, 1980; Yoshikami, George and Hagins, 1980) is thought to be associated with a cytoplasmic increase in Ca^{2+} in vertebrate preparations. To date, an unequivocal demonstration of cytoplasmic Ca^{2+} increases in rod outer segments has not been demonstrated. Several questions must be considered regarding H^{+} and Ca^{2+} intracellular changes before their functional consequences can be established. 1) Quantification of the intracellular changes; 2) the time course of the changes; 3) the stoichiometry of the changes with light; 4) the buffer capacity of the cells for H^{+} and Ca^{2+}; and 5) the locale of the change in the cell.

The present paper summarizes some results of experiments on Balanus photoreceptors that have been addressed to these questions.

METHODS

The Balanus eye is a simple ocellar eye consisting of three large photoreceptors about 100 μM in diameter (Fahrenbach, 1965). For study, the photoreceptors are isolated by removing the back layer of pigment epithelium and tapetal cells to expose the photoreceptors. The preparation is placed corneal side down on a light source for illumination and continuously suffused with artificial saline. The photoreceptors are penetrated under visual control with microelectrodes. Techniques used to investigate the properties of the cell have been described previously : 1) voltage-clamp analysis (see for example, Brown et al., 1970; Brown and Cornowall, 1975); 2) ion-sensitive electrodes (see Brown, 1976; Saunders and Brown, 1977; Brown, Pemberton and Owen, 1976); 3) indicator dyes (see Brown and Rydqvist, 1980; 1981). The microspectrophotometer used in conjunction with indicators is of the same type described by Change (1972) and Brinley and Scarpa (1975).

RESULTS

Light-Initiated Membrane Current

The top row of records in Fig. 1 shows membrane potential changes obtained from a photoreceptor cell at three different light intensities. Saturating light intensities produce a receptor potential that consists of peak transient phase followed by a steady phase that is sustained for the duration of the illumination. Reducing the intensity reduces the potential change and the response assumes a more rectangular time course. Not shown in these records, is a long-lasting hyperpolarization that ensues after strong flashes of light (Koike, Brown and Hagiwara, 1971). In each column below the membrane potential changes are voltage-clamp records of light-initiated membrane current (LIC) obtained at the same three light intensities and at the potential levels indicated adjacent to each trace. At a holding potential of -38 mV, it can be seen that the LIC with a bright light consists of a large transient current followed by a smaller steady current. The inward current becomes more rectangular as the light intensity is reduced. When the membrane potential was shifted to approximately +30 mV (fourth row of records), the light-induced inward membrane current is abolished indicating that the null current is obtained at the same membrane potential regardless of light intensity. In the bottom row of records, a large step change in the membrane potential level (to approx. +45 mV) shifts the light-induced current from inward to outward. From these results, it is concluded that: a) there is a light-initiated inward membrane current associated with the receptor potential; b) features of the inward membrane current qualitatively resemble the membrane potential changes; c) the zero-current potential is independent of light intensity and d) that the peak transient phase and steady phase of the receptor potential have the same reversal potential.

Effects of Calcium

Extracellular Ca^{2+} changes. It has been shown that the light-induced membrane current is proportional to the external Na^+ concentration; however, a small residual inward current was observed even when Na^+ concentration was reduced to zero (Brown et al., 1970). In the same study it was demonstrated that this residual current could be attributed to a Ca^{2+} current (Fig. 14, from Brown et al., 1970). Even though there appears to be a small inward Ca^{2+}

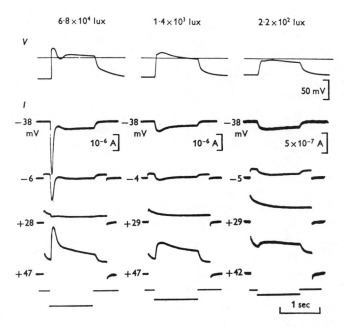

Fig. 1.   Top row. Membrane potential changes (V) recorded from
          Balanus photoreceptor at three different intensities of
          illumination (indicated above each record). Zero membrane
          potential is indicated by the horizontal lines. I Voltage-
          clamp records of membrane current during step changes of
          membrane potential from -38 mV to the level indicated to
          the left of each record. Steps of illumination (bottom
          traces) were applied during the changes of membrane poten-
          tial; inward current is displayed downward. (Figure from
          Brown et al., 1970).

current initiated by illumination, by far the greatest effect of Ca^{2+}
is a modification of the Na^+ conductance of the membrane during
illumination as shown in Fig. 2. The inset shows voltage traces
(V) and current traces (I) at three different external Ca^{2+} concentrations (top to bottom): 32, 20, and 2 mM Ca^{2+}. At light intensity
used in this experiment the voltage response is saturated at all
three light intensities but changes in time course can be noted
in the voltage traces. A clear difference due to Ca^{2+} is obtained
from the voltage-clamp records which show that the light-induced
inward current is systematically increased as the external Ca^{2+} is
reduced. The current-voltage relation of the membrane shows this
is especially marked at membrane potential levels around the resting

level. As the membrane was depolarized systematically to more positive potentials, the light-induced currents became more similar
and reverse at approximately the same membrane potential. At the
lowest Ca^{2+} concentration there was evidence of a small shift in
the null-current potential. This is consistent with other results
indicating that the membrane behaves as a reasonably good Ca^{2+} electrode in Na^+-free solutions. However, as these results show, with
a full complement of Na^+, the major effect of a lower external Ca^{2+}
concentration is an increase in the light-induced membrane conductance.

Intracellular Ca^{2+} changes. Intracellular Ca^{2+} changes in Balanus photoreceptor can be detected with Ca^{2+} ion-sensitive electrodes
(Ca-ISE) of the type described by Brown, Pemberton and Owen (1976).
Figure 3 shows Ca^{2+} changes recorded with a Ca-ISE (V_{Ca}) in conjuc-
tion with the light-induced potential change recorded with conventional 3M KCl electrode (E_m). It can be seen by comparison of the
V_{Ca} and E_m trace (top records) that during the steaky phase of the
receptor potential the Ca^{2+} electrode records a steady increase in
potential superimposed upon the membrane potential change. The
increase in Ca^{2+} with light is more easily seen by referring to the
result obtained from a different cell in the lower part of the
figure where a differential recording is made between the Ca-ISE
and the membrane potential recording electrode ($V_{Ca}-E_m$). It can
be seen in this trace that moderate light produced about a 5 mV
change in the Ca^{2+} potential. This translates to an increase of C_{Ca}^i
from pCa 7 to about 6.5 in this cell. At higher light intensities
pCa is raised to about pCa 6 from the resting level. The potential
difference recorded with the Ca^{2+} electrode from inside to the
outside of the cell can be seen in the top half of the record upon
removal of the Ca^{2+} electrode. The Ca^{2+} change is approximately
170 mV in this cell and the resting membrane potential at the time
of withdrawal was about 40 mV. This yields a net potential drop
for the Ca^{2+} electrode of about 130 mV. This potential drop would
correspond to a resting intracellular Ca^{2+} concentration of less
than 100×10^{-9}M. Calibration solutions for the Ca-ISE contained
about 0.75 mM Mg^{2+}, which is very close to the Mg^{2+} concentration
that has been evaluated in these cells with Eriochrome Blue (Brown
and Rydqvist, in preparation).

Injection of CaCl from a micropipette can produce a transient
increase in intracellular Ca^{2+} with concomitant effects on the
resting potential and the light-induced potential changes across

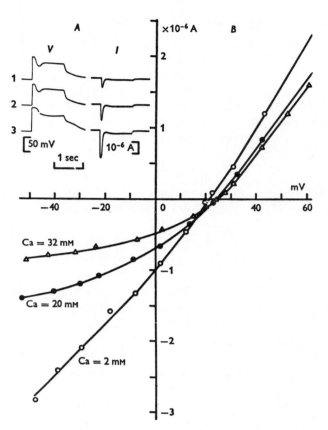

Fig. 2.   A.   Membrane potential changes (V) and membrane current (I)
elicited by light at 3 different Ca^{2+} concentrations:
(1) 32 mM, (2) 20 mM and (3) 2 mM.   B.   Light-initiated
membrane current vs. membrane potential measured 5 msec
after the onset of light at the Ca^{2+} concentrations
indicated adjacent to each curve.   (Figure from Brown,
et al., 1970).

the membrane.   This was first shown in <u>Limulus</u> ventral photoreceptor
by Brown and Lisman (1975) who iontophoresed Ca^{2+} into the cell.
An experiment in <u>Balanus</u> photoreceptor is shown in Fig. 4 in which
CaCl is pressure-injected into the photoreceptor and the C_{Ca}^{i} change
is monitored with a Ca-ISE.   Two injections were made and the second
raised Ca^{2+} to pCa 5.3 (C_{Ca}^{i} = 5 x 10^{-6}M).   The resting membrane
potential of the cell initially depolarized and then hyperpolarized.
Associated with the increase in intracellular Ca^{2+} was a diminishing

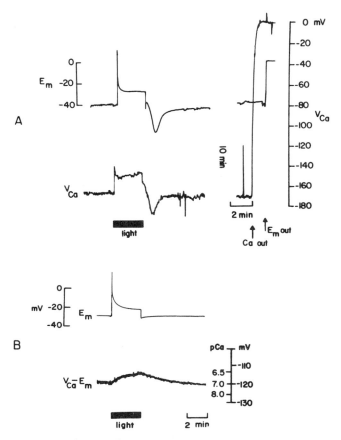

Fig. 3. Records obtained with Ca-ISE from two cells (A and B).
         Cell A: Record obtained single-ended from Ca^{2+} electrode
         to show potential differences of conventional KCl-filled
         microelectrode (top trace) and Ca-ISE (bottom trace) upon
         withdrawal of the electrodes at the end of the experiment.
         Note that light (bar) increases V_{Ca} even though sustained
         phase of receptor potential is steady. Cell B: Differen-
         tial recording of Ca^{2+} electrode and membrane potential
         changes ($V_{Ca}-E_m$) elicited by light. Light initiated a 7
         mV positive change in $V_{Ca}-E_m$.

amplitude of the receptor potential which recovered with a long time
course.   Thus, an increased intracellular Ca^{2+} can reduce the light-
induced membrane potential changes of the cell; however, the eleva-
tion in Ca^{2+} must be almost two decades to elicit the changes described above.

Effects of pH

Extracellular and intracellular pH changes. Extracellular
acidification of the Balanus photoreceptor produces only small
effects on membrane conductance and on the receptor potential.
Figure 5A shows membrane potential changes on a protracted time
base when the external saline was changed from pH 7.5 to pH 5.25
with phosphate buffer. Inward-going current pulses were being
passed across the membrane between each light flash to monitor
changes in membrane conductance. Phosphate buffer applied for a
period of about 1 minute resulted in a slight decrease of membrane
conductance and a slight transient increase in the amplitude of the
receptor potential. On the other hand, iontophoresing small amounts
of protons or bicarbonate ions from an intracellular microelectrode
produces quite marked long-lasting effects on the receptor potential.
Figure 5B shows that acid injected into the cell produces a reduction in the amplitude of the receptor potential and bicarbonate
(trace C) iontophoresed into the cell augments the amplitude of the
receptor potential.

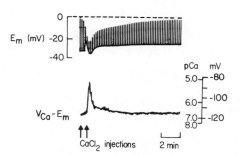

Fig. 4. Membrane potential changes and intracellular Ca^{2+} changes
         produced by pressure-injection of $CaCl_2$. Upward deflec-
         tion of top trace shows receptor potentials elicited by
         750 msec light flashes. Ca^{2+} injection raised pCa from
         the resting level (7.0) to about pCa 5.

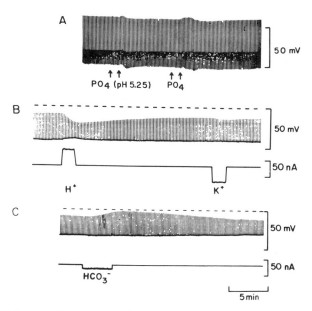

Fig. 5.   A: Effect of acid saline on the receptor potential and
          membrane conductance. The cell was penetrated with two
          KCl-filled micropipettes one of which was used to pass 5 nA
          hyperpolarizing current pulses across the cell membrane.
          The other micropipette was used to record membrane potential.
          Each upward deflection of the record corresponds to the
          receptor potential evoked by a 1 sec light stimulus at 10
          sec intervals between the hyperpolarizing pulses. The
          arrows indicate periods during which the cell was exposed
          to pH 5.25 phosphate buffered saline.
          B: Effect of intracellular injection of HCl on receptor
          potential. Upper trace: membrane potential recorded with
          a second KCl-filled micropipette. Each upward deflection
          correponds to the receptor potential evoked by a 450 msec
          light flash presented at 10 sec intervals. Lower trace:
          injection current passed between the barrels of a double-
          barrelled micropipette. One side was filled with 0.1M
          HCl, the other was filled with 3M KCl. Receptor bathed
          in 5% CO_2-HCO_3^- saline, pH 7.5.
          C: Intracellular injection of $KHCO_3$. Upper trace : mem-
          brane potential. Each upward deflection corresponds to the
          receptor potential evoked by a 450 msec light stimulus
          presented at 9 sec intervals. The interrupted line cor-
          responds to the reference potential (0mV). Lower trace:

(continued)

Fig. 5 (Continued)

      injection current passed between the barrels of a double-barreled micropipette. One side was filled with 0.1M KHCO$_3$, the other was filled with 3M KCl. Injection period is represented by a downward deflection of the current trace. (Figure from Brown and Meech, 1979).

    Effect of CO$_2$. Exposing the photoreceptor to a 5% CO$_2$-bicarbonate saline produces an intracellular acidification followed by an alkalinization of the cell after exposure to the experimental saline. This can be seen in Fig. 6. The intracellular changes of pH were followed by a glass pH microelectrode of the type described by Thomas (1974). The resting intracellular pH in this cell was about 7.3 and exposure to the CO$_2$ saline reduced the pH to about 7.1. There was a gradual creep back to the resting pH during application of the saline. Concomitant with the intracellular acidification is a reduction in the receptor potential that gradually recovers during the recovery of the intracellular pH. Replacement of the CO$_2$ saline produced an intracellular alkalinization and a rebound of the receptor potential. The receptor potential recovered with about the same time course as intracellular pH change. Thus, the receptor potential appears very responsive to subtle changes in the intracellular pH of the cell.

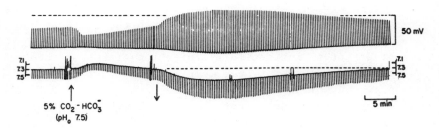

Fig. 6.   The effect of CO$_2$-HCO$_3^-$ saline on intracellular pH and the receptor potential. Upper trace: membrane potential; each upward deflection is a change in membrane potential elicited by an 800 msec light flash. Lower trace: pH$_i$; each downward deflection corresponds to the inverted receptor potential attenuated by the varactor bridge amplifier. Interval between light flashes: 18 sec. Upward arrow: onset of exposure to 5% CO$_2$-HCO$_3^-$ saline. Downward arrow: return to normal saline. The external pH (pH$_o$) was held constant at 7.5. (From Brown and Meech, 1979).

The buffer value of a buffer solution as defined by Van Slyke (1922) is:

$$BV = -\Delta B/\Delta pH \qquad (1)$$

where ΔB is the amount of base (or acid) added to the system and ΔpH is the resulting pH change. The buffer capacity of the system is often given in slykes (Woodbury, 1965) which is the number of millimoles of base or acid added to change a liter of the solution by one pH unit. The amount of bicarbonate (B) added to the cell system can be determined from the equilibrium condition of a CO_2-bicarbonate system.

$$[HCO_3^-] = 10^{pH-pK} \cdot [CO_2] \qquad (2)$$

Since the amount of base added to the system can be calculated and the pH change measured, it is possible to obtain an estimate of the buffer capacity of barnacle photoreceptor cytoplasm. This is shown in Fig. 7. HCO_3 levels were obtained for three different concentrations of CO_2: atmospheric, 2% and 5%. The solid curves are the pH-bicarbonate isopleths for a CO_2-bicarbonate solution. A line drawn through the data points obtained from this relation yields a slope of about -15 slykes which is about the same value that was obtained from a number of individual experiments using CO_2/HCO_3 saline with data extrapolated to zero-time (see Brown and Meech, 1979).

Effect of light on intracellular pH. Light elicits a small intracellular pH change in Balanus photoreceptors as illustrated in Fig. 8. pH changes were recorded with a glass pH-sensitive micro-electrode. The pH change was greatest when the receptors had been allowed to stabilize in the dark for a period of half an hour. The pH change is graded with light intensity as shown in Fig. 8, which shows pH changes elicited at three calibrated light intensities (see Figure legend). At light input of about 10^{11} photons per photoreceptor per second produces the near maximum pH change (A) since reducing the light intensity about 10-fold (B) elicits almost the same ΔpH_i. The maximum pH change observed with saturating light has been 0.3 pH unit in cells dark-adapted for at least 20 minutes.

Monitoring pH Changes With pH-Sensitive Dyes

Phenol Red. Experiments were conducted with cells injected with Phenol Red to improve on the time resolution of pH changes recorded with pH-ISE. Phenol Red is an attractive dye since it has

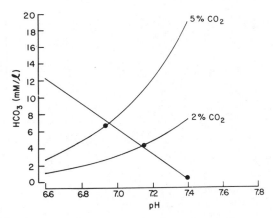

Fig. 7. P_{CO_2} isobars calculated from the Henderson–Hasselbach
          equation with P_{CO_2} held constant at the values indicated.
          The filled data points are from cellular measurements of
          cellular pH. The slope of the line through the data points
          is −15 mM HCO_3/pH unit per liter which is the estimated
          buffer value for this cell. (From Brown and Meech, 1979).

a good extinction coefficient in response to pH changes and is easily
injected into the cell. Figure 9A shows changes in absorbance of
an 0.5 mM Phenol Red solution containing 200 mM KCl. It can be seen
that absorbance decreases at 560 nm and increases at 430 nm as the
pH is decreased. There is an isosbestic point at about 470 nm.
There is essentially no absorbance change with pH beyond 625 nm.
Therefore, suitable wavelength pairs for the analysis of pH changes
in the cell could be 560 nm vs. 720 nm or 470 nm. Values of the
molar extinction coefficients are given in the Figure legend.
Figure 8B shows a mock experiment in the microspectrophotometer
with a pathlength of 0.1 mM to mimic cell diameter. Under these
idealized conditions, small changes in pH can easily be resolved.
The left ordinate gives the transmission of the solution in the
chamber containing normal saline (NBS) and 1 mM of Phenol Red at
two pH values added to the saline. On the right, absorbance values
are shown. Normal barnacle saline (NBS) was accorded a value of 0
absorbance. A change of pH by 0.4 units produced a ΔA of .087. It
would be anticipated from these model results that light-induced
pH changes should be easily resolved with a similar concentration
of Phenol Red in the cell .

     Figure 10 shows absorbance changes of a Phenol Red injected
cell. A glass pH electrode was also inserted into this cell. The
experiment began by injection of Phenol Red from the recording

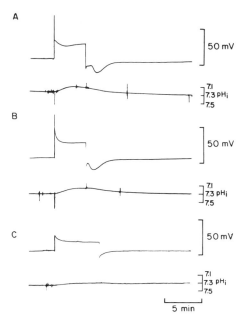

Fig. 8.   The effect of different light intensities on intracellular
          pH (lower trace) and membrane potential (upper trace).
          The period of illumination is indicated by the bar below
          each pair of traces.   The photon flux (520 nm photons/
          photoreceptor/sec) was: (A) 8.8 x 10^{10}; (B) 1.1 x 10^{10};
          (C) 1.1 x 10^9.   The cell was dark adapted for 15 min
          between light stimuli.   (From Brown and Meech, 1979).

pipette which contained 100 mM Phenol Red and 200 mM KCl (pH = 7.25).
The bottom two traces show absorbance changes at 560 vs. 720 nm
and at 490 nm, the isosbestic wavelength of the dye.   Injection of
the dye produced an absorbance increase at 490 and 560 nm.   Note
that a positive absorbance change is shown as a downward deflection
for the 560 nm trace.   From the extinction coefficient at 490 nm
and the measured absorbance change the calculated dye concentration
was 0.44 mM.   After injection of the dye, the 560 trace was shifted
to the pre-injection level.   About 3 minutes later, the cell was
exposed to a saline equilibrated with 5% CO_2.   It can be seen in
the top trace that the membrane potential depolarized slightly and
the receptor potential was reduced.   The ΔpH recorded with the pH-
ISE was 0.25 pH unit.   The calculated pH change from Phenol Red was
0.11 pH unit, from the dye concentration and the $\Delta\varepsilon^{pH}_{560}$.   A pathlength

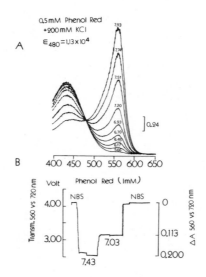

Fig. 9.   A: Changes in absorbance of a Phenol Red solution (0.5 mM)
          containing 0.2M KCl at different values of pH. Pathlength
          0.1 cm. $\varepsilon^{480} = 1.13 \times 10^4 M^{-1}$ cm^{-1}; $\Delta\varepsilon^{560} = 3.2 \times 10^4$ M^{-1}
          cm^{-1} pH^{-1}. B: Changes in trasmission (left ordinate) and
          absorbance (right ordinate) of a 1 mM Phenol Red solution
          in the dual wavelength microspectrophotometer. The wave-
          length pair 560 vs. 720 nm was chosen on the basis of the
          dye characteristics shown in Fig. 8; pathlength 0.01 cm.
          (Experiments conducted with B. Rydqvist).

of .01 cm was used for these calculations. These results are representative of many others obtained on this preparation which indicate that 1) Phenol Red gives indications of pH changes intracellularly, but the pH change is systematically smaller than changes
recorded with a pH microelectrode; 2) the time course of the absorbance change is more rapid than the time course of the pH change
recorded with the microelectrode. Thus, the dye appears to monitor
the time course of the pH change more accurately but the calculated
pH changes is usually 2 or 3 times less than the recorded change
with pH-ISE. One possibility for this difference is that the dye
binds to intracellular constituents and the concentration of the
dye available for complexation is overestimated from the absorbance
changes measured at 490 nm.

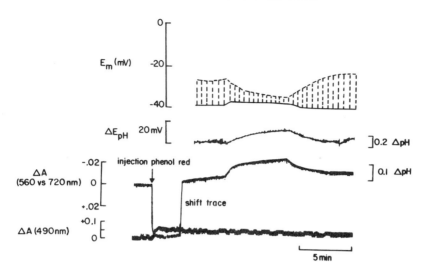

Fig. 10.   Effect of 5% CO_2 in normal saline on a <u>Balanus</u> photoreceptor injected with Phenol Red.   Upper trace: plot of
membrane potential (E_m) recorded with an electrode containing 100 mM Phenol Red and 200 mM KCl (pH = 7.25).
Second trace: pH_i recorded with a recessed-tip-pH-sensi-
tive electrode. Third trace: absorbance changes measured
differentially between 560 nm and 720 nm. Bottom trace:
absorbance change measured at 490 nm.   The concentration
of the dye in the cell was estimated by the change in
absorbance at 490 nm.   The pathlength was 100 μm. (Experiments conducted with B. Rydqvist).

<u>Arsenazo III</u>.   pH changes measured with AIII have been in
substantially better agreement with pH electrodes (Brown and
Rydqvist, 1980).   This suggests that at an equivalent concentration
(about 0.5 mM), the amount of AIII bound to cellular constituents
is not significant and that the parameters of the dye obtained
extracellularly can be applied to in-situ measurements.

One demonstration of the use of AIII as both a pH indicator
and a Ca^{2+} indicator is shown in Fig. 11 (Brown and Rydqvist, 1980;
1982).   In this case the cell was injected with 0.75 mM AIII.   Two
different wavelengths were monitored, 650 vs. 720 nm and 620 vs.
720 nm.   The former is most sensitive to Ca^{2+} and the latter is
most sensitive to pH changes.   If the extinction at both wavelengths
for Ca^{2+} and pH is known, it is possible to calculate the Ca^{2+}

change and pH change based on these absorbance measurements. Light
appears to elicit simultaneous pH and Ca^{2+} changes. This is shown
in the bottom trace for two different light intensities. The lowest
light intensity elicited a pH change of about 0.1 pH unit and a Ca^{2+}
change of approximately 3×10^{-7} M. The brighter light flash elicited a pH change of about 0.15 pH units and a Ca^{2+} change of about
8.5×10^{-7} M. These experiments have substantiated the results
obtained earlier with separate pH and Ca-ISE measurements.

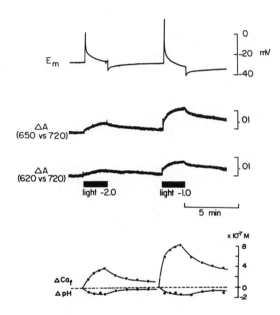

Fig. 11.   Changes in intracellular Ca^{2+} and pH based on simultaneous
           absorbance changes of AIII at two different wavelength
           pairs.   Top trace: membrane potential changes to two
           steps of light (bars) of different intensity.   Middle
           trace: change in AIII absorbance (ΔA) at 650 vs. 720 nm.
           Bottom trace: change in AIII absorbance at 620 vs.   720
           nm.   At the bottom of the Figure are calculated changes
           of intracellular Ca^{2+} and pH based on the differences
           of extinction of AIII at 650 and 620 nm for pH and Ca^{2+}.
           (Experiments conducted with B. Rydqvist).

DISCUSSION

The results described indicate that intracellular pH and Ca^{2+} changes both occur as a consequence of illumination in <u>Balanus</u> photoreceptors. The origin of these changes is presently unknown, but it is possible to describe several features of the changes.

A comparison of external pH and Ca^{2+} changes with intracellular changes indicate that small intracellular changes in the micromolar or submicromolar region can affect the receptor potential substantially whereas an equivalent change extracellularly exhibits little or no effect. Thus, there must be crucial sites that are available only at the inner membrane capable of subtle modification of membrane conductance.

The magnitude of the intracellular increases of H^+ and Ca^{2+} are small but measurable. Both ISE and dye indicators are in quite good agreement concerning the magnitude of the change with the possible exception of Phenol Red. Saturating light induces a pH change of about 0.3 pH units which represents a "visible" increase in intracellular protons of about 4×10^{-8} M (dark-adapted pH is about 7.4). This is a small change but considering the buffer capacity of the cell (about 15 slykes) it represents the residual of an intracellular H^+ change that would be in the millimole range if the cell was an unbuffered medium. It has been calculated that this increase represents about 100 H^+/photon incident on the cell (Brown and Meech, 1979). This could indicate that most of the protons are not evolved directly from the pigment bleach but at some later point in visual transduction, i.e. the protons are associated with a gain phase.

Indications are that Ca^{2+} is both present at a higher concentration and changes more with light than protons in the <u>Balanus</u> photoreceptors. The dark-adapted resting C_{Ca} is about pCa 7 measured with Ca-ISE or AIII measurements (Brown and Rydqvist, 1982). Bright light can raise pCa to about 6. This could indicate that Ca^{2+} is not as well buffered on a short time scale as H^+. There is some evidence to support this difference and indications are that Ca^{2+} has a lower stoichiometry with light than H^+ (Brown and Rydqvist, 1982). This suggests that both ions have a different origin in the transduction process and makes it less likely that they are associated with one another in a simple ligand system or in a simple exchange process (Brown and Meech, 1979).

ACKNOWLEDGEMENTS

The author wishes to acknowledge the collaboration of the
following investigators: Drs. S. Hagiwara, R.W. Meech, H. Koike and
B. Rydqvist. Technical assistance has been provided by T. Gillet
and S. Marron.

REFERENCES

Brinley, F.J. and A. Scarpa (1975). Ionized magnesium concentration
    in axoplasm of dialyzed squid axons, FEBS Letter 50, 82–85.
Brown, H. Mack (1976). Intracellular Na^+, K^+ and Cl^- activities
    in large barnacle photoreceptors. J. Gen. Physiol., 68, 281–
    296.
Brown, H., Mack and M.C. Cornwall (1975). Ionic mechanism of a
    quasi-stable depolarization in barnacle photoreceptors follow-
    ing red light, J. Physiol., 248, 579–593.
Brown, H. Mack, S. Hagiwara, H. Koike and R. Meech (1970). Membrane
    properties of a barnacle photoreceptor examined by the voltage-
    clamp technique, J. Physiol., 208, 385–413.
Brown, H. Mack and R.W. Meech (1975). Effects of pH and CO_2 on large
    barnacle photoreceptors, Biophys. J., 15 276 a.
Brown, H. Mack and R.W. Meech (1976). Intracellular pH and light
    adaptation in barnacle photoreceptor, J. Physiol., 263, 128 P.
Brown, H. Mack and R.W. Meech (1979). Light-induced changes of
    internal pH in a barnacle photoreceptor and effect of internal
    pH on the receptor potential, J. Physiol., 297, 73–94.
Brown, H. Mack, J.P. Pemberton and J.D. Owen (1976). A calcium-
    sensitive microelectrode suitable for intracellular measurement
    of calcium (II) activity, Anal. Chim. Acta, 85, 261–276.
Brown, H. Mack and B. Rydqvist (1980). Changes of intracellular
    Ca^{2+} in Balanus photoreceptors probed with Ca^{2+} microelectrodes
    and arsenazo III, Proc. of the Internat'l. Union of Physiol.
    Sci., 14, 339.
Brown, H. Mack and B. Rydqvist (1981). Arsenazo III-Ca^{2+}. Effect
    of pH, ionic strength and arsenazo III concentration on equi-
    librium binding evaluated with Ca^{2+}-ISE and absorbance meas-
    urements, Biophys. J., 36, 117–137.
Brown, H. Mack and B. Rydqvist (1982). Simultaneous changes of pH
    and Ca^{2+} in Balanus photoreceptors assayed by Arsenazo III and
    Ca-ISE, (in preparation).

Brown, J.E., P.K. Brown and L.H. Pinto (1977). Detection of light-induced changes of intracellular ionized calcium concentration in Limulus ventral photoreceptor using Arsenazo III, J. Physiol., 267, 299-320.

Brown, J.E. and J.E. Lisman (1975). Intracellular Ca modulates sensitivity and time scale in Limulus ventral photoreceptors, Nature, 258, 252-254.

Chance, B. (1972). Principles of differential spectrophotometry with special reference to the dual-wavelength method, Methods Enzymol., 3, 169-183.

Fahrenbach, W.H. (1965). The micromorphology of some single photo-receptors. Z. Zellforsch. mikrosk. Anat., 66, 233-254.

Gold, G.H. and J.I. Korenbrot (1980). Light-induced calcium release by intact retinal rods., Proc. Natl. Acad. Sci, 77, 5557-5561.

Koike, H., Mack Brown and S. Hagiwara (1971). Post-illumination hyperpolarization of a barnacle photoreceptor, J. Gen. Physiol., 57, 723-737.

Liebman, P.A. and E.N. Pugh (1981). Control of rod disk membrane phosphodiesterase and a model for visual transduction, in: "Current Topics in Membranes and Transport., Vol. 15: Molecular Mechanisms of Photoreceptor Transduction. W.H. Miller, ed., pp. 157-170, Academic Press, New York.

Millecchia, R. and A. Mauro (1969). The ventral photoreceptor cells of Limulus. III. A voltage-clamp study, J. Gen. Physiol., 54, 331-351.

Pinto, L.H. and S.E. Ostroy (1978). Ionizable groups and conductances of the rod photoreceptor membrane, J. Gen. Physiol., 71, 329-345.

Saunders, J.H. and H. Mack Brown (1977). Liquid and solid-state Cl^--sensitive microelectrodes. Characteristics and application to intracellular Cl^- activity in Balanus photoreceptor, J. Gen. Physiol., 70, 507-530.

Thomas, R.C. (1974). Intracellular pH of snail neurones measured with a new pH-sensitive glass microelectrode, J. Physiol., 238, 159-180.

Van Slyke, D.D. (1922). On the measurement of buffer values and on the relationship of buffer value to the dissociation constant of the buffer and the concentration and reaction of the buffer solution, J. Biol. Chem., 52, 525-570.

Woodbury, J.W. (1965). Regulation of pH, in: "Physiology and Bio-physics", T.C. Ruch and H.D. Patton, eds., pp. 899-934, W.B. Saunders: Philadelphia.

Yoshikami, S., J.S. George and W.A. Hagins (1980). Light-induced
    calcium fluxes from outer segment layer of vertebrate retinas,
    Nature, 286, 395-398.
Yoshikami, S. and W.A. Hagins (1971). Light, calcium and the photo-
    current of rods and cones, Biophys. J., 11, 47 a.

LIGHT-INDUCED VOLTAGE FLUCTUATIONS IN BARNACLE PHOTORECEPTORS

E. Kaplan, A. Mauro and S. Poitry

The Rockefeller University, N.Y.

INTRODUCTION

The transduction of light quanta into an electrical signal is not understood. However, in several arthropod photoreceptors this transduction process was shown to be associated with the appearance of discrete waves in the membrane potential, the so called 'quantal bumps' (in Limulus: Yeandle, 1957, and Adolph, 1964; in locust: Scholes, 1965; in the fly, Musca: Kirschfeld, 1965; in Drosophila: Wu and Pak, 1978). In the Limulus photoreceptors, where the quantal bumps were first observed, it was shown that the receptor potential is the superposition of the elementary responses which are initiated by the absorption of single quanta (Yeandle and Fuortes, 1964; Dodge et al, 1968). Wu and Pak reached similar conclusions for Drosophila photoreceptors (1978).

In sharp contrast to the photoreceptors mentioned above are other photoreceptors in which discrete waves were not observed. Among these are the photoreceptors in the lateral eye of the barnacle, Balanus eburneus (Shaw, 1972), the median eye of the giant barnacle B. nubilus (Hudspeth and Stewart, 1972), and the cephalopod eye of the squid, which shows no quantal bumps but in which light initiates voltage fluctuations (Hagins, 1965).

We report here the results of a study in which we looked for discrete waves in the lateral eye of the barnacle, Balanus eburneus. As others before us, we have been unable to see distinct quantal bumps, but the analysis of the light-induced fluctuations of the mem-

119

brane potential indicates that the light response of this photoreceptor, like the responses of those studied before, is generated by the
superposition of small elementary events which vary in amplitude
with light intensity. In this paper we present only voltage data.
We are now in the process of obtaining current measurements under
voltage-clamp conditions, measurements which will not be distorted
by the time constant of the membrane. These data will enable us to
measure the power spectrum of the light-induced fluctuations and
thus accurately estimate the amplitude, duration and rate of the
elementary changes in conductance.

METHODS

Barnacles were obtained from the Marine Biological Laboratory
in Woods Hole, Mass., or from the Gulf Speciment Laboratory in
Florida, and were stored in a large tank of filtered, circulated
artificial seawater, at a temperature of 5°C. The eyes were dissect-
ed, pinned to a Silgard dish and impaled with glass microelectrodes
(tip resistance: 20-40 MOhm) filled with 3M KCl. A high input
impedance, negative capacitance DC amplifier was used to record the
membrane potential. The amplified potential was plotted on a Gould
chart recorder (frequency response: 0-40 Hz) and taped for later
analysis on an FM tape recorder (frequency band: 0-2000 Hz). The
experiments were carried out at room temperature (approximately
21°C).

In the experiments in which we measured the frequency response
of the barnacle photoreceptor, we used a CRT (Tektronix 5100N), with
P31 phosphor, which has a broad emission spectrum, peaking at approximately 525 nm. The screen was uniformly illuminated, and its
raster was modulated by a microcomputer system (Milkman et al.,
1978), which also digitized (4 msec/sample), averaged and stored
the membrane voltage. The averaged records were then Fourier analyzed off-line on a PDP 11/45 computer.

RESULTS

Figure 1 compares the receptor potentials recorded from the
ventral photoreceptor of Limulus (right) and barnacle (left) to
increasing light intensities. The two recordings were carried out
one after the other in the same apparatus, so that corresponding
light intensities are identical. It is clear that the two preparations differ greatly: the Limulus membrane potential shows clear,

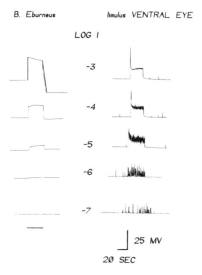

Fig. 1.   Comparison of light responses of a photoreceptor in the
          ventral "eye" of <u>Limulus</u> (right) with those from the bar-
          nacle photoreceptor (left). Sharp transient seen at light
          onset and offset is an artifact due to shutter action. It
          is interesting to note that the steady-state response of
          the barnacle photoreceptor at bright light exceed that of the
          <u>Limulus</u>. Similar results were recorded from other cells.
          The bar on the left indicates the duration of the light
          stimulus. It is absent on the right since light stimulation
          of fixed duration was not used to obtain there responses.

large discrete waves, whereas the barnacle responses are smooth and
continuous.

        However, if one looks at the barnacle response at a much higher
gain, one observes immediately that light initiates in this photoreceptor voltage fluctuations which last for as long as the light
is on. Figure 2a shows an example of the fluctuations recorded
from a typical cell. The responses were amplified, the high frequencies filtered out with a passive RC filter (cutoff: approximately
6 Hz), and the steady-state component of the response was eliminated
by a blocking capacitor (bottom trace). The top trace in Fig. 2a
is a low-gain, DC recording of the same response.

        Figure 2b shows the high-gain, AC recordings taken during dark-
ness, and in response to 3 light intensities. The figure shows that

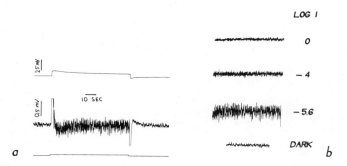

Fig. 2. a: The light response of a barnacle photoreceptor, shown
         in both low gain DC recording (top), and high gain AC
         recording (bottom), in which the high and low frequencies
         were eliminated by passive RC filters. The transient at
         the onset and offset of the light step is due to the ca-
         pacitive coupling. b: Membrane potential recorded from a
         barnacle photoreceptor at various light levels, indicated
         on the right. The voltage calibration is the same as for
         the bottom part of part a.

the amplitude of the light-induced fluctuations increases at first
with increasing light intensity, and then decreases at high light
levels. This behavior has important implications for the interpretation of our results, which will be discussed below.

    We note that the membrane potential of fully dark-adapted
barnacle photoreceptors is not perfectly smooth. Instead, one
observes continuous voltage fluctuations even in the absence of
light, in excess of the fluctuations due to the resistance of the
microelectrode itself.

    When the light is very bright (above O.D. = - 3) one observes
upon termination of the light step another type of voltage fluctuation, associated with the appearance of a post illumination hyperpolarization (PIH), which was shown by Koite et al. (1971) to result
from the activation of an electrogenic pump. The fluctuations during
ghe PIH are noticeably slower than the ones seen during dim and
intermediates light intensities. These fluctuations are not simply
due to the hyperpolarization (PIH) which follows bright illumination,
since hyperpolarizing the cell by passing current through the microelectrode fails to produce such fluctuations. Details of this
phenomenon will be deferred to a later report.

    The effect of increasing light intensity on the amplitude of
the voltage fluctuations is shown quantitatively in Figure 3, where

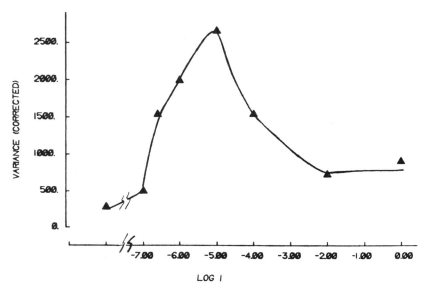

Fig. 3. The variance of the membrane potential recorded from a barnacle photoreceptor as a function of light intensity. The
variance in this figure was calculated from voltage records,
each 48 seconds long, which were digitized at intervals of
2 msec. The computed variance was corrected for the nonlinear summation of events as the membrane voltage approaches
its saturation level. In this plot the variance units are
arbitrary. Similar results were found in other cells.

the variance of the voltage is plotted <u>vs</u> the log of the light intensity. The decline of the variance after the initial rise is particularly significant, since it suggests that the elementary events
which give rise to the noise are becoming smaller under bright illumination. However, this conclusion might be considered premature,
because of the following argument. Light depolarizes the photoreceptor, bringing it closer to the equilibrium potential of its light
response. Therefore, as has been shown for Ach-induced fluctuations
at the neuromuscular junction (Kazt and Miledi, 1972), due to the
shunting effect of the passive conductance on the light-dependent
conductance, the variance would be expected to decrease under conditions which cause a large steady-state response, such as bright
illumination. To eliminate this distortion, the variance was corrected in the usual way, which assumes a resistive equivalent circuit for the membrane (Martin, 1955). We might add that this cor-

rection for nonlinearity can have only a minor effect on our results, since the mean steady-state depolarization, even at the brightest light intensity, was only about 1/2 of the maximum possible depolarization.

One might argue that the photoreceptors in the barnacle could actually be producing discrete waves, but that the time course of these waves is substantially slower than what has been observed in Limulus and other animals in which discrete waves have been seen, and therefore they summate to produce continuous fluctuations.

To check this possibility, we have measured the frequency response of the barnacle photoreceptor by stimulating it with sinusoidally modulated light (at several frequencies) from a uniformly illuminated CRT screen. The amplitude and phase of the fundamental Fourier coefficient of the response from a typical cell is shown in Figure 4. The luminance of the unmodulated screen depolarized the cell by approximately 10 mv, and the modulation depth in the experiment shown was 40%, in the linear range of both the CRT and the photoreceptor (as judged by the almost negligible harmonic distortion in the response.) Figure 4 shows that the response amplitude falls to 1/2 of its maximal value at approximately 3 Hz, which is not substantially different from the results obtained from Limulus. The barnacle photoreceptor is, therefore, not significantly more sluggish than the Limulus photoreceptor, and one must look elsewhere for an explanation to the absence of discrete waves in its membrane potential recordings.

In the few experiments we conducted on the lateral eye of the honeybee drone, we observed light-induced fluctuations similar to those in Balanus, and as in Balanus, no discrete waves could be seen in the voltage record.

DISCUSSION

The noise which light induces in barnacle photoreceptor resembles the Ach-induced noise which was observed in the neuromuscular junction by Katz and Miledi (1972). The unitary event which gives rise to the Ach noise is the all-or-none opening of an ionic channel, and the noisy membrane potential results from the superposition of many such events.

However, if the elementary event which produces the light-induced noise in the barnacle were an all-or-none event, like the opening of a two-state ionic channel which can only be open or closed,

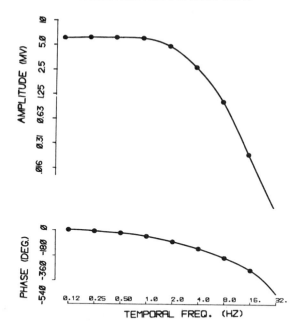

Fig. 4.   The temporal trasfer function of a barnacle photoreceptor.
The mean light level of the stimulus depolarized the receptor to a moderate level of 10 mv.   The modulation depth
was 40%, in the linear range of both the stimulating CRT
and the photoreceptor.   The response amplitude falls below 1/2 its maximal level when the modulation frequency
exceeds approximately 3 Hz.   Other cells gave similar results.

then the <u>amplitude</u> of the fluctuations cannot change when light intensity is increased.   More photons can only increase the <u>frequency</u>
of the events underlying the noise.   Since our data show that the
variance of the fluctuations <u>decreases</u> after an initial increase
as light intensity is increased, we must conclude that the elementary event (presumably-- the response to a single photon) represents
the cooperation of several, perhaps many, ionic channels.   As the
light becomes brighter, fewer channels participate in this quantal
response, and this reduction is the mechanism subserving light adaptation.   This conjecture is supported by futher analysis of the
voltage noise, which will be pubblished elsewhere.

If we estimate the duration of the elementary event from the
voltage transfer function, then by using Campbell's theorem and
the measured values for the mean and variance of the light response,

we estimate the amplitude of the elementary event to vary from a-
bout 32 microvolts to 10 microvolts at dim and bright light, respectively, and the corresponding rate to vary from 10^2 to 10^6/sec.

It is not clear why the eburneus photoreceptor fails to show
discrete waves when it is fully dark adapted. The electrical coupling among the photoreceptors in the eburneus eye must be at least
partially responsible for the attenuation of the elementary events,
as it is in vertebrate photoreceptors (Fain et al, 1976). However,
the coupling coefficients in barnacle (Shaw, 1972) are similar to
those found in the lateral eye of Limulus (Borsellino et al, 1965),
where the discrete waves are clearly observable.

The amplitude of the elementary event which we calculated
from our voltage recordings (approximately 30 microvolts) is close
to the 20 microvolts calculated by Hagins for the squid (1965),and
the 36 microvolts calculated by Payne (1981) for the locust, but
is somewhat smaller than the 80 microvolts found in the Drosophila
by Wu and Pak (1978). The difference, however, is small, and does
not seem to explain the apparent absence of discrete waves in the
membrane potential of the barnacle.

We should note here that in his Ph.D. thesis work M. Hanani
of The Hebrew University (personal communication) has found one
cell out of many which did show events similar to the discrete
waves seen in Limulus photoreceptors, although the amplitude was
considerably lower (approximately 0.5 mv).

REFERENCES

Adolph, A. R. (1964). Spontaneous slow potential fluctuation in the
    Limulus, photoreceptor, J. Gen. Physiol., 48, 297 – 322.
Borsellino, A., Fuortes, M.G.F. and Smith, T.G. (1965). Visual re-
    sponses in Limulus, Cold Spring Harbor Symp. Quant.Biol., 30,
    429 – 443.
Dodge, F. A., Knight, B. W. and Toyoda, J. (1968). Voltage noise
    in Limulus visual cells, Science, 160, 88 – 90.
Fain, G. L., Gold, H. G. and Dowling, J. E. (1976). Receptor coupling
    in the Toad retina, Cold Spring Harbor Symp. Quant. Biol., 40,
    547 – 561.
Fuortes, M. G. F. and Yeandle, S. (1964). Probability of occurrence
    of discrete potential waves in the eye of Limulus, J. Gen.
    Physiol., 47, 443 – 463.
Hagins, W. A. (1965). Electrical signs of information flow in pho-
    toreceptors, Cold Spring Harbor Symp. Quant. Biol., 30, 403 –
    418.

Hudspeth, J. and Stewart, A. (1977). Morphology and responses to light of the somata, axons, and terminal regions of individual photoreceptors of the giant barnacle, J. Physiol., 272, 1 - 23.

Katz, D. and Miledi, R. (1972). The statistical nature of the acetylcholine potential and its molecular components, J. Physiol., 224, 665 - 699.

Kirschfeld, K. (1966). Discrete and graded receptor potentials in the compound eye of the fly (Musca), in: "The functional organization of the compound eye", Bernhard, C. G. ed., pp. 291 - 309, Pergamon Press, Oxford.

Koike, H., Brown, M. H. and Hagiwara, S. (1971). Hyperpolarization of a barnacle photoreceptor membrane following illumination, J. Gen. Physiol., 57, 723 - 737.

Martin, A. R. (1955). A further study of the statistical composition of the end-plate potential, J. Physiol., 130, 114 - 122.

Milkman, N., Shapley, R. and Schick, G. (1978). A microcomputer-based visual stimulator, Behav. Res. Meth. and Instr., 10, 539 - 545.

Payne, R. (1981). Suppression of noise in a photoreceptor by oxidative metabolism, J. Comp. Physiol., 142, 181 - 188.

Scholes, J. (1965). Discontinuity of the excitation process in locust visual cells. Cold Spring Harbor Symp. Quant. Biol., 30, 517 - 527.

Shaw, S. R. (1972). Decremental conduction of the visual signal in barnacle lateral eye, J. Physiol., 220, 145 - 175.

Wu, C. F. and Pack, W. L. (1978). Light - induced voltage noise in the photoreceptor of Drosophila melanogaster, J. Gen. Physiol., 71, 249 - 268.

Yeandle, S. (1957). Studies on the slow potential and the effects of cation on the electrical responses of the Limulus ommatidium, Thesis, The Johns Hopkins University, Baltimore.

THE EARLY RECEPTOR POTENTIAL: ITS MODE OF GENERATION, APPLICATION TO STUDY OF PHOTORECEPTORS, AND FUNCTIONAL SIGNIFICANCE

V.I. Govardovskii

Institute of Evolutionary Physiology and Biochemistry

Leningrad, USSR

INTRODUCTION

The early receptor potential (ERP) was first recorded by Brown and Murakami from the monkey fovea in 1964. This fast response, which has almost zero latency, can be detected when the retina is stimulated with brief, intense flashes that bleach a considerable amount of visual pigment. The discovery of the ERP gave rise to a great deal of experiments, in the hope that the ERP might be a "missing link" between the photolysis of rhodopsin and photoreceptor excitation. It was suggested that the ERP could be converted by some kind of potential-sensitive membrane system into the late receptor potential which, as we now know, does transmit excitation along the cell (Brown & Murakami, 1964; Cone, 1965; Pak & Ebrey, 1965, and many others).

Shortly afterwards it became clear, however, that the ERP evoked by physiologically intense stimuli was too small to produce any noticeable effect. During the next decade the ERP came to be considered as an epiphenomenon generated by rhodopsin photolysis, and it was used as a tool for studying the photoreceptor properties and visual pigments in situ (Arden, 1969; Cone & Pak, 1971). More recently several attempts have again been made to include the early receptor potential in the main chain of events leading to photoreceptor excitation (Bolshakov et al., 1979; Trissl, 1979; Cafiso & Hubbell, 1980; Bennet, Michel-Villaz & Dupont, 1980). It is worthwhile, therefore, to review the present knowledge of the mechanism of ERP generation in order to asses the role of the ERP in visual tranduction.

1. <u>General properties of the response</u>

    The early receptor potential can be recorded using the conven-
tional electroretinographic technique of placing electrodes on each
side of the retina (Fig. 1a). In order to produce a measurable ERP
the stimulating flash should be strong enough to bleach a significant amount of the visual pigment, typically a few percent or more.
Employing the averaging technique, Debecker and Zanen (1975) were
able to record an ERPs 0,3 μV in amplitude with a flash which
bleached 0.04% of the visual pigment, which is still far beyond the
physiological level of illumination. However, provided the flash
intensity is high enough, ERP may reach 1-2 μV in amplitude and
exceed other components of the electroretinogram, due to fact that
the ERP amplitude, unlike that of the a- or b-wave, is strictly
proportional to the number of rhodopsin molecules bleached. The
response reaches saturation only when the flash intensity is sufficient to bleach all the pigment and/or when the probability that a
molecule of pigment will catch two or more quanta becomes significant (Cone, 1965; Hodgkin & O'Bryan, 1977).

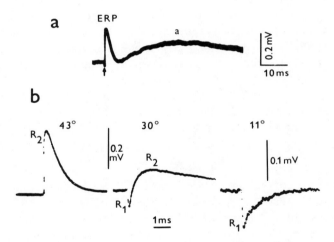

Fig. 1. (a) The initial part of the frog electroretinogram produced
         by an intense 0,2-ms flash (arrow). The a-wave and the
         early receptor potential. (b) Separation of the ERP compo-
         nents is isolated perfused albino rat retina by temperature
         variations. Note the contrary to usual electroretinographic
         convention, in this and the following figures cornea-nega-
         tive deflections are upward.

At normal body temperature in mammals the ERP consists almost entirely of a cornea-negative wave. When the temperature is lowered this wave decreases in amplitude and becomes slower, while the response becomes biphasic with an initial cornea-positive peak (R_1 component) blending into the negative wave (R_2) (Pak & Cone, 1964) (Fig. 1b).

Rapid electrical responses similar to the ERP are not confined to the photoreceptors and have been detected in other light-absorbing tissues, e.g. in retinal pigment epithelium, frog skin and green leaves (for review, see Arden, 1969; Cone & Pak, 1971). In some cases the response is of thermal origin. The heating of a cell by a strong flash causes changes in its membrane potential (Hagins & Mc Gaughy, 1967; Cone & Pak, 1971). In specialized photoreceptor organelles the mechanism of ERP production should be different, however, since the light intensity necessary to evoke an ERP in the retina is 2-3 orders of magnitude lower than in the pigment epithelium (Cone & Pak, 1971).

One of the most remarkable properties of the ERP is that it is insensitive to gross changes in chemical environment and tissue metabolism. It persists in mammalian preparations when the animal is killed, and is resistant to anoxia and metabolic inhibitors such as cyanide and dinitrophenol. Gross changes in the ionic mileu, which would suppress any usual neuronal activity, hardly affect the ERP. In fact, the response amplitude tends to rise when KCl, RbCl or NH_4Cl are substituted for NaCl in the external solution. Complete substitution of the ions by sucrose greatly enchances the ERP by increasing extracellular resistance. Thiol-blocking agents and short formaldehyde fixation as well as pH changes in the range 4.5 - 8.7 fail to affect the ERP (Brindley & Gardner-Medwin, 1966; Pak, Rozzi & Ebrey, 1967; Arden & al., 1968). Thus, it seems clear that the ERP cannot be produced by changes in the ionic permeability of the cell membrane.

On the other hand, the ERP appears to be intimately related to the events occuring during the photolysis of rhodopsin. The ERP spectral sensitivity curve matches the visual pigment absorbance, and the ERP is suppressed by background illumination in proportion to the fraction of rhodopsin bleached (Cone, 1965). Urea treatment, which denatures the rhodopsin without affecting its main absorption band, abolished the ERP (Giulio & Petrosini, 1973). Similar effects are produced by warming retinas to 58°C for several minutes, which preserves rhodopsin unbleached but leads to the loss of its orientation in the membrane (Cone & Brown, 1967).

It has been concluded that the ERP is produced by charge displacement within the rhodopsin molecule itself or within its near
environment, during the bleaching (Cone, 1965, 1967; Hagins & Mc-
Gaughy, 1967; Arden et al., 1968). Such a displacement in a direction perpendicular to the plane of the membrane acts as a current
generator, charging the membrane capacitance and producing an extracellular current and voltage drop. Two main questions relating to
the ERP are: i) which membrane in photoreceptors is the current generator, and ii) what stages of visual pigment photolysis are responsible for the two ERP components?

2. Sources of the ERP in cones and rods

In vertebrate cones, visual pigment-bearing discs are invagi-
nations of the plasma membrane of the outer segment. Hence, charge
displacement across the disc membrane will evoke a current flowing
through the extracellular space, inner segment membrane and cell
cytoplasma and thereby produce an extra and intracellular electrical
response. This mode of ERP generation applies to invertebrate photoreceptors as well, since their rhabdomeric microvilli are processes
of the cell membrane and are therefore topologically equivalent to
cone discs.

The situation for rods is rather different. Most of the rod
discs are closed structures which are completely detached from the
surface membrane of the outer segment (Cohen, 1968, 1970). External
currents produced by the two opposite membranes of each disc should
cancel each other and render the rod discs incapable of generating
any extradiscal response, either extracellular or intracellular.
Some response could appear if there were a certain asymmetry in the
pile of discs, e.g. owing to its particular orientation to incident
light. The polarity of the ERP should then be found to depend on
the direction of illumination, which is not the case (Brindley &
Gardner-Medvin, 1966). It has also been supposed that the extracellular ERP might be generated by the "total charge difference
between the two poles of the pile of discs, which results from the
absorption gradient of the photons along the rod" (Bennett et al.,
1980). The most likely sources of the rod ERP, however, appear to
be rhodopsin molecules located in the surface membrane of the outer
segment (Arden, 1969; Cone & Pak, 1971; Hagins & Rüppel, 1971).
This was proved in experiments exploiting the dichroic properties
of the photoreceptor membrane (Govardovskii, 1975, 1976).

As well known, light absorption by rod discs reaches its maximum when the E-vector of the light wave is oriented parallel to the discs, because the chromophoric groups of the rhodopsin molecules lie within the plane of photoreceptor membrane (Wald et al., 1963). Rolling up the membrane like the outer segment surface membrane produces a dichroic structure whose absorption coefficient is maximum when light has its electric vector parallel to the axis of the cylinder (Moody & Parriss, 1961). Therefore the rod discs and surface membrane, when illuminated "side on", should exibit dichroism of the opposite sign. This can serve as a means of differentiating between the two. When the retina was illuminated by a polarized light beam perpendicular to the outer segment axes, the cones produced a maximum ERP in response to a stimulus polarized in the disc plane, whereas in rods, the largest ERP was produced by flashes polarized along the photoreceptor axes. Hence, the response in rods was generated by the light absorbed in the surface membrane (Govardovskii, 1975).

The fact that the sources of the rod ERP are rhodopsin molecules localized within the surface membrane was demostrated even more convincingly using the registration of photoinduced dichroism (Govardovskii, 1976). Dark-adapted rat retinas were illuminated by two weak test flashes polarized in mutually perpendicular directions. ERP amplitudes were equal for flashes of equal intensities (Fig. 2a). A strong flash of linearly polarized light was then delivered; it predominantely bleached the rhodopsin molecules whose absorbing dipoles lay parallel to the E-vector of the flash light. Immediately following the flash rods became dichroic, which could be ascertained by the imbalance of the responses to the test flashes. The ERP response to a test flash was weaker when the flash was polarized parallel rather than normal to the bleaching light (Fig. 2b). The dichroism disappeared with a time constant of about 1 sec. (Fig. 2c-d). This long-lived dichroism is an indication that the rod ERP should be attributed to a source other than discs, because photoinduced dichroism of disc membranes is known to decay through rotational diffusion of rhodopsin - within a characteristic time of ca. 20 μsec (Cone, 1972). In surface membrane, on the other hand, dichroism will vanish due to lateral diffusion around the outer segment, which can take several seconds (Fig. 2).

The dichroic ratio obtained in the above experiment (1.24 $\pm$ 0.02 for a conditioning flash bleaching 45% of the rhodopsin) almost coincides with the value predicted theoretically (1.25). This means

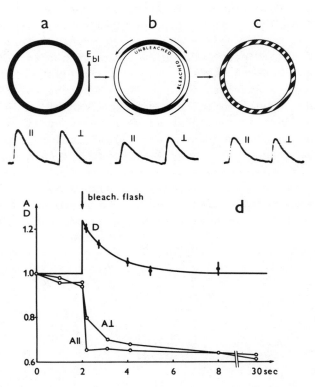

Fig. 2 (a–c) The appearance and decay of photoinduced dichroism of
the surface membrane of rat retinal rod outer segments, as
demonstrated by responses to test flashes polarized in two
mutually perpendicular directions. The responses before
(a), and 0,18 (b) and 6 s (c) after delivering a polarized
bleaching flash (E_{bl}). ‖ and ⊥ are directions of polarization of test flashes with respect to the bleaching flash.
(d) Time course of response amplitudes to the test flashes
(A‖, A⊥) obtained in a single experiment. Transient photoinduced dichroism (D) decays with a time constant of 1.25
sec. Each point is the mean of 8 experiments ± s.e.m. The
medium was Ringer: 0,32 M sucrose: glycerol ≃ 1:4:5 brought
to a refraction index of 1,408 in order to decrease light
scattering. Temperature: 37°C

that the contribution of discs to ERP is negligible compared to that of surface membrane.

The relaxation time also gives an estimate of the diffusion constant for lateral Brownian motion of the rhodopsin within the surface membrane. The value obtained ($1.6 \pm 0.5 \cdot 10^{-9}$ cm^2 sec^{-1}, Govardovskii, 1976) is similar to that for disc membranes ($3 \div 5 \cdot 10^{-9}$ cm^2 sec^{-1}, Liebman & Entine, 1974; Poo & Cone, 1974; Takezoe & Yu, 1981).

3. Stages of rhodopsin photolysis underlying the R_1- and R_2- components of ERP

Attribution of ERP components to definite stages of rhodopsin photolysis poses some difficulties. Clearly the events following the metarhodopsin I – metarhodopsin II transition are too slow to contribute to the ERP. The R_1-component is temperature resistant and can be recorded down to $-35°C$ (Pak & Ebrey, 1965). R_1 must therefore originate not later than at the lumirhodopsin – metarhodopsin I conversion. Since the R_2-component is strongly temperature-dependent and vanished near $0°C$, when meta I – meta II transition is blocked, it may be generated by this process. However, the time course of either R_1 or R_2 does not follow the kinetics of any reaction in photolysis sequence (Arden et al., 1968; Arden, 1969; Cone & Pak, 1971).

It is evident that the time course of the ERP depends both on the kinetics of the corresponding molecular transition and on the passive electric properties of photoreceptor cell. Hagins and Rüppel (1975) developed a cable model of the rat retinal rod which when stimulated by an exponential impulse with a time constant of 350 μsec (equivalent to meta I – meta II transition at $37°C$, according to Hagins & Rüppel, 1971) transforms it into a response similar to the R_2-component of the ERP. The result is not quite conclusive, because a complex electrical network can produce something like the R_2 response from almost any input, and Hagins' and Rüppel's model, which includes some 20 parameters, seems to be complex enough to do that. On the other hand, the model of Hodgkin and O'Bryan (1977), who treat the cell as a single integrating RC-circuit, is clearly oversimplified.

It appears possible for the kinetics of events underlying the ERP to be determined without any a priori assumptions as to the properties of the generation mechanism apart from its well-established linearity (Govardovskii, 1978). In fact, the response V(t) of a linear system to an arbitrary input $f(t)$ can be predicted from its impulse response $g(t)$:

$$V(t) = \int_0^t f(\tau) \, g(t - \tau) \, d\tau$$

The impulse response $g(t)$ is the response of the system to an infinitely short unit impulse, $\delta(t)$. Since the molecular transitions which might contribute to R_1, have characteristic times between 1 psec and 50 µsec (Abrahamson & Wiesenfeld, 1972) they approximate fairly well the delta-function. Therefore the R_1-component of the ERP represents, in fact, the impulse response $g(t)$ of the ERP-shaping system. Given $g(t)$ and $V(t)$, one can find $f(t)$ and reconstruct the process producing the ERP.

It is easy to make calculations by computer. However, the problem can be solved more clearly by means of an analog model which resembles the electrical structure of the photoreceptor (Govardovskii, 1975, 1978). In the model (Fig. 3a), a retinal rod is represented by the capacitance C_o and resistance r_o of the surface membrane of the outer segment, connected to the capacitance C_i and resistance r_i of the inner segment membrane through the resistances of the extracellular space r_e and receptor cytoplasm r_c. The current fed to the outer segment membrane should be proportional to the rate of the molecular transitions contributing to the ERP. The "R_1"-input is therefore connected to the model through the RC-circuit producing a brief, exponential current pulse. It decays with a time constant of 15 µsec, corresponding to that observed when a light flash is used to excite a real ERP. When a voltage step is applied to the "R_2"-input, the variable resistor r_T and capacitor C_T produce a current pulse of the opposite polarity. By adjusting r_T it is possible to simulate the temperature dependance of the rate of the first-order reaction which is supposed to underlie the R_2 component. "Temperature" variations do not affect the total charge displacement across the outer segment membrane. Voltage drops along the extracellular space (between points 1 and 0 in the model, Fig. 3a) represent the ERP.

At first, the signal was fed to the "R_1"-input, and the circuit parameters were adjusted to simulate the ERP recorded from the rat retina at 10°C. This ERP consisted almost entirely of the R_1 component. Then the signal was connected to the "R_2"-input and the value of r_T as well as the ratio of the R_1 and R_2 component amplitudes were matched so as to reproduce the ERP for an intermediate temperature, e.g. 30°C. Some additional adjustments of the "photo-

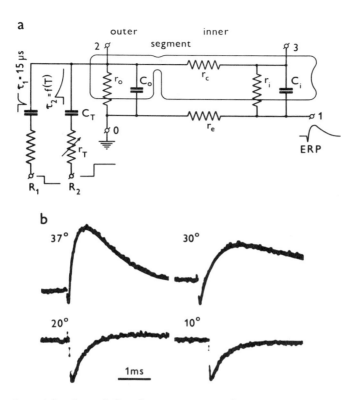

Fig. 3 (a) Electrical model of ERP generation. For explanation see
text.
(b) Model simulation of the ERP generated by the isolated
rat retina at different temperatures. Superimposed are real
ERP recordings (noisy curves) and model responses (smooth
curves). Medium: physiological solution with 89 Ohm·cm specific resistance. Bandpass: 0,1 Hz - 20 kHz 15 µs flash.

receptor" parameters were necessary in order to take account of a
minute fraction of R_2 present in the ERP generated at 10°C. After
this procedure, changing the r_T-value alone was enough to simulate
any waveform of the ERP generated by the retina within the temperature range between 10° and 45°C (Fig. 3b).

    The Arrhenius plot for the R_2-producing reaction is given in
Fig. 4, where the open circles represent the experimental values
for the rate constant obtained by means of the model. The time
constant $\tau \simeq 600$ µsec at 37°C and activation energy $E_A = 31$ kcal/mol
(130 kJ/mol) are in fairly good agreement with the spectrophotome-

tric data for meta I - meta II transition in the bovine photoreceptor membranes (Sengbush & Stieve, 1971; Applebury et al., 1974; Rapp,
1979).

In recent years some approaches to measuring the electrical responses from rod disc membranes have been developed. Rhodopsin films
and disc membranes have been attached to thick, artificial hydrophobic membranes (Trissl, 1979; Bolshakov et al., 1979), and the potential difference across the wall of the photoreceptor membrane vesicles has been monitored by means of a potential-sensitive dye (Bennet et al., 1980) and by spin-labeled hydrophobic ions (Cafiso &
Hubbell, 1980). Light-induced potentials observed in the experiments are thought to be analogous to the ERP generated by the plasma
membrane. Time constants of the rising phase of the response measured by Bennett et al. (1980) and by Cafiso & Hubbell (1980) fit the
model rather well (Fig. 4). Trissl's (1979) data, obtained with
rhodopsin-containing lipid-hexane films, deviate strongly from the
other results. This seems to result from the influence of detergent,
which is known to modify the photolysis kinetics (Abrahamson & Wiesenfeld, 1972). It should be noted, however, that the molecular transitions responsible for the generation of the R_2-component of the ERP
may be not completely identical to the metaI - meta II conversion detected spectrophotometrically. The meta II formation is likely to be
a multi-stage process, and the kinetics of charge displacement and
spectral changes may be slightly different (Bennett et al., 1980).

The R_1-component should appear not later than at the bathorho-
dopsin - lumirhodopsin conversion, because the lumi - meta I transition takes seconds at sub-zero temperatures (Abrahamson & Wiesenfeld,
1972), when the fast R_1 can still be recorded.

The overall significance of the results obtained with the model
should not depend on the choice of its specific form. By virtue of
its ability to produce an appropriate impulse response, the model
should permit the identification of the kinetics of the processes
involved in ERP generation. Moreover, since the model reproduces a
simplified version of the rod electrical structure, it could be used
for approximating the photoreceptor membrane parameters as well
(Govardovskii, 1978).

4. The nature of the charges moved and the magnitude of their displacement

ERP currents originate due to light-induced charge displacements across the rhodopsin-containing membrane. Charge movement

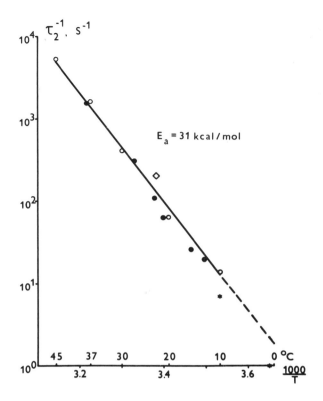

Fig. 4   Arrhenius plot for the rate constant of R_2-producing reaction. Open circles: measurements from the model of Fig. 3.
Filled circles: spectrophotometric data for metarhodopsin I
decay from Rapp (1979). Asterisks: rate constant for the
rising phase of the photovoltage measured in photoreceptor
membrane vesicles (Bennett et al., 1980). Square: the same
from Cafiso and Hubbell (1980).

may occur within the membrane as a result of conformational changes
of rhodopsin molecules (Cone, 1967; Hagins & Mc Gaughy, 1967, Arden,
1969) or may be produced by transferring charged particles through
the membrane – media interface (Cone, 1967; Cafiso & Hubbel, 1980).
In particular, it is tempting to relate the R_2-component to a
well-known proton uptake during meta I – meta II transition (Cone,

1967; Bolshakov et al., 1979; Cafiso & Hubbell, 1980). The protons
are bound on the cytoplasmic side of the membrane and should produce
a potential of the appropriate polarity. The time course of the
transmembrane potential change of the vesicles prepared from disc
membranes follows protonation kinetics. However, the two processes
differ markedly with respect to pH- and temperature dependance (Bennett et al., 1980). Apparently the proton uptake is not a main current source, even though protonation and charge transfer may result
from a common molecular mechanism.

The magnitude of the charge displacement during the ERP can be
found from the product of membrane capacitance and potential difference. The model shown in Fig. 3a enables easy "intracellular recordings" and measurements of the potential difference across the outer
segment membrane. The amplitude of the intracellular ERP can be
scaled by means of the extracellular response to a flash of known
intensity. Provided there is no leackage through r_o, r_e and r_c, a
full bleach will produce a 15 mV R_2-component. A similar value
(20 mV) follows from the intracellular recordings from cones
(Murakami & Pak, 1970; Hodgkin & O'Bryan, 1977) and from measurements of the rod membrane vesicle response (Bennett et al., 1980;
Cafiso & Hubbell, 1980). Assuming that the specific capacitance
of the membrane is approximately 1 mF/cm^2 and the rhodopsin density
$2.5 \cdot 10^4$ molecules per μm^2 (Liebman, 1972), one obtains a value of
0.05 elementary charges displaced per molecule of rhodopsin bleached
(supposing that the charge is transferred across the whole membrane
thickness). The 0.5 charges per rhodopsin bleached obtained by
Hagins and Rüppel (1971) is an overstimate because their assumed
value for rhodopsin density ($6 \cdot 10^3$ μm^{-2}) was too low.

During the R_1 component, there are approximately 0.006 elementary charges transferred per molecule of rhodopsin bleached
(Govardovskii, 1978).

Thus, if one or two charged groups were moving during rhodopsin
bleaching, their displacement in the direction perpendicular to the
membrane by as little as 1 - 5 Å could produce the ERP.

5. Energy relations in ERP generation and visual excitation

Several attempts have been made recently to revitalize the
idea of the triggering role of the ERP in visual transduction.
It was speculated that the ERP-induced potential difference across
the disc membrane might increase the permeability of potential-de-

pendent calcium channels, thus releasing the putative intracellular
messenger into the cytoplasm (Bolshakov et al., 1979; Cafiso & Hubbel,
1980). It was also suggested that the ERP might modulate the activity of potential-sensitive enzymes participating in the messenger
turnover (Bolshakov et al., 1979; Cafiso & Hubbell, 1980; Bennett
et al., 1980).

However, the earlier doubts about the possible functional significance of the ERP expressed, for exemple, by Arden (1969) and
Cone & Pak (1971) can be now confirmed by reliable quantitative es-
timations. It can be easily calculated that absorption of one quantum per disc and transfer of $q = 0.05$ elementary charge ($8 \cdot 10^{-21}$ C)
across the disc membrane of a surface area equal to cm^2 (as is the
case with bovine or rat rods) should produce a potential difference
of $V = 1.6 \cdot 10^{-7}$ Volt. The ERP energy would then be equal to
$qV/2 = 6.4 \cdot 10^{-28}$ Joule, which is 9 orders of magnitude lower than
the energy of visible quanta ($\sim 4 \cdot 10^{-19}$ J) and 7 orders of magnitude
lower than the energy of thermal motion ($kT \simeq 4 \cdot 10^{-21}$ J). Thus, the
energy of the ERP generated by physiological stimuli is incommensu-
rable with the membrane thermal noise and cannot produce any effect.
It is worthwhile noting that the efficiency of transformation of the
light energy into the ERP is extremely low, never exceeding 10^{-9} for
a threshold stimulus and rising up to $2.5 \cdot 10^{-5}$ only for a full bleach.

Therefore the ERP must be an epiphenomenon which cannot play any
meaningful role in visual transduction, although the ERP-generating
mechanism itself may lie in the main excitatory sequence.

6. Two mechanisms of ERP production: a possible difference between vertebrate and invertebrate photoreceptors

The charge on the membrane capacitance ($q = CV$) can be changed
either by charge transfer or by varying the capacitance C, e.g.
through changing membrane thickness or dielectric constant. In vertebrate photoreceptors the former mechanism seems to operate, since
the rod and cone ERPs are insensitive to the ionic environment and
to metabolic inhibitors which profoundly affect the transmembrane
potential V. In photoreceptors of Limulus, however, the ERP amplitude depends on the membrane potential. The polarity of the ERP
be reversed by depolarization (Smith & Brown, 1966). This would
imply that the ERP in Limulus is generated either by permeability
changes or is due to significant alterations of dielectric properties
of the photoreceptor membrane. This interesting point is worthy of
further study.

7. The ERP as a tool for photoreceptor studies

Despite its lack of functional significance, the ERP may serve as a powerful tool for investigating visual pigments and photoreceptor membrane properties, as well as for evaluating the electrical parameters of photoreceptors. The most obvious applications for the ERP lie in the studies of processes of visual pigment bleaching and regeneration within the retina, as well as in obtaining spectral sensitivity curves. The close connection found between the ERP and visual pigment photolysis, the linear relation between the response amplitude and the pigment concentration, and the absence of neural interactions between various receptor types at the ERP level enable even complex mixtures of visual pigments to be easyly analyzed (see e.g., Goldstein & Wolf, 1973; Govardovskii & Zueva, 1977).

Cone (1967) used the ERP for demonstrating photoreversible conversion of the products of rhodopsin photolysis in rods. This approach, together with the reconstruction of the ERP-generating reaction kinetics (Fig. 3-4), can be applied to in situ studies of the photolysis of cone visual pigments which still remain obscure. As an another example, the use of the ERP in the study of the Brownian motion of rhodopsin molecules within the rod surface membrane has already been described (Fig. 2).

The most promising application, however, would be investigation of the electrical parameters of photoreceptor's membranes. The time course of the ERP strongly depends on the passive electrical properties of the cell, in particular on the conductances of the outer and inner segment membranes. It is difficult to distinguish between these membranes by intracellular recordings, even in specimens with large cells. The use of a simple electric model (Fig. 3) permits their discrimination, since the increase in conductances of the inner and outer segments influences the kinetics of the ERP in opposite ways (Fig. 5a). For example, Yoshikami and Hagins (1973) found that lowering Ca^{++} activity in the bathing medium to 10^{-7} M led to generation of a distorted ERP with a shortened , biphasic R_2 component. In the model shown in Fig. 3 this distorted ERP may only be reproduced by an approximately 5-fold decrease in R_o with a simultaneous increase in R_i. Hence, lowering the extracellular calcium concentration really increases the conductance of the outer segment membrane, as postulated by the "calcium hypothesis". This result has not yet been obtained by a more direct method.

It is hoped that instead of being the object of attempts to

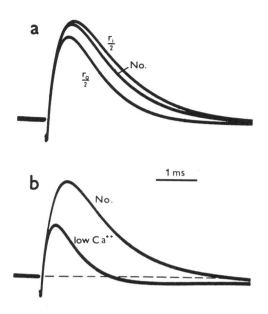

Fig. 5 (a) Changes in ERP waveform produced by a two-fold decrease
        in the resistances of the outer (r_o) or inner (r_i) segment
        membranes. Recordings from the model of Fig. 3.
        (b) Model simulation of an "abnormal" ERP recorded in low-
        -calcium Ringer by Yoshikami and Hagins (1973). The short-
        ened, biphasic ERP can be qualitatively reproduced by the
        model of Fig. 3a by means of a 5-fold decrease of the outer
        segment membrane resistance and a simultaneous two-fold
        increase of the inner segment resistance.

incorporate it into the process of visual excitation, the ERP will
find more realistic applications as a useful tool for photoreceptor
research.

REFERENCES

Abrahamson E.W., Wiesenfeld J.R. (1972). The structure, spectra
    and reactivity of visual pigments, in: "Handbook of sensory
    physiology", v. 7/1, Dartnall, H.J.A., ed., p. 69-121.,
    Springer-Verlag, Berlin - Heidelberg - New York.
Applebury M.L., Zuckerman D.M., Lamola A.A., Jovin T.M. (1974).
    Rhodopsin. Purification and recombination with phospholipids
    assayed by metarhodopsin I - metarhodopsin II transition, Bio-
    chemistry 13, 3448-3458.
Arden G.B. (1969). The excitation of photoreceptors, in "Progress

in biophysics and molecular biology", Butler J.A.V. and Nobel
D., eds., p. 373-421, Pergamon Press, Oxford - New York.

Arden G.B., Bridges C.D.B., Ikeda H., Siegel I.M., (1968). Mode of
generation of the early receptor potential, Vision Res., 8,
3-24.

Bennett N., Michel-Villaz M., Dupont Y., (1980). Cyanide dye measurement of a light-induced transient membrane potential associated with the metarhodopsin II intermediate in rod-outer-segmen
membranes, Eur. J. Biochem., 111, 105-110.

Bolshakov V.I., Drachev A.L., Drachev L.A., Kalamkarov G.R., Kaulen
A.D., Ostrovsky M.A., Skulachev V.P. (1979). Common properties
of bacterial and visual rhodopsins: conversion of the light
energy into the electric potential, Dokl. Akad. Nauk SSSR, 249,
1462-1466 (In Russian).

Brindley G.S., Gardner-Medvin A.R. (1966). The origin of the early
receptor potential of the retina, J. Physiol., 182, 185-194.

Brown K.T., Murakami M. (1964). A new receptor potential of the
monkey retina with no detectable latency, Nature, 201, 626-628.

Cafiso D.S., Hubbell W.L. (1980). Interfacial charge separation in
photoreceptor membranes. Photochem, Photobiol., 32, 461-468.

Cohen A.I. (1968). New evidence supporting the linkage to extracellular space of outer segment saccules of frog cones but not
rods, J. Cell Biol., 47, 424-444.

Cohen A.I. (1970). Further studies on the question of the patency
of saccules in outer segments of vertebrate photoreceptors,
Vision Res., 10, 445-453.

Cone R.A. (1965). The early receptor potential of the vertebrate
eye, Cold Spring Harb. Symp. Quant. Biol., 30, 483-490.

Cone R.A. (1967). Early receptor potential: photoreversible
charge displacement in rhodopsin, Science, 155, 1128-1131.

Cone R.A. (1972). Rotation diffusion of rhodopsin in the visual
receptor membrane, Nature New. Biol., 236, 39-43

Cone R.A., Brown P.K. (1967). Dependance of the early receptor
potential on the orientation of rhodopsin, Science, 156, 536.

Cone R.A., Pak W.L. (1971). The early receptor potential, in:
"Handbook of sensory physiology", v. 1. Loewenstein W.R.,
ed., p. 345-365, Springer-Verlag, Berlin - Heidelberg - New
York.

Debecker J., Zanen A. (1975). Intensity function of the early
receptor potential and of the melanin fast photovoltage in
the human eye, Vision Res., 15, 101-106.

Giulio L., Petrosini L. (1973). Effect of urea on the early receptor potential, Vision Res., 13, 489-492

Goldstein E.B., Wolf B.M. (1973). Regeneration of the green-rod pigment in the isolated frog retina, Vision Res., 13, 527-534.

Govardovskii V.I. (1975). On the sites of generation of the early and late receptor potentials in rods, Vision Res., 15, 971-981.

Govardovskii V.I. (1976). Lateral diffusion of rhodopsin within the surface membrane of rat retinal rod, Biofizika, 21, 1019-1023 (In Russian).

Govardovskii V.I. (1978). The mode of generation of the early receptor and electric model of retina rod, Biofizika, 23, 514-519 (In Russian).

Govardovskii V.I., Zueva L.V. (1977). Visual pigments of chicken and pigeon, Vision Res., 17, 537-543.

Hagins W.A., Mc. Gaughy R.E. (1967). Molecular and thermal origins of fast photoelectric effects in the squid retina, Science, 157, 813-816.

Hagins W.A., Rüppel H. (1971). Fast photoelectric effect and the properties of vertebrate photoreceptors as electric cables, Feder. Proc., 30, 64-68.

Hodgkin A.L., O'Bryan P.M. (1977). Internal recording of the early receptor potential in turtle cones, J. Physiol., 267, 737-766.

Liebman P.A. (1972). Microspectrophotometry of photoreceptors, in: Handbook of sensory physiology, v. 7/1. Dartnall, H.J.A. ed., p. 481-528, Springer-Verlag, Berlin - Heidelberg - New York.

Liebman P.A., Entine G. (1974). Lateral diffusion of visual pigment in photoreceptor disc membranes, Nature, 247, 457-459.

Moody M.F., Parriss J.R. (1961). The discrimination of polarized light by Octopus: a behavioural and morphological study, Z. vergl. Physiol., 44, 268-291.

Murakami M., Pak W.L. (1970). Intracellularly recorded early receptor potential of the vertebrate photoreceptors, Vision Res., 10, 965-976.

Pak W., Cone R.A. (1964). Isolation and identification of the initial peak of the early receptor potential, Nature, 204, 836-838.

Pak W.L., Ebrey T.G. (1965). Visual receptor potential observed at sub-zero temperatures, Nature, 205, 484-486.

Pak W.L., Rozzi V., Ebrey T.G. (1967). Effect of changes in the chemical environment of the retina on the two components of the early receptor potential, Nature, 219, 109-110.

Poo Mu-Ming, Cone R.A. (1974). Lateral diffusion of rhodopsin in the photoreceptor membrane, Nature, 247, 438-441.

Rapp J. (1979). The kinetics of intermediate processes in the photolysis of bovine rhodopsin - II. The intermediate decay sequence from lumirhodopsin$_{497}$ to metarhodopsin$_{380}$ II, <u>Vision Res.</u>, 19, 137–141.

Rüppel H. (1975). Membrane structure and transduction mechanism of visual receptors, <u>in</u>: "Photoreceptor optics". Snyder A.W. and Menzel R., eds. p. 499–512, Springer–Verlag, Berlin – Heidelberg – New York.

v. Sengbush G., Stieve H. (1971). Flash photolysis of rhodopsin. II. Measurements on rhodopsin digitonin solutions and fragments of rod outer segments, <u>Ztschr. Naturforsch</u>, 26, 861–862.

Smith T.G., Brown J.E. (1966). A photoelectric potential in invertebrate cells, <u>Nature</u>, 212, 1217–1219.

Takezoe H., Yu H. (1981). Lateral diffusion of photopigments in photoreceptor disc membrane vesicles by the dynamic Kerr effect, <u>Biochemistry</u>, 20, 5275–5281.

Trissl H.W. (1979). Light–induced conformational changes in cattle rhodopsin as probed by measurements of the interface potential, <u>Photochem. Photobiol.</u>, 29, 579–588.

Wald G., Brown P.K., Gibbons I.R. (1963). The problem of visual excitation, <u>J. Opt. Soc. Amer.</u>, 53, 20–35.

Yoshikami S., Hagins W.A. (1973). Control of the dark current in vertebrate rods and cones, <u>in</u>: "Biochemistry and Physiology of Visual Pigments", Langer H., ed., p. 245–255, Springer––Verlag, Berlin – Heidelberg – New York.

SOME BASIC INFORMATION ABOUT THE LIGHT RESPONSE OF FROG RODS

P. B. Detwiler
University of Washington
Department of Physiology and Biophysics
Seattle WA 98195
U.S.A.

The frog eye has been a standard preparation for vision research for more than a century. It has provided fundamental information about receptor photochemistry, the origin of the ERG and the properties of ganglion cells. In light of its history, it is surprising there is so little information about the cellular electrophysiology of the frog retina. This is particularly true of frog photoreceptors, which, to my knowledge, have been studied with intracellular electrodes on only one occasion (Toyoda, et al., 1970). As a result, there are several gaps in our understanding of their fundamental physiology. The aim of the present work was twofold: first to assess the practicality of using intracellular electrodes to study the frog retina and second, to answer some basic questions about the light response and spatial properties of frog rods.

METHODS

Frogs, _Rana_ _pipiens_ or _Rana_ _catesbeiana_, were dark adapted overnight and then decapitated. Under dim red light, an eye was removed from the pithed head, hemisected and the posterior half placed in a petri dish containing oxygenated frog Ringer solution. A stream of Ringer solution along with gentle dissection was used to separate the ret ina from the pigment epithelium. The retina, with the receptor side up, was floated onto a monofilament nylon mesh (210 μm opening, Small Parts Incorporated, Miami, Florida) and transferred to the recording chamber. Oxygenated profusion fluid flowed past the vitreal side of the retina at the rate of about five milliliters per minute. The receptor surface was kept moist by capillarity. Glass microelectrodes filled with 4M potassium acetate and having resistances between 200 and 400 megohms were connected to an electrometer amplifier. Before lowering an electrode onto the receptor side of the retina, it was centered in the output of an optical stimulator using a remote grid system that allowed the receptors to be maintained in their original dark adapted state. The stimuli were most commonly flashes 20 ms in duration of 520 nm light having an unattenuated irradiance of 2.4×10^3 erg sec^{-1} cm^{-2}.

RESULTS

When an intracellular electrode was advanced into the retina, a characteristic sequence of events took place. Within a short distance of the receptor surface, cells with a resting potential of about 40 millivolts were impaled. These were identified as rods on the basis of the kinetics of their responses to a dim and bright flash, their spectral properties, and their extreme sensitivity to light adaptation. Moderate to large potential shifts were observed as the electrode was advanced deeper into the retina, but these were associated very rarely with a light response. It thus appeared that rods were the only cells in the frog retina that could be recorded reproducibly with intracellular electrodes. In all cases (total of 43), these were red (λ_{max} = 502 nm) as opposed to green (λ_{max} = 433 nm) rods (Liebman and Entine, 1968). This sampling bias is most likely due to the fact that the red rods are larger and outnumber the green rods by about five to one. There were no clear differences in the results obtained with Rana pipiens and bullfrog retinas, but in general the recordings from bullfrog rods were felt to be slightly more stable.

Responses to Flashes: Figure 1 shows how the light response changed shape as a large diameter flash was increased from 3.95×10^{-1} to 3.86×10^3 photons μm^{-2}. With increasing flash, the time to the peak of the response decreased from 600 milliseconds to 75 milliseconds. The brightest flashes produced a maximum hyperpolarization of about 35 mV. The initial peak of these responses was followed by a slowly decining plateau. In these respects, the flash responses are the same as those described for other types of rods with one exception. The response to a bright flash included a dip or notch as the potential decayed from the peak to the plateau (Figure 1 inset). This was not seen in all cells but was commonly observed in the "best" cells, i.e. the ones that gave light responses

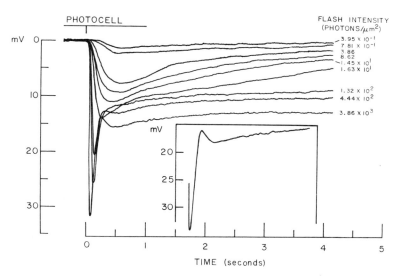

Fig. 1   Intensity series using a large spot (radius 529 μm).
          Tracings show the responses to 20 milliseconds, 520 nm,
          flashes of the intensities shown. The insert displays,
          on the same voltage and time scale, the "dip" during the
          peak to plateau transition of the response to the brightest
          flash.

greater than 25 mV. The "dip" in some ways resembles an oscillation
and might be produced by a voltage dependent conductance(s) in the
inner segment membrane.

Sensitivity: The absolute flash sensitivity of the most sensitive
rod was 12.6 mV photon^{-1} μm^2. In order to calculate the size of
the response evoked by the photoisomerization of a single rhodopsin
molecule, an effective collecting area was estimated (see Baylor &
Hodgkin, 1973; Baylor & Fettiplace, 1975). Since the retina was
illuminated from the receptor side, the geometric collecting area
of the rod, given by the cross-sectional area of the outer segment,
was 28 μm^2. The probability that a photon landing on the outer
segment will be absorbed in a pigment molecule and trigger photoisomerization resulting in hyperpolarization was assessed in the following manner. From Figure 1 of Liebman and Entine (1968), the
specific axial density of the frog red rod for 520 nm light (the
wave length used in the present experiment) was 0.0125/μm. The
probability for absorption along the 45 μm (mean of 10 measurements)
long outer segment is 0.73. This, combined with a quantum efficiency

for isomerization of approximately 0.65 (Dartnall, 1972) gives a
total probability of 0.47 that a photon incident on the outer segment will produce a voltage response. Thus the effective collecting area is 13.1 μm^2 and the peak hyperpolarization produced by a
single photoisomerization is about 1 mV. This particular calculation was made using <u>Rana</u> <u>pipiens</u> red rods, but essentially the same
result would be expected for bullfrog red rods since they are about
the same size and are thought to contain the same photopigment.

<u>Electrical Spread</u>: Since Baylor, Fuortes, and O'Bryan's (1971)
demonstration of electrical coupling between turtle cones, much evidence has accumulated to show that rods in the turtle and toad
retina are joined by passive electrical connections (Fain, 1975;
Schwartz, 1976; Copenhagen & Owen, 1976; Leeper, et al., 1978; Gold,
1979). Consequently, I thought it would be interesting to know
the extent and properties of electrical coupling in frog rods.
This was done by using a method introduced by Lamb (1976) and Lamb
& Simon (1976), in which a long, narrow (5 μm wide) strip of light
is flashed at various distances from the impaled cell. Moving the
strip of light away from the recorded cell caused the response to
get smaller and reach peak earlier. The shortening of the time to
peak indicates that the high frequency components of the response
spread with less attenuation through the coupled network than the
low frequency components. In this respect, the frog rod network
acts like a high pass filter and thus resembles the rod networks
in the snapping turtle and toad (Detwiler, et al., 1978 & 1980;
Owen & Torre, 1980). In Figure 2, the logarithm of the peak amplitude of the response is plotted against the position of the stimulating strip of light. The amplitude of the response declines exponentially with distance. The strip displacement over which the
potential fell to 1/e gave the space constant, λ , which is a convenient measure of the degree of electrical coupling. In the network of red rods in the frog, λ varied from 9 to 16 μm with a mean
value of 12 μm (see Table 1). This is much smaller than those
measured in the rod networks of the snapping turtle and toad where
respective values of 50 μm and 19 μm have been reported (Detwiler,
et al., 1980; Gold, 1979). Because of this large difference, it
seemed important to use some other method to obtain λ. This was
done by measuring the dependence of the response on the diameter of
a circular spot of light. Lamb (1976) has shown that the voltage
 V(0) at the center of an illuminated circle is

$$V(0) = V_{max} \left\{ 1 - \left(\frac{d}{2\lambda} \ K, \ \frac{d}{2\lambda}\right)\right\} \tag{1}$$

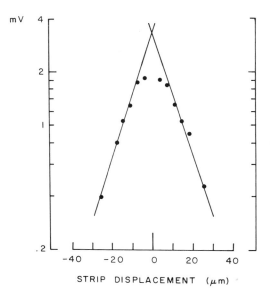

Fig. 2.   Spatial profile determined with a strip of light. Peak
           response amplitude as a function of strip displacement
           is plotted on semilogarithmic coordinates. The slope
           of the straight line, fitted to the points by eye, rep-
           resent space constants of 12 and 13 μm for negative and
           positive displacements respectively. Each point is the
           mean of four responses. All stimuli delivered 1.32×10^2
           520 nm photons/ μm^2.

where Vmax is the voltage response evoked by diffuse illumination,
d is the spot diameter, and K_1 is a modified Bessel function of the
first order. For these experiments, a dim, small (10 μm) diameter
spot was centered on the impaled cell and the flash responses were
recorded as the diameter of the spot was increased. The change in
response size with spot diameter is plotted in Figure 3. The solid
curve graphs the above equation where   was adjusted to provide a
fit to the experimental data. Table 1 shows that there was excellent agreement between the   values obtained using a long narrow
strip of light and those obtained using a circular spot of light.

These results support the conclusion that the space constant
for electrical spread in the frog red rod network is about 12 μm
and thus much smaller than the length constants measured in rod networks from other animals. Since λ is a measure of the extent of

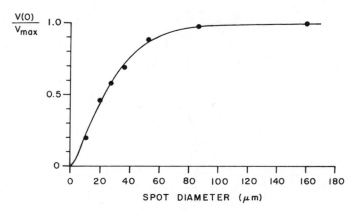

Fig. 3.   Change of response with spot size. The peak response
                amplitude, normalized to the maximum response produced
                by full-field illumination, is plotted against the di-
                ameter of the stimulating spot. Each point is the mean
                of at least two responses. The solid curve is equation
                (1) with λ=9.2 μm. All stimuli were 520 msec. flashes,
                of 16.3,520 nm photons/μm^2.

electrical coupling, and an effect of coupling is to decrease the
fluxuations in potential due to the random absorption of light quanta, one might expect frog rods to be noisier than turtle and toad
rods. This did not appear to be the case. In one rod, which was
thought to be noisier than most, the dark noise, defined as the volt
age variance in darkness minus the voltage variance in bright light
(Lamb & Simon, 1976), was 0.14 mV^2; a similar value has been reported for strongly coupled rods and cones in turtle. The random noise
in a coupled network depends on the ratio of λ and the mean cell
spacing, D (Lamb & Simon, 1976). In order to know if the frog rod
λ was compatible with their level of dark noise, D was estimated
by measuring the density $N = \dfrac{1}{D^2}$ of red rods. This was done using published photomicrographs of retinae where red and green rods
could be clearly distinguished (Plate 1, Denton & Wyllie, 1955;
Figure 2, Nilsson, 1964b; Plate 1, Baumann, 1977). The density of
red rod ranged from 3.97 x 10^{-2} μm^{-2} to 2.78 x 10^{-2}μm^{-2} with a mean
value of 3.46 x 10^{-2} μm^{-2} corresponding to D = 5.37 μm. The λ/D
ratio in 11 rods (Table 1) ranged from 1.8 to 2.6 with a mean of
2.2. This value of λ/D would reduce the dark noise by more than
50 fold relative to that expected to be present in an electrically
uncoupled cell (Lamb & Simon, 1976). The short λ of the frog rod

network is thus consistent with the observed level of dark noise.

DISCUSSION

The results of this brief paper indicate that the cells in the frog retina that can be studied most easily with intracellular electrodes are red rods. The general properties of these receptors are basically the same as those described for rods in other types of lower vertebrates (Schwartz, 1973; Cervetto et al., 1977; Detwiler, et al., 1980). They have a high sensitivity to light, such that a single photoisomerization gives about one millivolt potential change. The kinetics of the light response increases with light intensity and a bright large area flash of light produces a response with a prominent peak and plateau phase. In addition red rods in the frog retina are electrically coupled together and form electrical network that exhibit the properties of a high pass filter.

The most striking result in this study was that the mean space constant for electrical spread in the red rod network is much shorter than that measured in any other type of photoreceptor, yet the cells do not have an unusual amount of dark noise. This discrepancy is adequately explained on the basis of receptor density which gave a λ/D value of 2.2 and an expected 50 fold reduction in noise. It is interesting to note that the value of λ/D for frog red rods is very close to the mean values of 2.5 reported for both turtle and toad rods (Detwiler, et al., 1980; Gold, 1979). The similarity of these ratios in three different animals suggests that the space constant for a coupled receptor network might be scaled according to cell spacing in order to obtain an optimum level of noise reduction. If this is the case, one could use receptor density to estimate the mean λ for a coupled photoreceptor network. Examples of considerations of this type are shown in Table 2. These estimates assume a square receptor array and that the desired λ/D value for rods is 2.4 (the mean of turtle, toad and frog values) and 1.4 for cones (the mean value reported for red and green turtle cones by Detwiler & Hodgkin, 1979). There are no intracellular electrophysiological studies of the cells listed in Table 2 (see, however, Gold, 1979). Consequently, the tabulated length constants should, at best, be considered highly speculative. With this reservation in mind, note that the expected length constants for green rods and single cones are about 40% smaller in Rana pipiens than in Bufo marinus. In this regard, it is interesting that the measured length constants for red rods in these two animals also differs by 40%. If blue sensitive cones in the central region

Table 1: Comparison of space constants measured with a strip and circle of light

Animal	Cell#	STRIP			CIRCLE		$\bar{\lambda}$	λ/D
		$\lambda(-)$	$\lambda(+)$	λs	λc	$\lambda s/\lambda c$		
Rana pipiens	1	12.7	13.8	13.3	14.0	0.95	13.7	2.55
"	2	9.4	10.9	10.2	9.0	1.13	9.6	1.79
"	3	10.9	15.6	13.3	-	-	13.3	2.48
"	4	11.3	12.4	11.9	11.0	1.08	11.5	2.14
"	5	12.4	11.6	12.0	12.0	1.00	12.0	2.23
Rana Catesbiana	6	13.8	13.8	13.8	-	-	13.8	2.57
"	7	9.2	9.2	9.2	9.8	0.94	9.6	1.79
"	8	9.5	12.9	11.0	11.5	0.96	11.3	2.10
"	9	12.3	13.3	12.8	13.0	0.98	12.9	2.40
"	10	11.9	8.8	10.4	11.0	0.95	10.7	2.00
"	11	12.0	14.4	13.2	13.0	1.02	13.1	2.44
	Mean			11.9	11.6	1.00	12.0	2.23

All λ values are given in μm; $\lambda(-)$ and $\lambda(+)$ refer to space constants measured for positive and negative displacements respectively; λs is the mean of $\lambda(-)$ and $\lambda(+)$; λc is
determined from fitting eqn. 1 to data on variation of response with spot size; $\bar{\lambda}$ is the
mean of λs and λc; λ/D is $\bar{\lambda}$ divided by D, the mean cell spacing.

Table 2: Speculative space constants based on receptor density

Animal	Photoreceptor Type	N	λ(μm)	Reference
Rana pipiens	Green Rod	8.03×10^{-3}	27	Nilsson (1964b)
	Single cone	1.56×10^{-2}	11	
Bufo marinus	Green Rod	2.80×10^{-3}	45	Fain (1976)
	Single cone	4.70×10^{-3}	20	
Macaque Monkey	Blue Cone (Central)	32^{*}	45	DeMonasterio et al. (1981)
	Blue Cone (Peripheral)	65^{*}	91	
Human	Rod (Central)	1.60×10^{-1}	6	Osterberg (1935)
	Rod (Peripheral)	6.00×10^{-2}	10	

N is receptor density per μm^2; λ calculated by multiplying $\sqrt{1/N}$ by 2.4 for rods and 1.4 for cones; * gives mean blue cone separation in μm.

of the primate retina are coupled, they would be expected to have
a moderately long space constant. Such extensive coupling could
be mediated by interreceptor contacts (Dowling & Boycott, 1966)
and is not inconsistent with the visual resolution mediated by
blue-sensitive cones in man (Brindley, 1953). The shortest length
constants in Table 2 belong to human rods in the central retina.
The predicted value of 6   µm is half the value measured for red
rods in Rana pipiens, which fits with the fact that human rods are
about one half the diameter of frog rods.

REFERENCES

Bauman, Ch. (1977). Boll's phenomenon, Vision Research 17, 1325 –
    1327.
Baylor, D. A., and Fettipalce, R. (1975). Light path and photon
    capture in turtle photoreceptors, J. Physiol. 248: 433 – 464.
Baylor, D.A., Fuortes, M. G. F., and O'Bryan, P. M. (1971). Recep-
    tive fields of single cones in the retina of the turtle, J.
    Physiol., 214, 265 – 294.
Baylor, D.A., and Hodgkin, A. L. (1973). Detection and resolution
    of visual stimuli by turtle photoreceptors, J. Physiol., 234,
    163 – 198.
Brindley, G. S. (1953).   The effects on colour vision of adaptation
    to very bright lights, J. Physiol., 122: 332 – 350.
Cervetto, L., Pasino, E., and Torre, V. (1977). Electrical responses
    of rods in the retina of Bufo marinus, J. Physiol., 267, 17–51.
Copenhagen, D. R., and Owen, W. G. (1976).   Coupling between rod
    photoreceptors in a vertebrate retina, Nature, 260: 57 – 59.
Dartnall, H. J. A. (1972). Photosensitivity, in "Handbook of the
    sensory physiology" (Dartnall, H.J.A., ed.), pp. 122 – 145
    Springer-Verlag, New York.
DeMonasterio, F. M., Schein, S. J., and McCrane, E. P. (1981).
    Staining of blue-sensitive cones of the Macaque retina by a
    fluorescent dye, Science, 213, 1278 – 1271.
Denton, E. J., and Wyllie, J. H.(1955).   Study of the photosensi-
    tive pigments in the pink and green rods of the frog, J.
    Physiol., 127, 81 – 89.
Detwiler, P. B., and Hodgkin, A. L. (1979). Electrical coupling
    between cones in turtle retina, J. Physiol., 291, 75 – 100.
Detwiler, P. B., Hodgkin, A. L., and McNaughton, P. A. (1978).
    A surprising property of electrical spread in the network of
    rods in the turtle retina, Nature, 274, 562 – 565.

Detwiler, P.B., Hodgkin, A. L., and McNaughton, P. A. (1980). Temporal and spatial characteristics of the voltage response of rods in the retina of the snapping turtle, J. Physiol., 300, 213 - 250.

Dowling, J.E., and Boycott, B.B. (1966). Organization of the primate retina: electron microscopy, Proc. Roy. Soc. B., 166, 80 - 111.

Fain, G. L. (1975). Quantum sensitivity of rods in the toad retina, Science, 18, 838 - 841.

Fain, G. L. (1976). Sensitivity of toad rods: dependence on wave length and background illumination, J. Physiol., 261, 71 - 101.

Gold, G. H. (1979). Photoreceptor coupling in retina of the toad, Bufo marinus. II. Physiology, J. Neurophys., 42, 311-328.

Lamb, T. D. (1976). Spatial properties of horizontal cell responses in the turtle retina, J. Physiol., 263, 239 - 255.

Lamb, T. D., and Simon, E. J. (1976). The relation between intercellular coupling and electrical noise in turtle photoreceptors, J. Physiol., 263, 257 - 286.

Leeper, H. F., Norman, R. A., and Copenhagen, D. R. (1978). Evidence for passive electronic interations in red rods of toad retina, Nature, 275, 234 - 236.

Liebman, P. A., and Entine, G. (1968). Visual pigments of frog and tadpole (Rana pipiens), Vision Res., 8, 761 - 775.

Nilsson, S. E. G. (1964a). An electron microscopic classification of the retinal receptors of the leopard frog, J. Ultrastruct. Res., 10, 390 - 416.

Nilsson, S. E. G. (1964b). Interreception contacts in the retina of the frog (Rana Pipiens), J. Ultrastruct. Res., 11, 147 - 165.

Osterberg, G. (1935). Topography of the layer of rods and cones in the human retina, Acta Ophtal. Suppl., 6, 1 - 103.

Owen, W. G., and Torre, V. (1980). Ionic mechanism underlying the high-pass filtering of small signals by the rod network of the toad, Bufo marinus, J. Physiol., 308, 78 p.

Schwartz, E. A.(1973). Responses of single rods in the retina of the turtle, J. Physiol., 232, 503 - 514.

Schwartz, E. A.(1976). Electrical properties of the rod synctytium in the retina of the turtle, J. Physiol., 272, 217 - 246.

Toyoda, J., Hashimoto, H., Anno, H., and Tomita, T. (1970). The rod response in the frog as studied by intracellular recording, Vision Res., 10, 1093 - 1100.

RECOVERY FROM LIGHT-DESENSITIZATION IN TOAD RODS

L. Cervetto, V. Torre, E. Pasino, P. Marroni
and M. Capovilla

Istituto di Neurofisiologia del C.N.R., Pisa, Istituto
di Anatomia e Istologia Veterinaria, Pisa, Istituto di
Scienze Fisiche, Genova, Italy

INTRODUCTION

The visual system of vertebrates possesses a remarkable property whereby a fairly good discrimination of light changes occurs
over a wide range of ambient intensities (about 8 log units). Much
of this adaptability is attributed to the existance within the same
retina of two receptor types (rods and cones) with distinct functional properties and sensitivities (see Gouras, 1972).

Changes in the sensitivity and dynamic range of photoreceptors
when exposed to an adapting field have been extensively investigated
(Boynton & Whitten, 1970; Werblin, 1970; Normann & Werblin, 1974;
Kleinschmidt & Dowling, 1975; Fain, 1976; Normann & Perlman 1979).
Although there has been considerable discussion as to how these
changes take place, little is known about the mechanism of adaptation (Donner & Hemila, 1978; Bastian & Fain, 1979; Lamb, McNaughton
& Yau, 1981). The aim of the present paper is to analyse the effects
of prolonged illumination on flash sensitivity of toad rods. We
shall show that in rods both steady and repetitive light stimulation
initiate a sequence of changes in light sensitivity that develops
during exposure to the adapting field. Recently Capovilla, Cervetto, Pasino & Torre, (1981), showed that the sodium current, which
is initially suppressed by light, may be partially restored upon
prolonged illumination. This observation appears relevant to the
problem of light desensitization and adaptation in rods. The

existence of long-term, light dependent processes that control the sodium permeability of the rod membrane provides some clues to the nature of the phototransductive process.

Results similar to some of those presented here have also been obtained independently in turtle cones and frog rods by P.B. Detwiler (personal communication).

METHODS

Experiments were performed on the isolated retina of Bufo marinus.

The methods for preparation, perfusion, electrical recording and light stimulation are given in a previous paper (Capovilla et al. 1981). In the experiments to be described below, we used an infrared image converted (Find-R-scope, F J W Industries) for both dissection of the retina and control of the light spot and micro-electrode position, using a source of light with wavelengths longer than 700 nm. The intensity of the stimulating light is expressed in terms of estimated photoisomerizations per rod (Rh*), using an effective collecting area of 30 μm^2 (Fain, 1976; Cervetto et al. 1977).

NOMENCLATURE

Sensitivity. The flash sensitivity S_F is defined as the maximal hyperpolarization V_{max} produced by a single photoisomerization in an isolated rod. It is calculated by dividing the peak hyper-polarization of response in the linear range, during full field illumination, by the estimated number of photons absorbed by the rod. We define $_D S_F$ as the sensitivity in the dark adapted condition and $_L S_F$ as the sensitivity in the presence of a background light.

Desensitization. We define desensitization the decrease in S_F in the presence of a background of light, expressed as $1 - _L S_F / _D S_F$.

Recovery from desensitization. As shown below, the sensitivity falls to a lower value shortly after the initiation of a background of light. If the background illumination is maintained long enough the sentitivity may partially recover. This latter phenomenon will be named "recovery from desensitization" and it is meant to be different from the recovery of sensitivity after the offset of a backgroung of light.

RESULTS

Desensitization

Fig. 1 illustrates the influence of steady backgrounds of light of increasing intensity on rod voltage sensitivity. The records in C show linear range responses obtained from the same rod in darkness and in the presence of backgrounds of increasing intensity (3.4, 210 and 850 Rh^* sec^{-1}). In this experiment a background equivalent to 3.4 Rh^* sec^{-1} reduced the flash sensitivity of the rod from 1.6 mV/Rh^* (value in dark adapted conditions) to 1.25 mV/Rh^*. Backgrounds of 210 Rh^* sec^{-1} further reduced the flash sensitivity to 0.13 mV/Rh^*. When the background illumination was raised to 850 Rh^* sec^{-1} the flash sensitivity dropped to 0.030 mV/Rh^*. The desensitization $(1 - S_{L.F}/S_{D.F})$ is plotted as a function of the intensity of the conditioning background in A. It is seen that flash sensitivity was halved by backgrounds of light producing on average 6 Rh^* sec^{-1}, and was reduced at least one order of magnitude when the intensity of the background was raised to above 400 Rh* sec^{-1} (see also Bastian & Fain, 1979). The time to the peak of photoresponses is plotted as a function of the intensity of the background in B. It is seen that even very dim backgrounds (2.3 Rh^* sec^{-1}) are effective in decreasing the time to peak of voltage photoresponses. With bright backgrounds (above 10 Rh^* sec^{-1}) the time-to-peak of the photoresponses reaches a minimum value of about 300 msec.

The time course of the desensitization in rods is analysed in Fig. 2. Superimposed records in A are responses to a test flash producing on average 7.5 RH* delivered in darkness (dotted record) and at different time after the onset of a conditioning background whose intensity was estimated at about 6 Rh^* sec^{-1}. Results from five distinct experiments are illustrated in B. The desensitization is plotted as a function of the time between the onset of the background light and the test flash. Changes in the time to peak of the flash response in darkness and at different times during the background illumination are illustrated for the same five rods in C. It is seen that the process of desensitization is not directly related to the level of the membrane potential set by the background illumination. Desensitization starts with the onset of the background and continues to develop for about 1 sec after the maximum level of potential has been reached. The overall time taken by the process to reach a steady state is about 2 sec from the onset of the background.

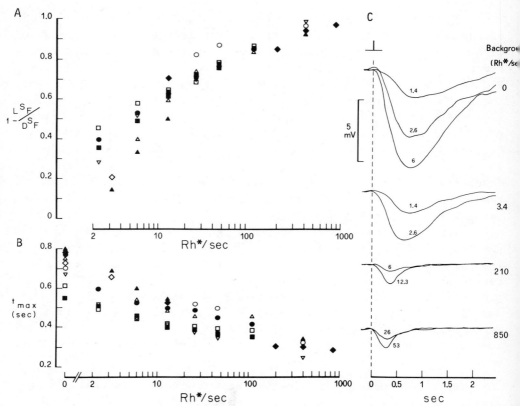

Fig. 1. Effects of steady backgrounds of different intensity (Rh* sec^{-1}) on the flash sensitivity of 9 rods. The desensiti-zation $1 - (_LS_F/_DS_F)$ is plotted againist the intensity of the background in A. The time to peak (t_{max}) is plotted as a function of background intensity in B. In C are the responses to flashes of different intensities obtained in darkness and in the presence of backgrounds of increasing intensitiy. The light intensities expressed in Rh* flash^{-1} are reported close to each record. The figures reported at the right hand side indicate the intensity of the back-ground illumination. Flash duration, 20 msec; wavelength, 510 nm.

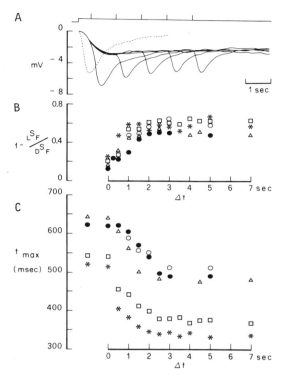

Fig. 2.   A: time course of desensitization produced by a 6 Rh* sec^{-1}
background. Dotted trace: flash response in dark adapted
conditions. Desensitization (B) and time to peak (C) as
function of the time Δt from the beginning of background
illumination (t=0) for 5 rods. Test flash: 7.5 Rh* at 510
nm. Flash duration: 20 msec.

Recovery from desensitization

    In studying the influence of backgrounds of increasing inten-
sity on the flash sensitivity another property emerged, namely
a partial recovery from desensitization. During exposure to backgrounds producing from 2.5 to 46 Rh* sec^{-1} the S_F decreased within
the first 1-3 sec to a value that remained unchanged for the subsequent several minutes. When the intensity was raised to 106 Rh*
sec^{-1} or more, however the flash response evoked 2 sec after the
onset of the background was always smaller than responses evoked
60 secs later in the same conditions of illumination. The average
value of the flash sensitivity determined in 11 rods was 1.2 mV/Rh*

in dark adapted conditions and decreased to 80 $\mu V/Rh^*$ 3.5 secs after
the onset of a background delivering 106 Rh^* sec^{-1}. However, 20
secs after the onset of the background the S_F had increased to 120
$\mu V/Rh^*$.

Fig. 3 illustrates the recovery from desensitization produced
by a background of light. In the uppermost record, responses to
flashes of 47.6 Rh^* are repeated every 2.65 sec, superimposed on a
steady background light of 838 Rh^* sec^{-1}. The same experiment is
repeated with brighter flashes in the lower three traces. Superimposed responses to different test flashes at a given time after
the onset of the background are shown at an enlarged time scale in
B. The value of the flash sensitivity was 3 $\mu V/Rh^*$ 1.8 sec after
the onset of the background, 11 $\mu V/Rh^*$ after 7.1 secs and 15 $\mu V/Rh^*$
after 25.6 sec. Recovery from desensitization is negligible when
the intensity of the adapting field corresponds to less than about
10^2 Rh^* sec^{-1}.

Qualitatively similar results were also obtained when the
intensity of the adapting field was raised to 1.3 x 10^4 Rh^* sec^{-1},
which is well beyond the intensity that produces a saturated
response.

Owen & Sillman, (1973) noted that during repetitive stimulation of the frog retina the aspartate isolated PIII component of
the electroretinogram (the late receptor potential) was first
suppressed and subsequently recovered.

Fig. 4 illustrates the results of an experiment in which a
rod was stimulated by trains of flashes of different intensities
delivered with different repetition rates. It is seen that flashes
subsequent to the first of each series evoked smaller responses or
no responses at all. The suppression was more marked when the
intensity of the flashes was increased and the interval between then
was decreased. Like the effects of dim backgrounds, the depressive
influence of repetitive flashes did not appreciably recover when
the estimated number of total Rh^*/sec was less than 100. The time
necessary for recovery and the extent of the recovery depended on
both intensity and repetition rate of flashes.

The time course of recovery of flash responsiveness is compared
for steady-state (A) and repetitive stimulation (B) in Fig. 5. The
record in A shows responses to a 464 Rh^* test flash delivered at
different times superimposed on a steady light equivalent to 378
Rh^* sec^{-1}. In B the same cell was stimulated with a flash equiva-

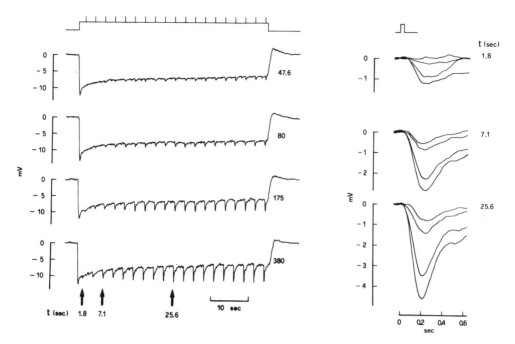

Fig. 3. Recovery from desensitization. Left column: responses to a test flash repeated every 2.65 sec superimposed on a steady background of light equivalent to 838 Rh^* sec^{-1}. The light intensities of flashes expressed in Rh^* are reported close to each record. Right column: responses to flashes equivalent to 47.6, 80, 175 and 380 Rh^* $flash^{-1}$ at different times (1.8, 7.1, and 25.6 sec) from the onset of the background light. Flash duration, 20 msec; wavelength, 510 nm.

lent to 464 Rh^* repeated every 1.228 sec for an equivalent flux of 377.8 Rh^* sec^{-1}. It is seen that several flashes subsequent to the first failed to evoke any response at all. During the subsequent minute, however, the flash response recovered to a substantial fraction of the control amplitude. The time course of recovery is similar in both A and B. In both cases the recovery is associated with acceleration of the falling phase of light responses. As with constant background recovery during repetitive stimulation is negligible with dim flashes (less than about 50 Rh^* $flash^{-1}$).

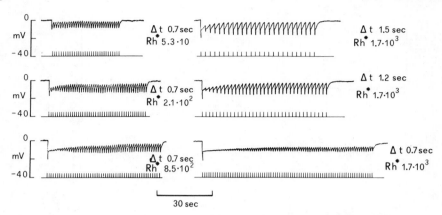

Fig. 4.   Rod responses to repetitive flashes.   Left column responses
          to sequences of flashes of increasing intensity (53, 210,
          850 Rh*/flash) repeated every 0.7 sec.   Right column,
          sequences of flashes equivalent to 1700 Rh*/flash delivered
          at progressively shorter intervals (Δt = 1.5; 1.2 and 0.7
          sec).

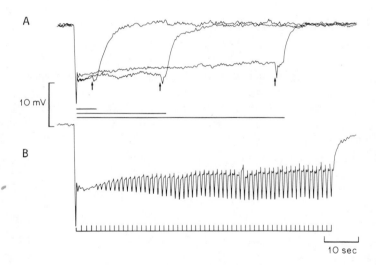

Fig. 5.   A: responses of a rod to a test flash delivered at differ-
          ent times during exposure to backgrounds (Rh* sec^{-1} = 378)
          of increasing duration.   The test flash (Rh* = 464) was
          delivered at times indicated by the arrows. Bars at the
          bottom signal the duration of the background illumination.
          B: responses to a flash (Rh* = 4.64 x 10^2) delivered every
          1.228 sec.

Kinetic changes during the process of recovery

Changes in the time scale of photoresponses induced by background illuminations are well known (Fuortes & Hodgkin, 1964; Baylor
& Hodgkin, 1974; Bastian & Fain, 1979). In analyzing the process
of recovery from desensitization we observed that in addition to an
increase of sensitivity changes in kinetics occur as well. Responses
of a rod to repetitive flashes (Δt = 1.2 sec) are illustrated on a
faster time scale in Fig. 6. It is seen that, after an initial
suppression, the amplitude of the flash response increased in parallel with both membrane depolarization and acceleration of its falling
phase (observe the slope of broken lines traced for a better visual
appreciation of the rate of response decay).

Fig. 7 illustrates results from an analysis of the falling phase
of responses to step of light of progressively longer duration.
Records superimposed in A are responses to five steps of light of
different duration (3, 5, 13, 25, 50 sec). It is seen that the
decay of the membrane potential from the plateau to the resting
level is drastically accelerated as the time of exposure to light
is prolonged (see also Coles & Yamane, 1975). The falling phase
of the response to the longest step appears rather complex with subsequent oscillations. A feature similar to this was also described

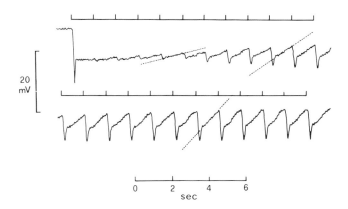

Fig. 6.   Responses to repetitive flashes (6.7 x 10^2 Rh[*], Δ t = 1.2
           sec). The same record continues from the upper to the
           lower trace. Broken lines are drawn for a better apprecia-
           tion of the rate of decay of membrane potential to the
           resting level. Raised bars at the top of each record monitor
           the flashes. Flash duration, 20 msec; wavelength, 510 nm.

in responses of turtle cones (Baylor & Hodgkin, 1974). The time
constant (τ) of the decay of membrane potential from the plateau
is described in detail in Fig. 7 B. After a light step of 3 to 5
sec the membrane potential relaxed towards the resting state with
a τ, of 0.6 sec that decreased to 0.28 sec with a step of 13 sec and
to 0.15 sec with a step of 50 sec. A progressive acceleration of
the falling phase was also observed in voltage responses to repetitive flashes during periods of recovery, so that during the interval
between two successive flashes the membrane potential could approach
more closely the dark resting potential (see Fig. 6).

Dark adaptation and recovery from saturation

To obtain information on the mechanism that control the amplitude of voltage response, light desensitization and recovery, it may
be helpfull to analyse the effects of interrupting the repetitive
stimulation with periods of darkness. Such an experiment is illustrated in Fig. 8. A sequence of flashes equivalent to 3.5 x 10^3
Rh*/flash was delivered with a Δ t = 1 sec. The beginning of the
experiment is indicated by the record at the top. During the first
sequence of repetitive flashes the rod responses were initially suppressed, but within 40 sec response recovered up to 30% of the
initial amplitude. During this interval the rod depolarized by 5

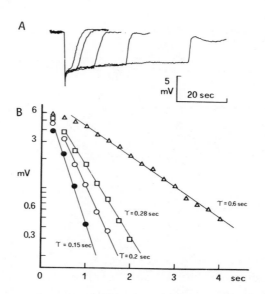

Fig. 7.   A: responses to steady illumination (106 Rh* sec^{-1}) of
          different duration (3, 5, 13, 25, 50 sec). B: relaxation
          toward the dark resting level of responses to steps of
          light of increasing duration. Wavelength, 510 nm.

mV and the response amplitude to the first two flashes of the second
sequence increased. Intervals of darkness of 5-20 secs were sufficient to elicit a substantial recovery of response amplitude. Observe, however, that in these conditions the first flash of the
sequence did not suppress the rod responsiveness to the subsequent
flashes. After a dark interval of 40 sec the peak amplitude had
nearly recovered, but responses to the subsequent flashes were
detected much earlier. This suggests that after 40 sec the rod was
still under the effects of the previous stimulations even though
the response amplitude was near to the control value. The original
conditions were restored only after intervals of darkness of 8
minutes or more. In general the process of recovery that occurs
during prolonged exposure to light, once established, seems to be
more persistent than the depressive influences of light on the
amplitude of the photoresponse. One may conceive that the processes
controlling the peak of the light responses and light desentitiza-
tion are distinct from the process that controls recovery during
prolonged illumination.

Possible mechanisms underlying the process of recovery

So far the process of recovery described above has been implic-
itly attributed to events occurring within the outer segment of
rods, i.e. closely related with the phototransductive process.
This assumption, however, needs some support. Fain (1976) reported

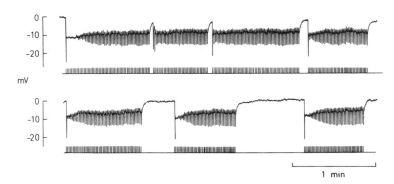

Fig. 8. Responses to a flash (Rh* = 3.5x10^3) repeated with Δ t =
1 sec. The repetitive stimulation is interrupted by in-
tervals of complete darkness of increasing duration. The
record at the upper row continues in the lower row. Intervals of darkness are monitored by notches in the bars
at the bottom of the record. Flash duration, 20 msec;
wavelength, 510 nm.

that 36% of photoreceptors in the toad retina are cones; there are
also indications that under certain conditions cones contribute to
rod responses (Schwartz, 1975; Copenhagen & Owen, 1976; Fain, 1976).
The extent of such contribution is reportedly small, but one cannot
exclude that with bright illumination cone responses might appreciably influence the rod membrane potential. The experiment illustrated in Fig. 9 was performed to test this possibility. A background
of 495 nm light of 840 Rh[*] sec^{-1} was used as a conditioning stimulus.
The rod responsiveness was then tested with flashes of monochromatic
light of 470, 510 and 630 nm at different times from the onset of
the conditioning illumination (records at the top). The results
show that the recovery is largely independent of wavelength, thus
ruling out that an input from cones significantly contributes to
this process. A similar conclusion can also be drawn from experiments with repetitive stimulation (records at the bottom).

When rods were exposed to solutions containing small amounts
of cesium (2mM) or high concentrations of potassium (10 mM), conditions both known to decrease the contribution of potential and time
dependent conductances to the rod photoresponse (see Fain, Quandt,
Bastian & Gerschenfeld, 1978; Capovilla, Cervetto & Torre, 1980).
The voltage responses closely resembled current responses (Yau,

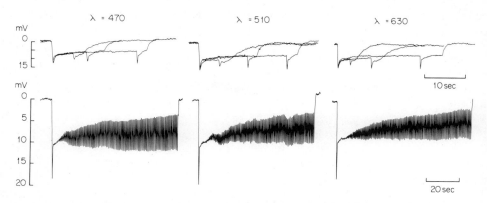

Fig. 9.   Effect of wavelength on recovery from desensitization.
          Upper row: responses to test flashes of different wave-
          length obtained at different times after the onset of a
          background of 495 nm light whose intensity is 840 Rh[*]
          sec^{-1}. Flash intensity: 1.3 x 10^{11} photon x cm^{-2} x sec^{-1}
          (λ = 510 nm); 3.19 x 10^{11} photons x cm^{-2} x sec^{-1} (λ = 470
          nm); 5.2 x 10^{13} photons x cm^{-2} x sec^{-1} (λ = 630 nm). Lower
          row: responses to repetitive flashes whose intensity is the
          same as above, Δ t = 1 sec. Flash duration, 20 msec.

Baylor & Lamb, 1979). As illustrated in Fig. 10, under similar
conditions the recovery is not hindered, thus suggesting that the
contribution of voltage and time dependent conductances is not
essential to this process and that the observed phenomena likely
reflect events occurring at the outer segment. In the presence of
cesium the extent of recovery was usually more pronounced that in
normal Ringer, suggesting perhaps that under normal circumstances
the presence of voltage and time dependent conductances may limit
the process of recovery.

DISCUSSION

Results in this paper show that the flash sensitivity (S_F) of
rods, which initially is depressed by backgrounds of light, partially
recovers during prolonged illumination. Qualitatively similar effects can be induced by sequences of repetitive flashes. Conceivably
these phenomena play a significant role in the ability of the visual
system to operate efficiently over an extended range of ambient
intesities. They also show that in the presence of bright saturating fields the ability of rods to signal light changes is only tem-
porarily suppressed and, if the exposure to a bright field is sufficiently long, rods again become capable of efficiently signalling

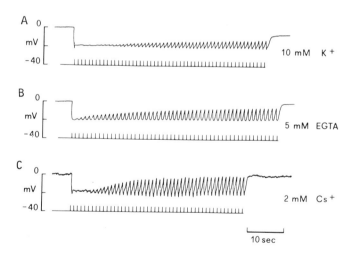

Fig. 10. Effects of repetitive stimulation with flashes (Rh[*] 1.7x
10^3 photon, Δt = 1 sec) in three different rods in different conditions; A: In the presence of 10 mM K[+]; B: 5 mM
EGTA; C: 2 mM Cs. Flash duration, 20 msec, wavelength,
510 nm.

light events, thus expanding their dynamic range.

As with the process that occurs during dark adaptation, the changes in sensitivity associated with prolonged exposures to steady light are likely to reflect multiple mechanisms involving factors different than pigment depletion and pigment regeneration (see Grabowsky & Pak 1975).

As mentioned earlier the process of recovery from desensitization becomes apparent in rods when the total flux of the adapting field is of the order of 10^2 Rh* sec^{-1}, which is below the saturation level of voltage responses. The amount of pigment that a similar flux can bleach in 10 sec is a negligible fraction (about 1 x 10^{-6}) of the total number of molecules contained in the outer segment (see Liebman & Entine 1968). Therefore, neither rhodopsin depletion nor the effects of self-screening (see Goldstein & Williams, 1966) can easily explain desensitization and recovery. Recovery was observed with background intensities of up to about 10^4 Rh* sec^{-1} which is well above the saturation level. Under such conditions more than one Rh* is likely to occur in a single disk and the processes involved may become exceedingly complex.

Developing the general idea (Baylor & Fuortes, 1970; Cone 1973) that an internal transmitter is activated by light and blocks ionic channels, Baylor, Hodgkin & Lamb 1974, a, b) proposed for turtle cones a kinetic model in which the concentration of a blocking substance (Z_1) is controlled by two sequences of transformations. The first sequence consists of five linear reactions that lead to a buildup of Z_1, while another sequence leads to inactivation of Z_1 throught several step. Assuming that the reaction which transforms Z_1 into the inactive product is autocatalytic, they were able to explain light desensitiztion in cones. The scheme, however, is explicitly intended to account for events associated with illumination lasting no more than a few seconds. Interestingly enough, the validity of a scheme similar to the one proposed for cones might be easily extended to also cover the phenomena associated with prolonged illumination described above. This can be done simply by introducing a factor capable of modifying the equilibrium constants of the reactions in the inactivation of Z_1 (see Cervetto et al., 1977). The experiment illustrated in Fig. 6 indicates that following repetitive stimulation, periods of darkness that allow a substantially recovery of the flash sensitivity leave the time course of the recovery profoundly modified with respect to the original dark-adapted condition. The dissociation between these two properties could be explained by supposing that a substance R_1 ia activated upon prolonged illumination. In this scheme R_1 is different from Z_1 in that it does not reduce the light sensitive conductance and is removed very slowly. Moreover the observation that the decay of membrane potential at the offset of a constant background is accelerated as the time of illumination is prolonged (see Fig. 7) leads to the suggestion that the hypothetical substance R_1 exerts its effect by accelerating some of the reactions of the removal of Z_1, possibly k_{12} and/or k_{23}.

In essence these modifications are equivalent to saying that the process must be coupled to some exergonic process. The assumption that phenomena of adaptation may require energy seems a reasonable proposition. However we should emphasize that while it may be convenient to attempt an explanation of the observed phenomena within the framework of an already formulated scheme, other models based on different hypotheses may explain the results reported above as well.

In a previous paper, Capovilla, et al. (1981) showed that a light-sensitive sodium current is partially restored upon prolonged illumination. In analyzing the effects of changing the concentration of external Na^+ on the process of recovery we have observed a close correlation between the extent of recovery and the membrane hyperpolarization induced by low external Na^+. This supports the idea that during prolonged illumination a process develops in rods that leads to an increased light sensitive conductance.
length and background illumination. J. Physiol., 261, 71–101

REFERENCES

Bastian, B.L. & Fain, G.L. (1979). Light adaptation in toad rods: requirement for an internal messenger which is not calcium. J. Physiol. 297, 493–520.

Baylor, D.A. & Fuortes, M.G.F. (1970). Electrical responses of single cones in the retina of the turtle. J. Physiol. 207, 77–92.

Baylor, D.A. & Hodgkin, A.L. (1974). Changes in time scale and sensitivity in turtle photoreceptors. J. Physiol. 242, 729–758.

Baylor, D.A., Hodgkin, A.L. & Lamb, T.D. (1974 a). The electrical response of turtle cones to flashes and steps of light. J. Physiol. 242, 685–727.

Baylor, D.A., Hodgkin, A.L. & Lamb, T.D. (1974 b). Reconstruction of electrical responses of turtle cones to flashes and steps of light. J. Physiol. 242, 759–791.

Boynton, R.M. & Whitten, D.N. (1970). Visual adaptation in monkey cones: recordings of late receptor potentials. Science, 170, 1423-1426.

Capovilla, M., Cervetto, L. & Torre, V. (1980). Effects of changing external potassium and chloride concentrations on photoresponses of Bufo bufo rods. J. Physiol. 307, 529-551.

Capovilla, M., Cervetto, L., Pasino, E. & Torre, V. (1981). The sodium current underlying the responses to light of toad rods. J. Physiol. 317, 223-242.

Cervetto, L., Pasino, E. & Torre, V. (1977). Electrical responses of rods in the retina of Bufo marinus. J. Physiol. 267, 17-51.

Coles, J.A. & Yamane, S. (1975). Effects of adapting lights on the time course of the receptor potential of the anuran retinal rod. J. Physiol. 247, 189-207.

Cone, R.A. (1973). The internal transmitter model for visual excitation: some quantitative implications, in: "Biochemistry and Physiology of Visual Pigments", ed. Langer, H. pp. 275-282. Berlin: Springer.

Copenhagen, D.R. & Owen, W.G. (1976). Functional characteristics of lateral interaction between rods in the retina of the snapping turtle. J. Physiol. 259, 251-282.

Donner, K.O. & Hemila, S. (1978). Excitation and adaptation in the vertebrate rod photoreceptors. Medical Biology, 56, 52-63.

Fain, G.L. (1976). Sensitivity of toad rods: dependence on wavelength and background illumination. J. Physiol., 261, 71-101.

Fain, G.L., Quandt, F.N., Bastian, B.L. & Gerschenfeld, H.M. (1978). Contribution of a cesium sensitive conductance increase in the rod photoresponse. Nature, Lond. 272, 467-469.

Fuortes, M.G.F. & Hodgkin, A.L. (1964). Changes in time scale and sensitivity in the ommatidia of Limulus. J. Physiol. 172, 239-263.

Goldstein, E.B. & Williams, T.P. (1966). Calculated effects of "screening pigments". Vision Res. 6, 39-50.

Gouras, P. (1972). Light and dark adaptation, in: Handbook of Sensory physiology, vol. VII/2, Physiology of Photoreceptor Organs ed. Fuortes, M.G.F., pp. 610-634. Berlin: Springer.

Grabowski, S.R. & Pak, W.L. (1975). Intracellular recordings of rod responses during dark-adaptation. J. Physiol. 247, 363-391.

Kleinschmidt, J. & Dowling, J.E. (1975). Intracellular recordings from gecko photoreceptors during light and dark adaptation. J. Physiol. 66, 617-648.

Lamb, T.D., McNaughton, P.A. & Yau, K.-W. (1981). Spatial spread of activation and background desensitization in rod outer segments. J. Physiol. 319, 463-496.

Liebman, P.A. & Entine, G. (1968). Visual pigments of frog and tadpole (Rana pipiens). Vision Res. 8, 761-775.

Normann, R.A. & Perlman, I. (1979). The effects of background illumination on the photoresponses of red and green cones. J. Physiol. 286, 491-507.

Normann, R.A. & Werblin, F.S. (1974). Control of retinal sensitivity: I. Light and dark adaptation of vertebrate rods and cones. J. gen. Physiol. 63, 37-61.

Owen, W.G. & Sillman, A.J. (1973). The suppression-recovery effect in the frog photoreceptor. Vision Res. 13, 2591-2594.

Schwartz, E.A. (1975). Cone excite rods in the retina of the turtle. J. Physiol. 246, 639-651.

Werblin, F.S. (1971). Adaptation in a vertebrate retina: intracellular recording in Necturus. J. Neurophysiol. 34, 228-241.

IONIC CURRENTS ACTIVATED BY VOLTAGE AND BY INTRACELLULAR CALCIUM:

A VOLTAGE CLAMP STUDY IN SOLITARY VERTEBRATE PHOTORECEPTORS

C.R. Bader and D. Bertrand

Départment de Physiologie Centre Médical Universitaire

21 rue Lombard 1211 Géneve 4 Switzerland

SUMMARY

Solitary rod inner segments were obtained by enzymatic dissociation of the tiger salamander retina. Individual membrane currents
were studied with the single-electrode voltage-clamp technique and
with pharmacological agents. Extracellular TEA blocked an outward
current which was activated, by depolarization and carried predominantly by potassium ions. Extracellular caesium blocked an inward
current which was activated by hyperpolarization and carried by
sodium and potassium ions. An inward calcium current was activated
by depolarization and could be blocked by extracellular cobalt.
Intracellular accumulation of calcium activates two other currents:
one is blocked by intracellular caesium and is most likely a calcium-
activated potassium current; the current remaining in the presence
of intracellular caesium is carried, in part, by chloride. The
five currents described can all be activated in the range of voltages
in which rod photoreceptors normally operate.

INTRODUCTION

The receptor potential of vertebrate photoreceptors in response
to light stimulation results from the interaction of several mechanisms. The initial signal, produced by a decrease in sodium permeability in the outer segment (Hagins, Penn & Yoshikami, 1970), is a
hyperpolarization of the cell (Tomita, 1965; Baylor & Fuortes,
1970). This change in membrane potential affects voltage-dependent

mechanisms, which in turn contribute to the shaping of the receptor
potential (Schwartz, 1976; Fain, Quandt, Bastian & Gerschenfeld,
1978; Detwiler, Hodgkin & MacNaughton, 1978; Baylor, Lamb & Yau,
1979; Bader, MacLeish & Schwartz, 1979). The study of these voltage-
dependent mechanisms is best achieved by using the voltage clamp
technique. In the intact retina, however, photoreceptors form a
syncytium (Baylor & Hodgkin, 1973; Fain, Gold & Dowling, 1975;
Schwartz, 1976; Copenhagen & Owen, 1976); currents can spread from
cell to cell, making it difficult to investigate with precision the
electrical properties of individual photoreceptors. This difficulty
can be overcome by studying solitary photoreceptors obtained by
enzymatic dissociation of the retina (Bader, MacLeish & Schwartz,
1978). Solitary photoreceptors survive several days in culture,
respond to light as do rods in the intact retina and can be voltage
clamped with one or two microelectrodes. Using this technique, the
current affected directly by the transduction process was investigated in previous experiments in the tiger salamander retina (Bader
et al., 1979).

     In collaboration with Dr. Eric Schwartz (Department of Phar-
machological Sciences, University of Chicago), we have begun in
Geneva an investigation of the voltage-dependent properties of tiger
salamander rod photoreceptors. Preliminary experiments indicated
that these properties were mainly if not exclusively localized in
the cell soma and synaptic pedicle. Therefore we used solitary
photoreceptors that lacked an outer segment (Fig. 1). For conven-
ience, we shall call these rods without outer "solitary inner segments". Solitary inner segments were found frequently among dissociated cells, their outer segment having been removed in the dissociation procedure. The ellipsoid body was always clearly visible
adjacent to the nucleus, and a synaptic process, which extended
from the soma, was present in most cells.

     The methods for obtaining these solitary inner segments and
for having them adhere to a substrate is described in detail elsewhere, together with the superfusion and recording procedures
(Bader, Bertrand & Schwartz, submitted). Briefly, retinae from
light adapted tiger salamanders (Ambistoma tigrinum) were lifted
from the underlying pigment epithelium and incubated in a solution
containing the proteolytic enzyme papain for 14 to 16 hr at 16°C.
After rinsing, retinae were triturated with a fine-bore Pasteur
pipette. Aliquots of the cell suspension were transfered on to a
coverslip coated with collagen with attached concavalin-A. Photo-

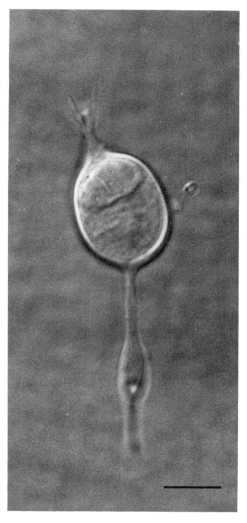

Fig. 1.   Solitary inner segment of a salamander rod photoreceptor.
          The outer segment was removed during the dissociation
          procedure. The bar represents 10 μm. The photographs
          were taken with a Zeiss 63x Planapochromat objective and
          Nomarski interference contrast optics.

receptors adhered to this substrate in 10 to 20 min and could subsequently be superfused without the agarose gel that was previosly
used to immobilize dissociated photoreceptors (Bader et al., 1978).

RESULTS

Previous studies on rods in the intact retina showed that
tetraethylammonium (TEA), caesium and cobalt affect their membrane
properties (Fain, Quandt & Gerschenfeld, 1977; Fain et al., 1978).
We attempted to investigate individual currents by superfusing
solitary inner segments with combinations of these 3 drugs. In this
manner three voltage-dependent currents could be identified. The
procedure was as follows (Fig. 2A): an inner segment was impaled
with a microelectrode and superfused with a solution containing
caesium (5 mM) and cobalt (3 mM). The rationale was that the two
drugs would selectively block certain channels and leave untouched
channels that might subsequently be blocked by adding TEA to the
medium. In this way the current that can be suppressed by TEA is
studied in isolation by using a simple subtraction procedure. For
example, in Fig. 2A the cell was first held in voltage clamp at
−72 mV and then stepped to +2 mV for 300 msec. After the initial
current required to discharge the membrane capacitance, the current
increased and reached a steady state (Fig. 2A, trace labelled Co,
Cs). The same cell was then superfused with a medium containing
TEA (30 mM) in addition to the two drugs and the depolarizing step
was repeated (Fig. 2A, trace labelled TEA+Co,Cs). In the presence
of the 3 drugs, the current necessary to mainain the cell at +2 mV
remained nearly constant. The difference between the two traces
in Fig. 2A reveals that depolarization of a solitary inner segment
activates an outward current that can be blocked by TEA. We shall
present evidence below that this current is carried mainly by potassium ions and therefore we call it I_K.

Fig. 2B illustrates an experiment in which a second current
was isolated using a different combination of the drugs. An inner
segment was superfused with TEA (to block I_K) and cobalt. The
potential of the cell was held in volgate clamp at −32 mV and stepped
for 300 msec to −100 mV. After the capacitative surge, the current
slowly increased (Fig. 2B, trace labelled TEA, Co). The same cell
was then superfused with the mixture of the 3 drugs, and it can be
seen that during the step to −100 mV the current remained essentially constant (Fig. 2B, trace labelled Cs+TEA, Co). The difference
between the two traces in Fig. 2B is an inward current that is

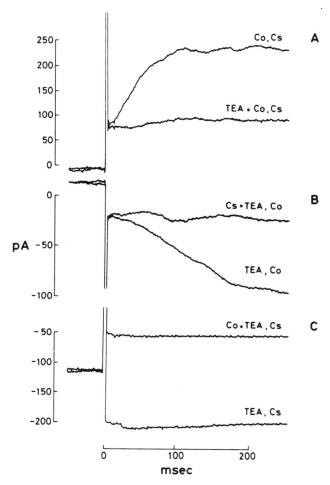

Fig. 2. Three voltage dependent-currents in rods. <u>A</u> Voltage and
        time-dependent current blocked by TEA. An inner-segment
        was impaled with a 4M K acetate filled pipette, superfused
        in a medium containing caesium (5 mM) and cobalt (3 mM) and
        maintained in voltage clamp at -72 mV. The current evoked
        when the voltage was stepped from -72 mV to +2 mV was re-
        corded (trace labelled Cs, Co). The solution was then
        changed to one containing TEA (30 mM) in addition to caesium
        and cobalt and the procedure repeated (trace labelled
        TEA+Cs, Co). <u>B</u> Voltage and time-dependent current sup-
        pressed by caesium. An inner segment was impaled with an
        electrode containing 4M K acetate and maintained in voltage
        clamp at -30 mV. The medium contained cobalt (3 mM) and
                                                        (continued)

activated by a hyperpolarization of the rod membrane. This inward current, called I_h, can be blocked by caesium ions and, as we shall see, is carried mainly by sodium and potassium ions.

Using a combination of TEA and caesium to block I_K and I_h, it was possible to study the current blocked by cobalt, presumably a calcium current. This current, however, turned out to be more complicated to investigate since an increase in intracellular calcium caused the activation of two other currents. In order to study the calcium current in isolation, inner segments had to be penetrated with electrodes containing the calcium chelator EGTA, which was injected intracellularly to prevent changes in the intracellular calcium concentration. Under these conditions, when a cell was superfused with a medium containing TEA and caesium, a depolarizing step of voltage from -70 to -5 mV for 300 msec caused the change in current illustrated in Fig. 2C (trace labelled TEA, Cs). Note that the activation of this current is too fast to be resolved by our single electrode voltage clamp apparatus. Superfusion of the same cell with a medium containing cobalt in addition to the two other drugs drastically changed the current required to hold the cell at -5 mV (Fig. 2C, trace labelled Co+TEA, Cs). Thus cobalt blocks an inward current that is activated by a depolarization of the cell membrane. As we shall see this current is carried mainly by calcium ions and we call it I_{Ca}. We did not find a significant inactivation of this current, at least for depolarizations up to -25 mV. This is also true when no EGTA is present intracellularly.

Figure 2 (continued)

TEA (30 mM). The potential was stepped from -30 mV for 300 msec (trace labelled TEA, Co). The same procedure was then repeated in a medium containing caesium (5 mM) in addition to TEA and cobalt (trace labelled Cs+TEA, Co). C Voltage-dependent current blocked by cobalt. An inner segment was impaled with an electrode containing EGTA, and superfused with a medium containing TEA (30 mM) and caesium (5 mM). Sufficient EGTA was injected to block the time-dependent outward current normally activated by calcium entry (see Fig. 6). The current required when the membrane potential was stepped from -70 mV to -5 mV was recorded (trace labelled TEA, Cs). The medium was then changed to one that containing cobalt (3 mM) in addition to TEA and caesium and the voltage step was repeated (trace labelled Co+TEA, Cs).

Identity of the ions carrying I_h, I_K and I_{Ca}

(a) I_h. We found that I_h was variable from cell to cell, suggesting that some intracellular or extracellular factor might modulate the amplitude of the current. A change in extracellular potassium from 2.5 to 5.0 mM increased I_h more than 3-fold in half the cells studied. The ability of potassium to increase and of caesium to block I_h suggested that this current was carried by

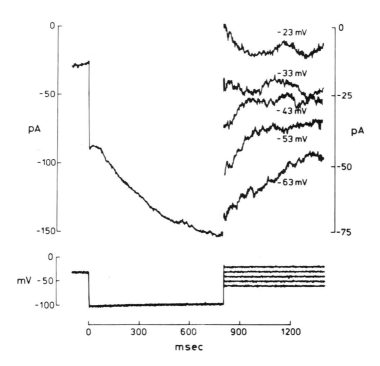

Fig. 3.   Reversal potential of I_h. An inner segment was superfused with a medium containing TEA (30 mM) and cobalt (5 mM) and maintained in voltage clamp at −30 mV. The potential was stepped from −30 mV to −102 mV for 800 msec to activate I_h and then stepped to several final holding levels. Tail currents recorded at 5 holding voltages are plotted. Tail currents reverse polarity at −33 mV. Note the difference in current scales for the hyperpolarizing step and for the tails.

monovalent cations. Studies of the reversal potential of I_h corroborated this notion. The procedure used to determine the reversal potential of I_h is illustrated in Fig. 3. A cell was superfused with a medium containing TEA and cobalt to block I_K and I_{Ca}. I_h was activated by applying a hyperpolarizing step in voltage clamp from -30 to -100 mV for 800 msec. Releasing the potential to less hyperpolarized values (the voltages are indicated in the Fig.) gave rise to tail currents. In this cell, tail currents reversed polarity near -33 mV. In 6 cells the reversal potential of I_h was -32 +/- 3 mV. Increasing extracellular potassium shifted the reversal potential in the depolarizing direction but the shift was less than expected if potassium was the only ion permeating the channel.

The possibility that sodium was carrying part of I_h (see Fain et al., 1978; Werblin, 1979) was confirmed by experimental in which choline replaced sodium in the medium. In a medium without sodium the reversal potential for I_h, measured in 7 cells, was -76 +/- 6 mV, a value close to the potassium equilibrium potential (see below). Thus, it appears that potassium and sodium are the major charge carriers for I_h.

(b) I_K. The reversal potential for I_K was determined in a similar manner as for I_h. Cells were superfused with a medium containing caesium and cobalt to block I_h and I_{Ca}, and I_K was activated by applying a large depolarizing voltage step. The voltage was then released to less depolarized levels and tail currents were recorded. In 7 cells the reversal potential for I_K was -72 +/- 4 mV. Changing the extracellular potassium 2- and 4-fold shifted the reversal potential to values close to the predicted values for a perfectly selective potassium electrode. We conclude therefore that I_K is carried essentially by potassium ions.

(c) I_{Ca}. There are several indications that this inward current is carried mainly by calcium ions. This current was not decreased by the total removal of sodium ions, which excludes sodium as a major charge carried. The apparent null potential was at a depolarized voltage (+45 mV), implying that the contribution of potassium can only be minimal (but see Reuter & Scholz, 1977 a). Substituting barium for calcium tended to increase the duration of action potentials recorded in current clamp conditions; this suggests that a divalent ion was the major charge carrier. Finally the suppression of I_{Ca} observed in the presence of cobalt or of D-600, points to calcium as the principal ion carrying I_{Ca}.

Steady state current-voltage relations for I_K, I_h and I_{Ca}

A detailed analysis of the kinetic properties of I_K, I_h and I_{Ca} has not yet been achieved. We shall therefore limit our description of the steady state properties of these currents. To determine steady state currents, each current was activated as seen above (see Fig. 2) and the amplitude measured at the steady state for different voltage steps. Data collected from many cells are plotted in Figs. 4 and 5. These current-voltage relations indicate that I_K, I_h and I_{Ca} can all be activated in the range of voltages in which photoreceptors normally operate.

In Fig. 4 the steady state current voltage relation for I_K is illustrated (9 cells). It is seen that I_K is activated by depolarizations above −60 mV. In Fig. 5A the current-voltage relation is shown for I_h; I_h is activated when rods are hyperpolarized below −30 mV. In Fig. 5B, two current-voltage curves are plotted. The filled circles represent the current recorded in the presence of TEA and caesium (I_K and I_h blocked); the open circles represent the current measured in the presence of all three drugs. The difference between the two sets of data in Fig. 5B is I_{Ca}. In this cell I_{Ca} starts to be activated when the cell is depolarized above −45 mV, goes through a maximum near −10 mV and decreases to zero near +50 mV. We have never observed a reversal of the calcium in any of the cells studied so far. The current-voltage relation for I_{Ca} has a negative slope between −45 mV and −10 mV. This negative slope is responsible for the generation of action potentials observed in the intact retina, in the presence of TEA (Fain et al., 1977).

Note that in the presence of all three drugs (Fig. 5B, open circles) the current-voltage relation is essentially linear between −75 and −20 mV, i.e. over this range of voltages the cell behaves as a passive resistor of high value (2.1 GΩ here).

Currents activated by a rise in intracellular calcium concentration

When rod inner segments were superfused with a medium containing TEA and caesium (to block I_K and I_h) but no EGTA was injected intracellularly to buffer the calcium concentration, the effect of a depolarization of the membrane was complex. Fig. 6 illustrates the effect of a step depolarization from −70 mV to +10 mV, in voltage clamp. Trace a was obtained in the presence of calcium and trace b was recorded when cobalt replaced calcium in the medium.

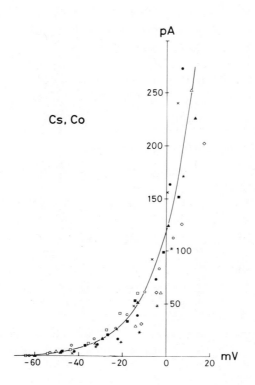

Fig. 4.   Steady state current-voltage relation for I_K in 9 cells
superfused with a medium containing caesium (5 mM) and
cobalt (3 mM). The membrane potential was held in voltage
clamp at -70 mV and stepped to several depolarized voltages
(Fig. 2$\underline{A}$ is an example at +2 mV). The difference at the
steady state between the currents recorded, at a given
voltage, in absence or presence of TEA is plotted on the
ordinate as a function of the voltage during the step.
The continuous line was computed from the empirical
equation :

$$I_K = g\ (V-E_K)\ (1+\exp((V-V'_K/V''_K))^{-3}$$

with E_K = -72 mV, g = 15 nS, V'_K = -33 mV and V''_K = 2.5 mV.

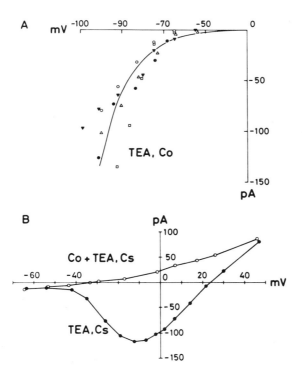

Fig. 5A. Steady-state current-voltage relation for I_h in 5 cells
          superfused with a medium containing TEA (30 mM) and cobalt
          (3 mM). The membrane potential was held at -30 mV and
          stepped for 800 msec to several hyperpolarized voltages
          (Fig. 2B is an example at -100 mV). The difference at
          the steady state between currents recorded, at a given
          voltage, in the absence or presence of caesium are plotted
          on the ordinate as a function of the voltage during the
          step. The continuous line was fitted by eye. B Voltage
          dependence of the steady-state calcium current. An inner
          segment was impaled with an EGTA-containing pipette and
          currents were measured as illustrated in Fig. 2C. The
          filled circles are from records obtained in a medium
          containing calcium (trace labelled TEA, Cs). The open
          circles were obtained when the same cell was superfused
          with a medium in which calcium was replaced with cobalt
          (trace labelled Co+TEA,Cs). The difference between the
          current recorded in the absence or presence of cobalt
          represents I_{Ca}.

From the comparison of the two records it can be seen that immediately after the beginning of the depolarization there is an inward
current, I_{Ca}. This inward current decays and becomes outward during
the course of the depolarizing pulse. For voltage changes giving
rise to an initial calcium current, the steady state current was
always outward, i.e. outward current always dominates the inward
calcium current at the steady state. When the potential is returned

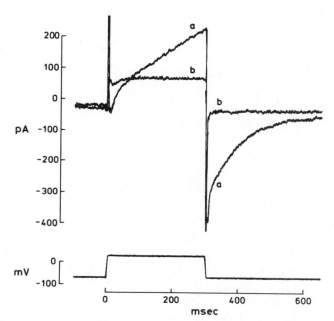

Fig. 6.   Effect of a depolarizing step in voltage clamp in the pres-
          ence of TEA and caesium.   A cell was superfused with a
          medium containing TEA and caesium to block I_K and I_h.   The
          membrane voltage was stepped from −70 mV to +10 mV for 300
          msec and the current was recorded (trace a).   The medium
          was then changed to one containing cobalt in addition to
          TEA and caesium and the same depolarizing step was repeated
          (trace b is the current).   When no EGTA is present intra-
          cellularly, the effect of a depolarizing step of voltage
          is complex (compare with Fig. 2C).

to -70 mV there is a long lasting tail of inward current. Such tails were never observed in the presence of intracellular EGTA. The outward current developing during the depolarizing voltage step is, in part, due to a calcium-activated potassium current ($I_{K(Ca)}$, see below). Such a current has been observed in a variety of neurons (Meech, 1978). The large inward tail current, however, is not likely to be carried by potassium ions for the following reasons; first, this tail current is large at -70 mV, i.e. at a potential close to the potassium equilibrium potential, where any current carried by potassium should be small; second, when caesium was injected intracellularly to block $I_{k(Ca)}$ (Tillotson & Horn, 1978), the outward current during a depolarizing step was considerably reduced but the inward current tail was not affected at potentials near -70 mV. This result is consistent with the hypothesis that another current than $I_{K(Ca)}$ is activated by a rise in intracellular calcium concentration. The magnitude and duration of the inward current tail were increased with an increase in duration of the depolarizing step. This is what one would expect from a mechanism activated by an accumulation of intracellular calcium during a depolarizing step.

We looked for a reversal potential for this calcium activated current. I_K and I_h were blocked with TEA and extracellular caesium and $I_{K(Ca)}$ was suppressed by intracellular injection of caesium. Thus only I_{Ca} and the unknown calcium-activated current were left. Fig. 7 shows the currents recorded during 2 depolarizing steps in voltage clamp. When the voltage was stepped from -70 mV to -27 mV, following the rapid initial inward current (identified as I_{Ca}), there was a slow increase in inward current. Such a current was seen only when caesium was present intracellularly. For a voltage step to -2 mV, the initial inward current (I_{Ca}) was followed by a slowly developing outward current. In this cell the polarity of the slowly developing current reversed polarity at -13 mV. In 15 cells the mean reversal potential was $-17.4 +/- 3.6$ mV, which is quite different from the calcium null potential ($+45$ mV). This calcium-activated current was seen in the absence of sodium and, from what we have just said, can not be carried by either potassium or calcium. When, however, the extracellular chloride concentration was reduced the reversal potential was affected. Reducing the chloride concentration 3-fold shifted the mean reversal potential to $-0.4 +/- 1.5$ mV. This shift from -17 to near 0 mV is less than the predicted shift for a chloride selective electrode. It is therefore likely that another ion besides chloride flows through the same channel, but we shall nonetheless call this calcium activated current I_{Cl}.

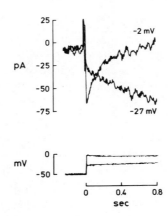

Fig. 7.   Reversal potential of the calcium-activated anion current
          I_{Cl}. An inner segment was superfused with a medium con-
          taining TEA (30 mM) and caesium (5 mM) and impaled with a
          pipette containing caesium. Injection of caesium blocked
          the calcium-activated potassium current $I_{K(Ca)}$. The mem-
          brane potential was stepped in voltage clamp from −50 mV
          to more depolarized levels. At potentials more hyperpo-
          larized than −20 mV a slowly increasing <u>inward</u> current was
          observed (the current for a step to −27 mV is shown); at
          potentials more depolarized than −10 mV a slowly increasing
          <u>outward</u> current was observed (the current for a step to
          −2 mV is shown). In this cell the slowly increasing cur-
          rent reversed polarity at −13 mV.

DISCUSSION

        Treating solitary rod inner segments with TEA, caesium and
cobalt in various combinations revealed the existence of three
different components of the total ionic current that flows through
their membrane. Each of the three pharmacological agents seemed
to block reversibly one current for which a reversal potential could
be found. A current activated by an increase in intracellular
calcium could be blocked by injecting EGTA into a cell and separated
into two distinct components by injecting caesium. The general
properties of the currents identified in rod inner segments are
summarized in Table 1.

        In our experiments, currents were studied one by one by com-
paring in the same cell records obtained before and after pharmacological block. Attwell & Wilson (1980) have also attempted to
analyze the ionic currents of solitary salamander rods. Their

TABLE   1

Summary of the general properties of identified currents
in rod inner segments.

$ This value represents the null potential. We did not
observe a reversal potential for I_{Ca}.

* This reversal potential was not measured but is assumed
to be equal to E_K.

** These agents blocked the corresponding currents when
injected <u>intracellularly</u>.

Current	Activation	Block	Reversal potential	Permeant ion
I_h	Hyperpolarization from −30 mV	Cs	−32 mV	Na^+, K^+
I_K	Depolarization from −70 mV	TEA	−72 mV	K^+
I_{Ca}	Depolarization from −50 mV	Co	+45 mV $^\$$	Ca^{2+}
$I_{K(Ca)}$	Increase in intracellular Ca concentration	Co Cs** EGTA**	−72 mV*	K^+
I_{Cl}	Increase in intracellular Ca concentration	Co EGTA**	−17 mV	$Cl^-, ?$

methods, however, was to compare records obtained from different
cells. This may, in part at least, be the reason why their conclusions are quite different from ours.

I_K in rods. The existence of a TEA-sensitive current in the
rod photoreceptor membrane was first reported in the intact retina
(Fain et al., 1977) and later on observed in solitary photoreceptors
from the tiger salamander retina (Werblin, 1979; Attwell & Wilson,
1980). We show here that this TEA-sensitive current is carried by
potassium ions. We find a reversal potential for I_K at -72 mV in
2.5 mM extracellular potassium. This value could be shifted by
changes in extracellular potassium concentration as predicted if
the channels for I_K were selectively permeable to potassium ions.
In a few experiments E_K was determined in intact, light-adapted,
solitary photoreceptors; the values found were in the same range
as those measured in inner-segments. Given the selectivity of the
channel for potassium we can estimate the intracellular potassium
concentration from E_K, using the Nernst equation; with a $[K]_O$ of
2.5 mM and an E_K of -72 mV the intracellular potassium concentration
would be 44.5 mM.

I_K is activated in the physiological range of voltages in
which photoreceptors operate. We found that I_K is already activated
at -60 mV and that at -30 mV a steady current of about 15 pA is
present. I_K does not seem to inactivate at potentials below zero
mV. It is therefore conceivable that a steady potassium current
flows through the membrane in the dark. This current will decrease
during the hyperpolarization produced by light and thus may contribute to the shaping of the voltage response to light.

The fact that I_K is activated at the resting voltage in the
dark may be important for the photoreceptor function. In darkness,
sodium ions enter the cell at the outer segment (Hagins et al.,
1970; Sillman, Ito & Tomita, 1969; Brown & Pinto, 1974). This
"generator current" can be 55 pA in tiger salamander rods (Bader
et al., 1979). Thus, sodium ions must be extruded, presumably
through a sodium-potassium pump. If we assume a Na/K exchange ratio
of 3/2 for the pump (Thomas, 1972), this implies that in darkness
36 pA of potassium ions (brought in by the pump) must leave the
cell. Inner-segments exposed to TEA, caesium and cobalt have high
resistances and exhibit only a small residual leakage current. If
this lekage current was carried entirely by potassium, the potassium
current in the presence of the drugs would not exceed 20 pA at -30

mV. We know, however, that in the presence of the three drugs the resting potential was between -20 and -30 mV (see Fig. 5$\underline{B}$, open circles), indicating that only a fraction of the leakage current can be carried by potassium. Thus, additional pathways have to be found to extrude the required amount of potassium. I_K may provide one pathway and the calcium-activated potassium current ($I_{K(Ca)}$) may provide another one. Our results suggest that these two currents could together produce the required potassium flux.

I_h in rods. The presence in the rod membrane of a current having some of the properties of I_h was inferred from pharmacological studies in the intact toad retina (Fain et al., 1978). Extracellular caesium was found to modify the shape of the response to a flash. Specifically, the decline from a peak to a plateau voltage observed after a bright flash was suppressed. In solitary photoreceptors, voltage clamp experiments demonstrated the existence of an inward current activated during a hyperpolarizing step of voltage (Bader et al., 1979; Attwell & Wilson, 1980). In the present study we have shown that the inward current activated by hyperpolarization can be blocked by adding caesium to the superfusion medium.

Previous experiments in the intact retina has suggested that the current activated by a hyperpolarization had its reversal potential near the resting membrane potential in darkness (Schwartz, 1976) and was carried in part by sodium ions (Fain et al., 1978). Measurements of the reversal potential of I_h tend to confirm these suggestions. The value of E_h was -32 mV under control conditions and could be shifted by changing the concentration of either sodium or potassium ions in the extracellular medium. In fact, when sodium was totally substituted with choline E_h became equal to the potassium equilibrium potential. Sodium and potassium appear thus to be the principal charge carriers for I_h. If we assume an intracellular potassium concentration in solitary inner segments of approximately 45 mM (see above), the intracellular sodium concentration may have to be as high as 50 mM, in order to satisfy the osmotic equilibrium. This would set the sodium equilibrium potential near $+5$ mV. The algebraic sum of the putative E_{Na} and of E_K (-72 mV) is -33.5 mV, a value close to E_h. This would suggest that sodium and potassium contribute nearly equally to I_h.

One feature of I_h that distinguishes it from other currents in rods is its variability in amplitude from cell to cell in the physiological range. The concentration of extracellular potassium can modulate I_h. This effect of potassium on I_h is similar to that observed in starfish eggs (Hagiwara, Miyazaki & Rosenthal, 1976). This increase in I_h is not only the result of a shift of the reversal potential E_h (increase in driving force), but is essentially due to an increase in conductance, as suggested by preliminary analysis of the relation between steady state conductance and voltage. The caesium-sensitive current of rods is thus similar to the inward-rectifying current observed in starfish eggs (Hagiwara et al., 1976). In both, a time-dependent increase in inward current follows hyperpolarization and is blocked by caesium. Moreover, a change in external potassium concentration affects both the driving force and the conductance. The two currents differ, however, in several respects. The current of starfish eggs is carried by potassium only and its activation kinetics follow a simple exponential time-course. The I_h current of rods is carried by potassium and sodium and its activation follows a sigmoid time-course. These currents are therefore similar but not identical. Similar currents have also been studied in tunicate eggs (Miyazaki, Takahashi, Tsuda & Yoshii, 1974) and vertebrate muscle (Horowicz, Gage & Eisenberg, 1968).

The kinetic properties of I_h suggest that this current is primarily responsible for the decline from the transient to the plateau observed during the response to a bright flash. One might speculate that the role of I_h is to drive the potential to less hyperpolarized levels so that the release of synaptic transmitter, presumably reduced during a light-induced hyperpolarization, can again be enhanced.

$\underline{I_{Ca}\ \text{and calcium-dependent currents in rods}}$. The presence in the rod membrane of a calcium current and of a calcium-activated potassium current was inferred from pharmacological studies on the intact toad retina (Fain et al., 1977, 1978; Fain, Gerschenfeld & Quandt, 1980; Fain & Quandt, 1980). The existence of a chloride translocating mechanism is suggested by recent work in rods (Capovilla, Cervetto & Torre, 1980) and in cones (Lasanky, 1981). The finding of a chloride current activated by a rise in internal calcium concentration was, however, unexpected.

It is generally accepted that vertebrate photoreceptors release their synaptic transmitter continuously in darkness (Trifonov, 1968; Cervetto & Piccolino, 1974; Kaneko & Shimazaki, 1976) by a calcium-dependent mechanism (Cervetto & Piccolino, 1974; Kaneko

& Shimazaki, 1976; Schwartz, 1976). The calcium current described
here may subserve this function. The membrane potential for photoreceptors in darkness (-30 to -45 mV) spans the foot of the current-
voltage curve of I_{Ca}. In addition, there seems to be little inactivation of the calcium current, so that a steady I_{Ca} may be present
in darkness. A hyperpolarization occurring during exposure to light
would thus be expected to decrease the calcium current and thereby
to reduce the release of synaptic transmitter.

For I_{Ca} to be able to play a role in the synaptic transmission
of rods, it is essential that I_{Ca} does not inactivate at resting
potential in darkness. The absence of inactivation of the calcium
current is not easy to prove because of the existence of currents
activated by an increase in intracellular calcium. In the presence
of EGTA, however, which suppresses these calcium-activated currents,
we could show that the calcium current remained activated at a
constant level for at least 30 sec and at a voltage of -30 mV (this
voltage is close to the resting voltage of rods in darkness). This
experiment would tend to exclude a voltage-dependent inactivation
of I_{Ca} (we cannot exclude that a partial inactivation did occur at
a rate faster than be resolved by our voltage clamp apparatus).

EGTA, however, might interfere with another type of inactivation described in certain invertebrate cells (Hagiwara & Nakajima,
1966; Kostyuk & Krishtal, 1977; Tillotson, 1979; Brehm, Eckert &
Tillotson, 1980), namely a calcium-mediated inactivation of I_{Ca} via
a rise in intracellular calcium concentration. The following
argument speaks against this possibility. When caesium was injected intracellularly, and only I_{Ca} and I_{Cl} were present, we could
measure a reversal potential for I_{Cl}, i.e. the current record during
a depolarizing step near -17 mV (see above) was flat; since at this
voltage only I_{Ca} should flow, this would indicate that I_{Ca} is not
affected by intracellular accumulation of calcium.

In darkness, five current may be activated: the generator
current (carried mainly by sodium), I_K, I_{Ca}, $I_{K(Ca)}$ and I_{Cl}. The
dark resting potential is determined by the balance between these
currents, in addition to the leakage current and the possible contribution of a sodium pump, that is likely to be electrogenic
(Thomas, 1972). The sodium current, I_{Ca} and possibly I_{Cl} tend to
depolarize the cell while I_K and $I_{K(Ca)}$ act in the opposite way
(in darkness, I_h can be considered as nearly inactivated). Since
calcium is involved directly or indirectly in at least three currents, the modulation of the calcium current by extracellular

factors or synaptic inputs can be expected to affect the membrane
potential of rods in darkness. Modulation of a calcium current by
a neurotransmitter has been described in other systems (Reuter and
Scholz, 1977 b; Dunlap and Fischbach, 1978). Effects of neurotransmitters, however, are not necessarily restricted to voltage-dependent
calcium channel (Pellmar, 1981). There is evidence that vertebrate
photoreceptors receive synaptic inputs from second order neurones
(Baylor, Fourtes & O'Bryan, 1971; Fuortes, Schwartz & Simon, 1973;
O'Bryan, 1973; Piccolino & Gerschenfeld, 1977). Conceivably, these
synaptic inputs may activate (or inactivate) channels in the photoreceptor membrane. These inputs may play a role at the synapse in
shaping the signal that is transmitted to second order neurones.

ACKNOWLEDGMENTS

     This work was supported by grants from the Swiss National
Science Foundation (3.301.0.78 and 3.625.0.80). The work was done
in collaboration with Dr. E.A. Schwartz from the Department of
Pharmacological and Physiological Sciences (University of Chicago).
During his 6 month stay in Geneva, Dr. Schwartz was supported by a
grant from the Roche Research Foundation.

REFERENCES

Attwell, D., & Wilson, M. (1980). Behavior of the rod network in
     the tiger salamander retina mediated by membrane properties
     of individual rod, J. Physiol., 309, 287-315.
Bader, C.R., MacLeish, P.R. & Schwartz, E.A. (1978). Responses to
     light of solitary rod photoreceptors isolated from the tiger
     salamander retina, Proc. natn. Acad. Sci. U.S.A., 75, 3507-
     3511.
Bader, C.R., MacLeish, P.R. & Schwartz, E.A. (1979). A voltage-
     clamp study of the light response in solitary rods of the
     tiger salamander, J. Physiol., 296, 1-26.
Baylor, D.A. & Fuortes, M.G.F. (1970). Electrical responses of
     single cones in the retina of the turtle, J. Physiol., 207,
     77-92.
Baylor, D.A., Fuortes, M.G.F. & O'Bryan, P.M. (1971). Receptive
     fields of cones in the retina of the turtle, J. Physiol.,
     214, 265-294.
Baylor, D.A. & Hodgkin, A.L. (1973). Detection and resolution of
     visual stimuli by turtle photoreceptors, J. Physiol., 234,
     163-198.

Baylor, D.A., Lamb, T.D. & Yau, K.-W. (1979). The membrane current of single rod outer segments, J. Physiol., 288, 589-611.

Brehm, P., Eckert, R. & Tillotson, D. (1980). Calcium-mediated inactivation of calcium current in Paramecium, J. Physiol., 306, 193-203.

Brown, J.E. & Pinto, L.H. (1974). Ionic mechanism for the photo-receptor potential of the retina of Bufo marinus, J. Physiol., 236, 575-591.

Capovilla, M., Cervetto, L. & Torre, V. (1980). Effects of changing external potassium and chloride concentrations on the photo-responses of Bufo bufo rods, J. Physiol., 307, 529-551.

Cervetto, L. & Piccolino, M. (1974). Synaptic transmission between photoreceptors and horizontal cells in the turtle retina, Science, 183, 417-418.

Copenhagen, D.R. & Owen, W.G. (1976). Functional characteristics of lateral interactions between rods in the retina of the snapping turtle, J. Physiol., 259, 251-282.

Detwiler, P.B., Hodgkin, A.L. & MacNaughton, P.A. (1978). A surpris-ing property of the electrical spread in the network of rods in the turtle retina, Nature, (Lond.), 274, 562-565.

Dunlap, K. & Fischbach, G.D. (1978). Neurotransmitters decrease the calcium component of sensory neurone action potentials, Nature (Lond.), 276, 837-839.

Fain, G.L., Gold, G.H. & Dowling, J.E. (1975). Receptor coupling in the toad retina, Cold Spring Harb. Symp. quant. Biol., 40, 547-561.

Fain, G.L., Quandt, F.N. & Gershenfeld, H.M. (1977). Calcium-dependent regenerative responses in rods, Nature, Lond., 269, 707-710.

Fain, G.L., Quandt, F.N., Bastian, B.L. & Gerschenfeld, H.M. (1978). Contribution of a caesium-sensitive conductance increase to rod response, Nature, Lond., 272, 467-469.

Fain, G.L., Gerschenfeld, H.M. & Quandt, F.N. (1980). Calcium spikes in rods, J. Physiol., 303, 495-513.

Fain, G.L. & Quandt, F.N. (1980). The effects of tetraethylammo-nium and cobalt ions on responses to extrinsic current in toad rods, J. Physiol., 303, 515-533.

Fuortes, M.G.F., Schwartz, E.A. & Simon, E.J. (1973). Colour-dependence of cone responses in the turtle retina, J. Physiol., 234, 199-216.

Hagins, W.A., Penn, R.D. & Yoshikami, S. (1970). Dark current and photocurrent in rat retinal rods, Biophys. J., 10, 380-412.

Hagiwara, S., Miyazaki, S. & Rosenthal, N.P. (1976). Potassium
    current and the effect of caesium on this current during a-
    nomalous rectification of the egg cell membrane of a starfish,
    J. Gen. Physiol., 67, 621-638.
Hagiwara, S. & Nakajima, S. (1966). Effects of the intracellular
    Ca ion concentration upon the excitability of the muscle fiber
    membrane of a barnacle, J. Gen. Physiol., 49, 807-818.
Horowicz, P., Gage, P.W. & Eisenberg, R.S. (1968). The role of the
    electrochemical gradient in determining potassium fluxes in
    frog striated muscle, J. Gen. Physiol., 51, 193S-203S.
Kaneko, A. & Shimazaki, H. (1976). Synaptic transmission from
    photoreceptors to bipolar and horizontal cells in the carp
    retina, Cold Spring Harb. Quant. Biol., 40, 537-546.
Kostyuk, P.G. & Krishtal, O.A. (1977). Effects of calcium and
    calcium-chelating agents on the inward and outward current
    in the membrane of molluscan neurones, J. Physiol., 270,
    569-580.
Lasansky, A. (1981). Synaptic action mediating cone responses to
    annular illumination in the retina of the larval tiger sala-
    mander, J. Physiol., 310, 205-214.
Meech, R.W. (1978). Calcium-dependent potassium activation in
    nervous tissues, Ann. Rev. Biophys. Bioeng., 7, 1-18.
Miyazaki, S., Takahashi, K., Tsuda, K. & Yoshii, M. (1974). Analysis
    of non-linearity observed in the current-voltage relation of
    the tunicate embryo, J. Physiol., 238, 55-77.
O'Bryan, P.M. (1973). Properties of the depolarizing synaptic
    potential evoked by peripheral illumination in cones of the
    turtle retina, J. Physiol., 235, 207-223.
Pellmar, T.C. (1981). Transmitter control of voltage-dependent
    currents, Life Sci., 28, 2199-2205.
Piccolino, M. & Gerschenfeld, H.M. (1977). Lateral interactions in
    the outer plexiform layer of turtle retinas after atropine
    block of horizontal cells, Nature, Lond., 268, 259-261.
Reuter, H. & Scholz, H. (1977 a). A study of the ion selectivity
    and the kinetic properties of the calcium-dependent slow
    inward current in mammalian cardiac muscle, J. Physiol., 262,
    17-47.
Reuter, H. & Scholz, H. (1977 b). The regulation of the calcium
    conductance of cardiac muscle by adrenaline, J. Physiol.,
    264, 49-62.
Schwartz, E.A. (1976). Electrical properties of the rod syncytium
    in the retina of the turtle, J. Physiol., 257, 379-406.

Sillman, A.J., Ito, H. & Tomita, T. (1969). Studies on the mass receptor potential of the isolated frog retina. II. On the basis of the ionic mechanism, Vision Res., 9, 1443-1451.

Thomas, R.C. (1972). Electrogenic sodium pump in nerve and muscle cells, Physiol. Rev., 52, 563-594.

Tillotson, D. & Horn, R. (1978). Inactivation without facilitation of calcium conductance in caesium-loaded neurones of Aplysia, Nature, Lond., 273, 312-314.

Tillotson, D. (1979). Inactivation of Ca conductance dependent on entry of Ca ions in moluscan neurones, Proc. natn. Acad. Sci. U.S.A., 76, 1497-1500.

Tomita, T. (1965). Electrophysiological study of the mechanisms subserving color coding in the fish retina, Cold Spring Harb. Symp. quant. Biol., 30, 559-566;

Trifonov, Y.A. (1968). Study of synaptic transmission between photoreceptor and horizonatal cell by electrical stimulation of the retina, Biofizica, 13, 809-817.

Werblin, F.S. (1979). Time- and voltage-dependent ionic components of the rod response, J. Physiol., 294, 613-626.

REGENERATIVE PHOTORESPONSES IN TOAD RODS

W.G. Owen[1] and V. Torre[2]

Physiological Laboratory
Downing Street
Cambridge CB2 3EG U.K.

INTRODUCTION

In a recent paper Fain & Quandt (1980) showed that addition of
TEA and/or Sr^{++} to the perfusate at a concentration of 10-20 mM
induced regenerative electrical activity in rods of the toad retina.
They interpreted the intracellularly recorded sustained oscillations
and spikes in terms of a regenerative Ca^{++} current associated with
channels in the plasma membrane of the rod photoreceptors. Experiments in which mechanically isolated rods (Werblin 1979, Attwell &
Wilson 1980) and enzymatically dissociated rods (Bader, McLeish,
Schwartz 1978, 1979) were voltage clamped, failed to reveal a region
with negative slope in the current-voltage relation, though Attwell
& Wilson (1980) have observed, in rods exposed to TEA, a region
with almost zero slope.

Only recently have recordings from the isolated <u>inner</u> segments
of the tiger salamander shown the existence of a regenerative Ca^{++}
current, (see Bader, Bertrand, this volume).

In this paper we analyse the effect of external TEA^{+} (tetraethyl
ammonium ions) on the electrical activity of rods in the isolated
perfused retina of the toad. We will present evidence from intra-

1. Department of Biophysics and Medical Physics University of
    California, Berkeley, California 94720, U.S.A.

2. Istituto di Scienze Fisiche, Viale Benedetto XV 6, Genova, Italy.

cellular recordings in intact rods that, in the presence of 15 mM
TEA, the current-voltage relation has a region of negative conductance between -37 mV and -30 mV.

METHODS

    Experiments were performed on the retina of the toad Bufo
marinus, a retina that can be easily separated from the retinal
pigmented epithelium and superfused with media of known ionic concentrations. After dark-adapting overnight, retinae were isolated
under infrared illumination and mounted receptor side up in a perfusion chamber. Rods were superfused with a Ringer solution containing: 132 mM Na^+, 2.6 mM K^+, 120.6 mM Cl^-, 22 mM HCO_3^-, 2 mM Ca ,
2 mM Mg^{++}, 5 mM glucose, buffered with a mixture of 5% CO_2 and 95%
O_2 to pH 7.6. Rods were stimulated from above with a circular spot
(1 mm diameter) of monochromatic light (498 nm) of duration 50 msec,
though in some experiments a narrow slit of light (11 μm x 1 mm) of
the same duration was used.

    Responses were recorded intracellularly with the aid of fine
glass microelectrodes filled with 4M potassium acetate. In some
experiments, double barelled electrodes were used to record intracellular voltage while injecting steps of extrinsic current. Voltage
responses were digitized at a sampling rate of 50 Hz. Subsequently
the data (X_1...... X_i......) were smoothed by a digital filter, in
which each output point y_i was equal to

$$\frac{1}{2\ N+1} \sum_{-N\ i}^{+N} X_i$$

    The value of N was between 0 and 4.

RESULTS

    Fig. 1 illustrates the effect on the electrical activity of a
rod of adding 10 mM TEA to the perfusate. The dark membrane potential depolarized by about 7 mV and the amplitude of the voltage
response to a brief bright flash of light (equivalent to 6200 Rh^*)
increased in amplitude. The membrane potential at the peak of the
response was slightly less negative than in control Ringer, while
the plateau to which the membrane potential relaxes following the
peak was virtually unchanged. The rising phase and the time course
of the relaxation from the peak to the pateau did not change in the
presence of external TEA (see Fig. 1b). In Fig. 1a it is shown that

after 60 seconds of treatment with TEA, the repolarizing phase of
the response to a bright flash of light exhibited sustained oscillations and the appearence of full spikes of about 30 mV. This electrical instability of the membrane potential is shown in greater
derail in Fig. 1c. The period of the oscillations was approximately
600 msec. In che great majority of impaled cells this oscillatory
behavior gradually declined and eventually stopped altogether. In
a few cases the remaining light responses were markedly distorted.

It has been suggested that addition of 15 mM TEA to the external
medium completely abolishes the outward rectification present in the
rod membrane (Werblin 1979, Fain & Quandt 1980). Attwell & Wilson
(1980), however, observed a reduction but not an abolition of the
outward rectification. In a first series of experiments we obtained
contradictory results, because in the presence of 15 (or more) mM
TEA we observed a decrease in the input impedance and a decrease
in the flash sensitivity of the rod to dim light flashes. When 5
mM TEA was used, however, we observed an increase both in the input
resitance and in flash sensitivity. We therefore performed a series
of experiments to establish the stoichiometry of TEA effects.

Stoichiometry of the action of TEA

We investigated the effect of TEA on the electrical properties
of rod photoreceptors by perfusing the retina with Ringer solutions
containing different concentrations of TEA.

Fig. 2 shows the effect of 20, 10 and 5 mM TEA on the dark
membrane potential and on the voltage response to a brief flash of
light equivalent to 7.5 Rh^*. In general, larger doses of TEA induced
larger membrane depolarizations in darkness. This is clearly seen
in the collected data presented in Table 1. The effect on the light
response was more complex. With 5 mM (Fig. 2d) and with 10 mM
(Fig. 2c) TEA the amplitude of the light response increased by about
30%. Higher concentrations of TEA, however, produced no further
increase in response amplitude as is illustrated in Fig. 2b. Indeed,
in many cases we observed a clear decrease, both in the amplitude
of the response and in the flash sensitivity of the rod (as in the
cell of Fig. 3 and Fig. 4).

In Table 2 we show the change in amplitude and time to peak of
the response to a brief flash of light equivalent to 7.5 Rh^* for
various TEA concentrations. It is clear that TEA prolongs the time
to peak of the light response and has a complex action on the rod
sensitivity.

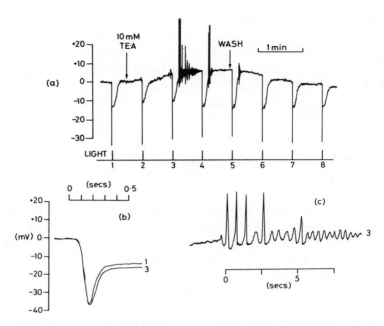

Fig. 1.   Effect of 10 mM TEA on the electrical activity of a rod.
(a)   Chart recording of the experiment; lower trace is the
light monitor.   (b)   Responses labelled 1 and 3 in (a)
shown in greater detail.   (c)   The repolarizing phase of
response labelled 3 in (a) shown in greater detail.   Dark
membrane potential −40 mV, monochromatic light of 498 nm.
Flash intensity equivalent to 6200 Rh[*]; flash duration
50 msecond.

Input resistance changes in TEA

It is useful to distinguish three components in the instantaneous (slope) membrane conductance $g_m(V)$. $g_m(V)$ has a voltage-and
time-independent component, g_m, that takes account of the fixed
part of the membrane conductance.   The second component, $g_m(V)$, is
the steady-state voltage-dependent conductance and represents the
sum of conductances of gated channels open at the membrane potential
V.   The third component is associated with the existence of regenerative current is X, E_x is its Nernst equilibrium potential and g_x
(V) is its steady state conductance, we have the additional term:

$$(V - E_x) \left. \frac{\partial g_x}{\partial V} \right|_V \tag{1}$$

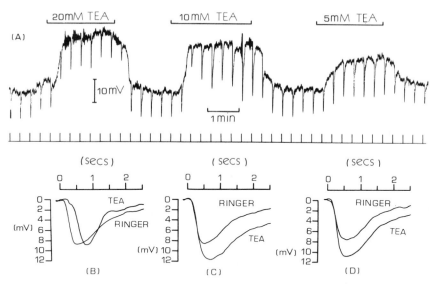

Fig. 2. Stoichiometry of the effect of external TEA. (a) Chart recording of the experiment. Upper bars indicate time of solution changes. Bottom trace is light artifact. (b) record labelled Ringer is the average of 5 responses recorded in control solution; record labelled TEA is the average of 5 responses recorded in the presence of 20 mM TEA. (c) Record labelled Ringer is the average response of 4 records recorded before changing the test solution; record labelled TEA is the average of 6 responses recorded in the presence of 10 mM TEA. (d) Record labelled Ringer is the average of 4 responses recorded before changing the test solution; record labelled TEA is the average of 5 responses recorded in the presence of 5 mM TEA. Dark membrane potential in Control Ringer -42 mV; monochromatic light 498 nm. Flash intensity equivalent to 7.5 Rh[*]. Flash duration 50 msec. Responses smoothed with a digital filter (see Methods) with N=3.

where $g_x(V)$ is gated by a single variable of H.H. type. This term may be negative and, if sufficiently large, may cause the total instantaneous conductance to become negative. The membrane potential will then become unstable and spikes or oscillations may occur. In the rod membrane the ion, X, is likely to be Ca^{++} (Fain & Quandt 1980; Bader, Bertrand, this volume). Our experiments are made under conditions which do not permit voltage - clamping the rods;

Table 1.

mM		ΔV_m	N of cells
5	TEA	5.7±.6	16
10	TEA	9.6±.9	8
15	TEA	10.1±1.	12
20	TEA	16.6±.4	5

Table 2.

Ringer			TEA		
V_{peak} (mV)	t_{peak} (msec)	mM	V_{peak} (mV)	t_{peak} (msec)	N of cells
4.3±.5	665±40	5	6.7±.6	798±108	12
4.5±.9	680±55	10	4.6±.8	843±106	3
4.3±.7	658±37	15	1.8±.5	1116± 90	9
5.5±.8	720±58	20	3.4±.9	1150± 73	3

V_{peak} average response to a flash equivalent to 14.06 Rh[*]/flash

they are electrically coupled in a network. Thus, any effect we
observe is likely to be due both to the direct action of TEA and
to membrane polarization.

To monitor simultaneously changes in sensitivity and changes
in the input resistance, we impaled rods with double barrel electrodes and stimulated the photoreceptor alternately with a dim flash
of light (equivalent to 5.8 Rh[*]) and with a pulse of current of
-.045 nA injected through the current-passing barrel. In the experiment shown in Fig. 3a the flash of light elicited a peak response
of 3.8 mV and the pulse of current a voltage deflection of about
8 mV. After adding 15 mM TEA to the perfusate, the light response
decreased to approximately 1 mV and the voltage deflection induced
by the current pulse dropped to 5.5 mV. All these changes were
reversible upon removal of TEA from the bathing medium. Fig. 3b
shows the same experiment repeated in the presence of 400 μM Co^{++}.
The addition of this divalent cation to the perfusate quickly hyperpolarized the dark membrane potential by about 6 mV and slowed the
time course of the photoresponse (Owen & Torre in preparation).

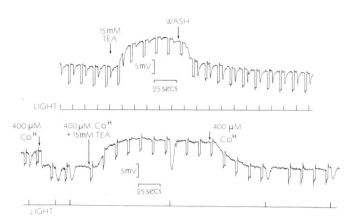

Fig. 3.   Effect of 15 mM TEA on input resistance and cell sensitivity.
Upper record: effect of 15 mM TEA on rod whose dark membrane potential was -42 mV. Lower record: effect of 15 mM
TEA in the presence of 400 μm Co^{++} on a rod, whose dark
membrane potential was -46 mV. Light stimuli as in Fig.
2. Current injected was -.045 nA.

When 15 mM TEA was added to the perfusate the dark membrane potential depolarized by about 11 mV and a clear increase both in the
input resistance and in the flash sensitivity was observed.

    These results can be interpreted by supposing that 15 mM TEA
in the external medium blocks some ionic channel, thereby decreasing
membrane conductance, while depolarization of the membrane causes
a compensating increase in membrane conductance. When the TEA-
induced membrane depolarization was counterbalanced by the action
of Co^{++} the blocking effect of TEA was clearly evident. This experiment also suggests, however, that applying 15 mM TEA from the
outside does not abolish the outward going rectification present
in the current-voltage relation of the rod since even in the presence
of 15 mM TEA the membrane conductance 12 mV above the dark membrane
potential is four times larger than the membrane conductance at the
dark membrane potential.

Regenerative photoresponses in the presence of TEA

    As illustrated in Fig. 1, we observed spikes and sustained
oscillations during the repolarizing phase of the rod's response
to a bright flash of light. This regenerative behavior can affect
the whole shape of the light response with surprising results.

When the retina was perfused with 15 mM TEA, the dark membrane potential decreased on average by 10.2 mV and the flash sensitivity decreased by 58%. Fig. 4 shows at two different scales a series of responses to brief flashes of light of increasing intensity from 5.8 Rh^* to 314.5 Rh^* recorded in the presence of 15 mM TEA. The responses to the two brighest flashes have been shifted down on the ordinate for a clearer presentation. In the lower part of Fig. 4 the initial phase of these responses is reproduced in greater detail.

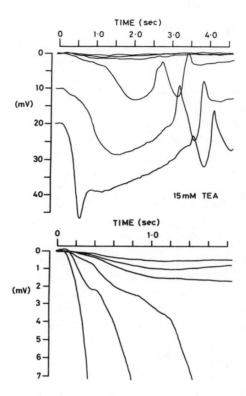

Fig. 4. Light response in the presence of 15 mM TEA. Monochromatic light 498 nm. Light intensity of flashes: 5.8, 12, 23, 55, 130, 314 Rh^*. Flash duration 50 msec. Each record is the average of 5 responses. The responses to the three dimmest lights have been smothed as described in Fig. 2. Dark resting potential in Control Ringer −38 mV, in the presence of 15 mM TEA −24 mV. In the upper panel the responses to the two brightest flashes have been shifted downward for a better discrimination. In the lower panel of the figure the initial phase of responses is reproduced in greater detail.

These light responses show some unusual features: a very low sensitivity (the rod of Fig. 4 had a sensitivity in control Ringer of .8 mV/Rh* while in the presence of TEA the sensitivity dropped to 70 μV/Rh*); the existence of a threshold 2 or 3 mV below the dark resting potential; two or three prominent, slow oscillations occurring during the repolarization to the resting potential. In what follows, we will try to explain the origin of these complex features. In the absence of voltage clamp data our explanation will be restricted to the simplest of possible mechanisms.

To explain the threshold behavior, best illustrated in the lower part of Fig. 4, following a suggestion of Professor Sir Alan Hodgkin, we suppose initially, that the current-voltage relation can be described by:

$$I = F(V) = aV + b V^2 \tag{2}$$

where a and b are constants and V is the displacement from the normal dark potential. The equation for the membrane potential is:

$$C \dot{V} = j - F(V) \tag{3}$$

where C is the total membrane capacitance and j the photocurrent. From (2) and (3), we obtain:

$$C \dot{V} = j - aV - bV^2 \tag{4}$$

Eq (4) can be solved analytically, when j is a constant. This analytical solution is useful for the understanding of the underlying mechanism. Eq (4) is solved by separating the variables and integrating. Let be $\Delta = -4 \ b - a^2$ when $\Delta < 0$ we have

$$V(t) = - \frac{a}{b} - \frac{\sqrt{-\Delta}}{2b} \ tgh \ (- \frac{\sqrt{-\Delta t}}{2c} + arctgh \ \frac{-a}{\sqrt{-\Delta}}) \tag{5}$$

when $\Delta = 0$ we have

$$V(t) = \frac{ac}{b(2C+at)} - \frac{a}{2B} \tag{6}$$

when $\Delta > 0$ we have

$$V(t) = - \frac{a}{2b} - \frac{\sqrt{\Delta}}{2b} \ tgh \ (\frac{t\sqrt{\Delta}}{2c} + arctgh \ \frac{-a}{\sqrt{\Delta}}) \tag{7}$$

From Eq. (5) - (7) it is clear that there is a threshold when $j = -a^2/(4b)$. When $j \geq -a^2/(4b)$ the voltage for $t \to \infty$ approaches the value of $-a/2b - \sqrt{-\Delta}/2b$ and when $j < -a^2 2b$ the voltage diverges towards infinity. When $j = -a^2/4b$ the voltage approaches the value of $-a/2b$ which is the voltage 'threshold'. When $j = -a^2/4b - \varepsilon$ and when ε is very small, the voltage V, before increasing very rapidly, remains for a rather long time near $-a/2b$. By decreasing ε appropriately we can prolong the "waiting" time around $-a/2b$ indefinitely.

From the analytical solution, it is clear that the voltage threshold is $V_T = -a/2b$ and the photocurrent that reaches the threshold is $j_T = -a^2/4b$. Choosing $V_T = -3$ mV (see Fig. 4) and $j_T = -10$ pA (the photocurrent that is produced by a flash of light equivalent to 30 Rh*) (T. Lamb, P. MacNaugthon & K.-W. Yau personal communication) we obtain $a = 6.6 \times 10^{-9}$ mho and $b = 1.1$ mho V^{-1}. The choice of the photocurrent is somewhat arbitrary and, in any case, is not essential to our argument. In agreement with Lamb, McNaughton & Yau (1981) and Owen & Torre (1982), we have chosen:

$$j = j_{max} \frac{1 - e^{-A} f(t)}{1 + K e^{-A} f(t)} \tag{8}$$

where $K = 1$, $f(t) = (e^{-\alpha t} - e^{-\beta t})^n$ and A is proportional to the light intensity. We assign the values, $j_{max} = -30$ pA, $\alpha = .5$ sec^{-1}, $\beta = 1.2$ sec^{-1} n=3 (Lamb MacNaughton & Yau 1981, Torre & Owen 1982) and assume a value of 30 pF for the membrane capacitance (Bader et al., 1979; Attwell & Wilson, 1980).

Fig. 5(a) shows the graphical solution of Eq. (4) for various values of A proportional to the light intensities used in Fig. 4. In Fig. 5(b) we have drawn the current-voltage relation used. The initial phase of the photoresponses shown in the lower part of Fig. 4 is satisfactory reproduced.

The current-voltage relation described by Eq. (2) is seen to be inadequate, however, when we consider the later phase of the photoresponse since it predicts that the potential will simply move to $-\infty$ & remain there. To prevent the voltage from reaching $-\infty$, the relation must be modified. The simplest way to do this is to introduce a cubic term in the function describing the current-voltage relation. Thus:

$$F(V) = a V + b V^2 + c V^3 \tag{9}$$

With a value for c of .55 10^{-4} mho V^{-2} the n-shaped I - V relation
shown in Fig. 5(a) is obtained. To account for the oscillations
seen during the repolarizing phase of light responses it is necessary
to introduce a mechanism able to inactivate with a delay the regenerative effect of the negative resistance. The simplest way is to
consider a circuit of the type shown in Fig. 6.

The set of equations now becomes:

$$C \ \dot{V} = \dot{j} - (a \ V + b \ V^2 + c \ V^3) - I_2 \tag{10}$$

$$L \ \dot{I}_2 = V - I_2/g_2 \tag{11}$$

where I_2 is the current flowing through the arm of the circuit with
the inductance. This circuit is identical with that proposed by
Fitzhugh (1969) to model the rhythmic activity in nerve axons and
muscle cells. The value of the inductance can be chosen so that,
in the limit of sinusoidal oscillations, the oscillatory period is
about 0.5 secs; i.e., $2\pi \ \sqrt{LC} \approx .5$ sec. Thus we choose L = .2 10^9

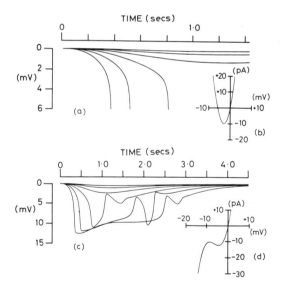

Fig. 5.   (a) Graphical solution of Eq. (4) with the I −V relation
          shown in (b). Parameter values reported in the text. (c)
          Graphical solution of Eqs. (10) and (11) with the I - V
          relation shown in (d). Parameter values reported in the
          text.

H and g_2 can be chosen to give a time constant of the same order;
i.e., $g_2 = 2. 10^{-9}$ mho. The values assigned to L and g_2 are of the
same order of magnitude as those used by Torre & Owen (1981) to explain the high-pass filtering of linear-range responses by the rod
network. Fig 6(c) shows the graphical solutions of Eq. (10) and Eq.
(11) with the chosen parameters. The essential features are well
reproduced: the threshold behavior and the oscillations at the end
of responses to bright flashes. This model is very useful in suggesting the existence of a region of negative conductance in the current-
voltage relation in the presence of 15 mM external TEA. The cell
of Fig. 4 had a dark membrane potential of -38 mV and under the
action of TEA the membrane depolarized in darkness to -24 mV. Thus
the region of negative conductance must lie between -34 and -27 mV.
In other cells this region was found between -37 and -30 mV. We
will now consider some of the complications of the circuit of Fig.
5. When $j = 0$, the system defined by equations (10) and (11) and
the current-voltage relation shown in Fig. 5(d) have only one stable
equilibrium position; the dark resting membrane potential. With a
step of constant current, j, the system can enter a region of instability, and the membrane potential will exhibit sustained oscillations. If j is further increased the system will again become
stable and the oscillations will disappear. When we illuminated the
cell whose flash responses are reproduced in Fig. 4, with a steady
light equivalent to 14.1 Rh*/sec (Fig. 7a), the membrane potential
hyperpolarized by about 11 mV, initiating a series of sustained
oscillations, whose amplitude grew for about 15 seconds reaching a
constant peak-to-peak amplitude of 20 mV and a period of approximately 750 msec (Fig. 7b).

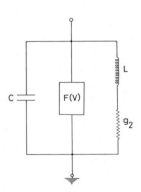

Fig. 6.   Equivalent electrical circuit used to explain the regen-
          erative behavior of rods membrane.

When the light intensity was increased to 26.2 Rh[*]/sec, the rod membrane initially hyperpolarized by 13 mV and subsequently exhibited only a few smaller oscillations. Finally with a light intensity equivalent to 63 Rh[*]/sec oscillations were no longer seen during the steady light though a few oscillations were observed at the end of the stimulus as the membrane repolarized through the region of instability. Figs. 7a and 7c also show clearly one inadequacy of the model. It is clear that the oscillations build up in time, while in the circuit of Fig. 6 the negative slope conductance is not time-varying.

In the presence of 15 mM of TEA the current-voltage relation has a region of negative slope-conductance, it is possible that the curve crosses the voltage axis (I=0) more than once. In this case, the dark membrane potential would have 3 equilibrium positions V_1 < V_2 < V_3. V_1 and V_3 would be stable equilibrium positions, while V_2 would be an unstable equilibrium position around which the membrane potential would exhibit sustained oscillations. It should then be possible to perturb the system in such a way that the membrane potential would jump from one stable to the other one, crossing the unstable position. The electronic coupling of rods causes their activity to be pooled, thereby promoting a synchrony in their dynamic behavior. In consequence, the electrical properties of rods in a coupled network are highly stable. Only in three cases have we observed a phenomenon that could be interpreted as a transition from one stable equilibrium state to another. This is shown in Fig. 8. We were recording a series of responses to flashed slits of light of intensity equivalent to 15.8 Rh[*]/rod, while bathing the retina in a Ringer containing 15 mM TEA. After 5 almost identical responses (top record in Fig. 8), we observed the response shown in the bottom part of Fig. 8   In this case, the membrane potential, at the cessation of the flash of light, instead of repolarizing back to the previous dark membrane potential, began to oscillate and finally reached a stable dark membrane potential 12 mV below the original level. We interpret this surprising result as a transition from one stable state to another one, crossing a region of instability.

Regenerative spread of excitation in presence of TEA

In a network of electrically coupled rods, the unidimensional space constant early in the response, λ_{in}, (Torre, Owen 1982; see also Detwiler this volume) is approximately proportional to the square root of the instantaneous membrane resistance. In all the

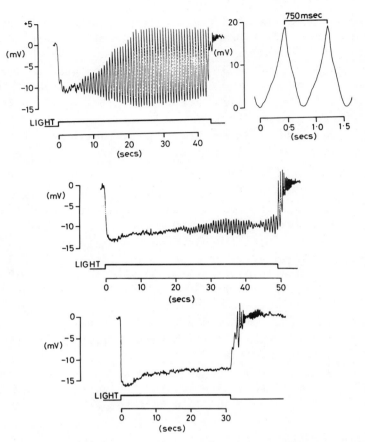

Fig. 7. Light induced oscillations in the presence of 15 mM TEA.
Same cell as in Fig. 4. Upper trace: monochromatic (498
nm) steady light equivalent to 14.1 Rh*/sec. On right two
of the sustained oscillations are reproduced in greater
detail. Middle trace: monochromatic (498 nm) steady light
equivalent to 26.2 Rh*/sec. Bottom trace: monochromatic
(498) steady light equivalent to 63 Rh*/sec.

experiments in which we compared λ_{in} in the presence of external
TEA with that in Control Ringer we consistently found it to be much
larger. If the measurement of the lateral spread of excitation is
performed in the linear range, then, according the theory developed
for the rod network, an increase in λ_{in}, indicates an increase in
the membrane resistance, provided that the coupling(s) resistance,
R_s, remains unchanged.

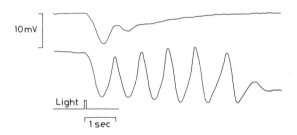

Fig. 8.   Transition of the dark membrane potential from one stable
           state to another stable state in the presence of 15 mM TEA.
           Light stimulus as in Fig. 2. Upper trace shows a typical
           light response in the presence of 15 mM TEA. Lower trace
           shows a sudden jump induced by the light, to another dark
           membrane potential.

        From the data of Fig. 4 it is clear that in the presence of
15 mM TEA$^+$ the linear range may be extremely narrow and as soon as
the region with negative resistance is reached non-linear phenomena
may appear. Fig. 9 shows the result of a "slit" experiment in normal
Ringer: here λ_{in} decreased from an initial value of 43 µm to a value
of 24 µm within 2 seconds. We then perfused the retina with 200 µM
Co^{++} and observed the reduction in high-pass filtering described
earlier: λ decreased from 30 µm to 25 µm during the photoresponse.
When 15 mM TEA$^+$ was added to the perfusate we obtained the series
of responses shown in Fig. 9b: responses recorded at 10, 30, 40,
50, 60, 70 µm from the centered position are reproduced. It is
clear that λ_{in} increased dramatically, the excitation spreading
much further early in the response than was evident in Control
Ringer. λ_{in} was around 135 µm compared to the control value of 45
µm. In the linear range an increase in λ_{in} from 45 to 135 µm would
indicate an increase in the slope membrane resistance of about 15
times. Such an increase was not consistent with the results of
current injection experiments using double-barreled electrodes. In
the experiment shown in Fig. 9 a light intensity equivalent to 28.7
Rh* was used. When the light intensity was reduced to 10.06 Rh* λ_{in}
decreased to 90 µm, showing clearly that we were outside the linear
range. We have not been able to measure the "instantaneous" length
constant in the linear range in the presence of 15 mM TEA, because
the linear range is so narrow. This regenerative lateral spread of
excitation can be easily explained by the circuit of Fig. 6. As
soon as the voltage response to the centered stimulus reaches the
threshold V_t, the excitation will be transmitted much further than
when the threshold V_t is not reached.

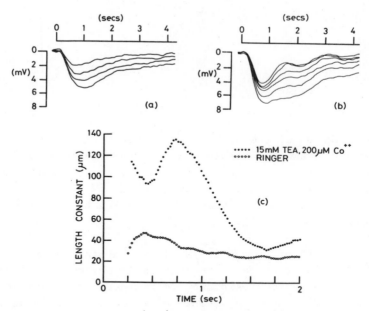

Fig. 9. The effect of 16 mM TEA[+] and 200 μM Co[++] on high pass filtering. a) in control Ringer. b) in the test solution. c)
the network length constant plotted as a function of time
from the records shown in (a) and (b).

Spikes in high Sr[++]

As already reported, photoreceptors can exhibit spiking activity when perfused with high external Sr[++] (Piccolino & Gershenfeld
1978, 1980; Fain, Quandt & Gerschenfeld 1977).

Addition of 10 mM (Sr[++]) to the perfusate caused a membrane
hyperpolarization of 3-4 mV leaving unaltered the level of the peak
and the plateau of a bright flash response. Sr[++] clearly affected
the waveform of the responses to dim light flashes by increasing
the time-to-peak and causing the appearance of one or two oscillations during the hyperpolarizing phase. Three minutes after the
addition of Sr[++] the membrane potential began to show spiking behaviour. Spikes of around 30-40 mV were observed. Addition of 100
μM Co[++] caused an additional hyperpolarization of a few mV and
blocked the spiking activity.

In Fig. 10 we reproduce the effect of 10 mM Sr^{++} on three different cells. Observe the different shape and frequency of firing of the spikes. In C a clear undershoot follows the spike. in B no undershoot i present; in A we see an overshoot followed by an undershoot. In none of these cells, spiking in the presence of 10 mM Sr^{++}, have we observed a slow depolarizing wave preceding spike initiation such as is typically seen in pacemaking neurons (Noble 1975). All of the oberved spontaneous spikes resembled transmitted spikes.

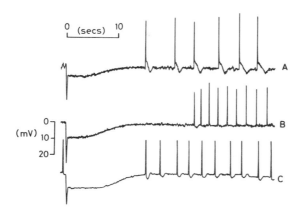

Fig. 10. Spontaneous spikes in the presence of 10 mM Sr^{++}. Light stimulus as in Fig. 1. Dark resting potential in control Ringer: -43 mV (A), -44 mV (B), -42 mV (C). Upon addition of 10 mM Sr^{++} the dark membrane potential hyperpolarized by about 5 mV in the three cells.

DISCUSSION

Our results confirm the notion that the rod plasma membrane contains a regenerative conductance, which is probably a Ca^{++} conductance (Fain et al. 1978, Fain & Quandt 1980, Bader et al. this volume).

We did not find that 15 mM TEA completely abolishes the outward-going membrane rectifications as claimed by Fain & Quandt (1980). Rather, we believe that TEA increases the membrane resistance but, at an external concentration of 15 mM, leaves the membrane conductance considerably higher at about -30 mV then at about -44 mV (see Attwell & Wilson 1980). In the presence of 15 mM TEA it was possible to demonstrate in many cells the existence of a region with negative conductance in the I-V relation. This region was found between -36 and -29 mV, (average values) in agreement with Fain et al. (1980).

Regenerative mechanism in rods

It is possible to reveal regenerative activity in toad rods by two different procedures: by external application of TEA^+ in concentrations between 5 & 15 mM or by addition of 10 mM of Sr^{++} to the extra cellular medium. However, the regenerative behaviour observed with the two substances differs in many respects.

First, TEA probably induces regenerative activity by decreasing the shunting membrane conductance, so that relative contribution of the negative component to the total membrane conductance becomes larger. By contrast, the addition of 10 mM Sr^{++} is believed to augment the current through the regenerative conductance, an effect that would be equivalent to increasing the driving force on this current. This would increase the absolute magnitude of the negative component of the total membrane conductance.

We note also an asymmetry in the position of the threshold of the regenerative behaviour in presence of TEA and in presence of Sr^{++}. In the great majority of cases, in the presence of TEA, membrane instability is most clearly evident during transient depolarization or when the membrane potential is hyperpolarized by light (see data of Fig. 1, 4, 7, 8, 9, 10), the latter because in 15 mM TEA the region of instability is negative with respect to the dark potential. In some instances, we observed instability of the membrane dark potential for a period of 2 - 4 minutes, though the membrane later became stable again. In the presence of Sr^{++} the region of membrane instability lies positive with respect to the dark potential. Photoresponses in 10 mM Sr^{++} did not show the threshold behaviour that we observed in the presence of 15 mM TEA (see Fig. 4). In agreement with this is the observation that spikes were more readily evoked by anode-break stimulation in the presence of Sr^{++} than in the presence of TEA. Perfusion with 100 μM of Co^{++} was sufficient to block the spikes induced by Sr^{++}, but did not always block all regenerative activity. This was true with concentrations of Co^{++} up to 200 μM (see the data of Fig. 9 for example). In some cases we perfused the retina with 200 μM Co^{++} obtaining the usual effect, as shown in Fig. 3. Yet the subsequent addition of 15 mM TEA induced clear oscillatory behavior, even in presence of 200 μM of Co^{++}. When after a few minutes we repeat this experiment, invariably no further oscillations were observed. This suggests that to completely abolish all regenerative behaviour it is necessary to use concentrations of Co^{++} larger than 200 μM.

The action of TEA

We obtained some evidence that TEA reduces the membrane conductance (see Fig. 3) but does not abolish the outward-going rectification. However, we have no direct evidence that external TEA blocks a voltage and time-dependent K^+ conductance. It is worth noting that the time- and voltage- dependent K^+ conductance that we believe to be responsible for high-pass filtering behaviour of the rod network (Torre & Owen 1981) was not abolished by the addition of 15 mM of external TEA. The action of TEA will not be clear until there exists reliable data obtained under voltage clamp in conditions where the external ionic concentration can be quickly changed.

REFERENCES

Attwell, D. & Wilson, M. (1980). Behaviour of the rod network in the tiger salamander retina mediated by membrane properties of the individual rods, J. Physiol., 309, 287-315.

Bader, C.R., MacLeish, P.R. & Schwartz, E.A. (1978). Responses to light of solitary rod photoreceptors isolated from tiger salamander retina, Proc. natn. Acad. Sci. U.S.A., 75, 3507-3511.

Bader, C.R., MacLeish, P.R. & Schwartz, E.A. (1979). A voltage-
    clamp study of the light response in solitary rods of the
    tiger salamander, J. Physiol., 296, 1-26.
Fain, G.L., Quandt, F.N. & Gerschenfeld, H.M. (1977). Calcium-
    dependent regenerative responses in rods. Nature, Lond.,
    269, 707-710.
Fain, G.L. & Quandt, F.N. (1980). The effect of TEA and cobalt
    ions on responses to extrinsic current in toad rods, J. Physiol.
    303, 515-533.
Fitzugh, R. (1969). Mathematical models of excitation and propaga-
    tion in nerve, in: "Biological Engeneering". H.R. Swann ed.,
    MacGraw-Hill, New York.
Piccolino, M. & Gerschenfeld, H.M. (1980). Characteristics and
    ionic processes involved in feed-back spikes of turtle cones,
    Proc. R. Soc. B, 206, 439-463.
Piccolino, M. & Gerschenfeld, H.M. (1978). Activation of a regen-
    erative calcium conductance in turtle cones by peripheral
    stimulation, Proc. R. Soc. B, 201, 309-315.
Noble, D. (1975). "The initiation of the Heartbeat", Clarendon
    Press, Oxford.
Torre, V. & Owen G.W. (1981). Ionic basis of high pass filtering
    of small signals by the rod retina of toad Bufo marinus, Proc.
    R. Soc. B., 212, 253-261.
Werblin, F.S. (1979). Time- and voltage- dependent ionic components
    of the rod response, J. Physiol., 294, 613-629.

SYNAPTIC RESPONSES OF RETINAL PHOTORECEPTORS

A. Lasansky

Laboratory of Neurophysiology, National Institute of
Neurological and Communicative Disorders and Stroke
National Institutes of Health, Bethesda, Maryland 20205
U.S.A.

The existence of a synaptic input to retinal receptors that antagonized the direct photoresponse was first described by Baylor, Fuortes and O'Bryan (1971). They observed that following a brief flash, the response of the turtle cones to a light spot of 600 μ radius exhibited a delayed depolarization not detectable in responses to a spot of 70 μ radius. This depolarizing effect could be isolated by stimulating the periphery of the receptive field during steady illumination of the center and was also elicited when horizontal cells were hyperpolarized by extrinsic current. Because of this finding, and the large receptive field of the surround effect, a negative synaptic feed back from horizontal cells to cones was postulated, its chemical nature indicated by the opposite polarity of the pre- and post-synaptic potential changes.

The hypothesis that the surround response is mediated by a chemical synapse received additional support from the observation that it is associated with a decrease in the resistance of the cone cell membrane (O'Bryan, 1973). Two depolarizing components were also described: and early spike-like transient followed by a slower wave. The former is more consistently elicited when the retina is perfused with media containing Sr^{++} or Ba^{++} and is therefore thought to represent a regenerative increase in Ca^{++} conductance (Piccolino and Gerschenfeld, 1980). The experiments on perfused retinae, however, did not give information on the ionic nature of the slow component.

A major obstacle to the study of the mechanism of generation
and functional role of the antagonistic surround responses is their
lability. As shown by Fuortes, Simon and Schwartz (1973), while the
depolarizing surround effect is often large immediately following
impalement of a cone by a microelectrode, its amplitude almost
always declines rapidly, although the direct photoresponse may
remain unchanged. When the feed back response finally reaches a
stable level, it is, with few exceptions, weak or almost negligible.
This final condition, presumably brought about by electrode-
inflicted injury, is illustrated in Fig. 1 by the responses of a
cone of the turtle Pseudemys scripta elegans to steps of illumination with two circles of different diameter. Although the larger
circle evoked hyperpolarizing responses with a steady phase of
slightly lower amplitude, the difference is minor and to some extent
can be ascribed to changes in extracellular currents.

A better demonstration of the surround response can be achieved
sometimes by illumination with annular patterns. Bright annuli,
while evoking a direct hyperpolarizing response due to light
scattering to the center of the receptive field, also may evoke a
depolarizing component of larger magnitude than what may have been
expected from comparing responses to circles of different diameter
(see Gerschenfeld and Piccolino, 1980). Furthermore, the brightness
of an annulus can be reduced until not enough light is scattered to
evoke a detectable central response. Under such conditions illumination of the surround results in virtually no change in membrane
potential (Fig. 2A), but the input resistance is decreased (Fig.
2B). This change in input resistance can be also detected with
other patterns of illumination (O'Bryan, 1973; Gerschenfeld and
Piccolino, 1980), but the use of a dim annulus has several
advantages. Thus, a clear decrease in input resistance (Fig. 2B)
may be observed in cones where comparison between the responses to
circles of light of different diameter suggests an almost negligible
surround effect (Fig. 1). As discussed below, the small amplitude
of the depolarizing component in the response to a large circle may
be ascribed to blocking of the surround effect by the hyperpolarization associated with the direct photoresponse.

In addition, experiments such as in Fig. 2 have unexpectedly
revealed that the feed back response is transient. Thus, when
illumination with a dim annulus was maintained, the change in the
cone input resistance declined and disappeared in several seconds
(Fig. 2D). This transient character was not due to loss or

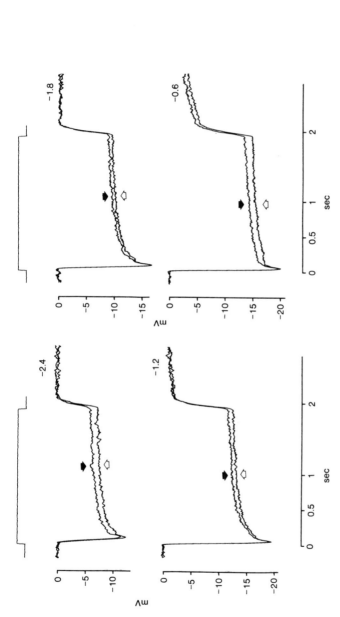

Fig. 1. Superimposed responses of a retinal cone of the turtle Pseudemys scripta elegans to steps of light with circles of 240 μ (open arrows) and 1100 μ (filled arrows) diameter. The responses to the larger circle have a steady phase of slightly lower amplitude. Intracellularly recorded from the isolated and oxygenated eyecup with a 3M-potassium acetate-filled electrode. The light was passed through an interference filter with peak transmission at 594 nm and its unattenuated flux (relative intensity 1.0) measured at the level of the retina was about 8.1×10^{14} photons sec^{-1} cm^{-2}. The duration of the stimulus, which starts at time zero, is shown above, and its relative intensity in each case is given in logarithmic units. Zero in the voltage scale corresponds to membrane potential in darkness.

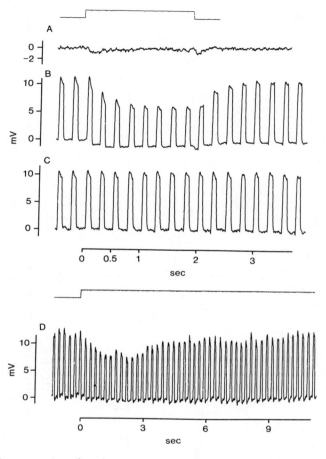

Fig. 2. Changes in the input resistance of turtle cones induced by
annular illumination. Experimental details as for Fig. 1. A, an
annulus (O.D., 1100 µ; I.D. 240 µ) at the relative light intensity
of -2.4 logarithmic units evokes virtually no change in membrane
potential. B, a train of pulses of depolarizing current (2.0×10^{-10}
A) was injected through the electrode during illumination with the
annulus at the same relative intensity as in A. The decrease in the
amplitude of the pulses during illumination indicates a loss in
membrane resistance. Average of three responses. C, a train of
pulses as in B, but in darkness. D, a long step of annular
illumination (relative intensity -2.4 log units) evoked an initial
decrease in input resistance in another cone. The effect gradually
disappeared even though the illumination was maintained. Depolarizing pulses of 1.3×10^{-10} A. Average of three responses.

deterioration of the surround effect, as such observations could be
repeated after a suitable interval in darkness (about 1 min.); Fig.
2D, for instance, represents the average of three responses.
Instead, it may be assumed that the decay of the surround effect
during sustained illumination reflects intrinsic properties of the
feed back synapse, since under those conditions the horizontal cells
remain steadily hyperpolarized.

Finally, since a dim annulus can evoke a decrease in input
resistance without an associated change in potential, it may be
inferred that the underlying response is an increase in permeability
to an ion that is passively distributed across the cone cell
membrane. This ion was shown to be Cl^- by the observation that the
amplitude of the surround response of salamander cones was markedly
increased when the recording microelectrodes where filled with a
potassium chloride solution, instead of the usual 4M potassium
acetate (Lasansky, 1981). The effects of such an injection of Cl^-
into a turtle cone are illustrated by the records in Fig. 3: while
the responses to a small light circle were still purely hyperpolarizing, those to a larger circle became predominantly depolarizing (Fig. 3A), even when the stimulus elicited a central response
of maximal amplitude (Fig. 3C). Illumination with an annulus was
followed by a graded depolarization, preceded by a brief hyperpolarization when enough light was scattered to the center to
elicit a direct response from the cone (Fig. 3B). The depolarizations had a slow rising phase and could outlast the stimulus by
more than 2 sec. Those evoked by the large circle had a higher
amplitude and lasted longer than those evoked by the annulus;
although the responses to the annulus were recorded after those
to the large circle, this observation cannot be ascribed to a
deterioration of the surround effect, since it was confirmed by a
subsequent response to the large circle (Fig. 3D). It would seem,
therefore, that in this instance central illumination facilitated
the surround response.

Observations of this kind, however, can be made only exceptionally, since the usual deterioration of the surround effect promtly
leads to a purely hyperpolarizing response to a large circle of
light, although one that still retains a more pronounced relaxation
than seen when the electrodes are filled with a potassium acetate
solution (Fig. 4A). Nevertheless, while these changes take place
the response to a dim annulus may remain stable or even increase
in amplitude (Fig. 4B). It would then seem that the deterioration

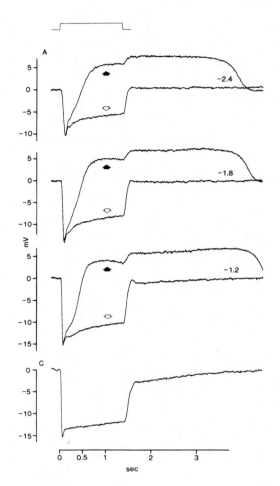

Fig. 3. Responses of a turtle cone to steps of light with various
patterns, recorded intracellularly with a 3M-potassium choloride-
filled electrode. Other experimental procedures as for Fig. 1. A,
superimposed responses to circles of 240 μ (open arrows) and 1100 μ
(filled arrows) diameter; the relative light intensity in each case
is indicated in logarithmic units. While the responses to the small
circle are hyperpolarizing, those to the large circle are diphasic.
B, responses to an annulus (O.D., 1100 μ; I.D., 240 μ) at the same

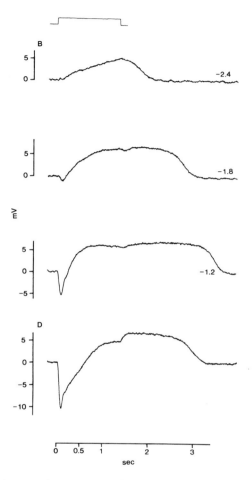

relative light intensities as in A. C, response to the small circle
at a relative light intensity of 0.6. log units. The peak amplitude
does not exceed that of the response to the brightest stimulus in
A, so that it can be seen that maximal amplitude had already been
reached. D, response to the large circle at a relative intensity
of −2.4 log units. This record was obtained after those in B,
which in turn had been obtained after those in A. The surround
component in D still reaches a higher amplitude and lasts longer
than the response to the annulus at the same light intensity.

of the surround effect consists only of its becoming more easily
blocked by the hyperpolarization associated with the direct
photoresponse.

This blocking action of hyperpolarization can be better
demonstrated with extrinsic current and has already been reported
by other authors (O'Bryan, 1973; Gerschenfeld and Piccolino, 1980).
As shown in Fig. 5, with increasing hyperpolarization the depolarizing response to an annulus, although initially increasing in
amplitude, showed a longer time-to-peak and was finally suppressed.
The records were then identical to those obtained with potassium
acetate-filled electrodes, so that it may be concluded that
hyperpolarization eliminated the synaptically induced increase in
Cl^- conductance, as also shown by the amplitude of the voltage drop
at the end of the current pulses in Fig. 5.

One possible interpretation of this observation is that the
synaptically activated Cl^- conductance is voltage-dependent. Nonlinear Cl^- conductances have been already described in other cells,
although not in nerve tissue (Gaffey and Mullins, 1958; Bennett,
1961; Grundfest, 1971; Fukuda, 1974; Fukuda, Henkart, Fischbach and
Smith, 1976), while voltage-sensitive channels are known to occur
in some synapses which, as those involved in horizontal cell feedback, give origin to slow responses (see Hartzell, 1981). Also as
in some of those synapses, the transmitter mediating the cone
surround responses may close ionic channels, since the Cl^- conductance is increased when horizontal cells hyperpolarize and presumably stop releasing transmitter (Lasansky, 1981).

An alternative mechanism for the generation of the cone
responses to annular illumination is suggested by the knowledge
that they also involve the activation of a voltage-dependent Ca^{++}
conductance (Piccolino and Gerschenfeld, 1980; Gerschenfeld and
Piccolino, 1980). This effect could be secondary to the depolarization resulting from the synaptic activation of the Cl^- conductance.
On the other hand, a Ca^{++}-activated anionic current has been
recently observed in retinal photoreceptors (Bader, Bertrand and
Schwartz, 1981). Thus, it would seem equally possible that the
primary synaptic effect is the opening of Ca^{++} channels and that
the voltage-sensitivity of the Cl^- conductance is secondary to
that of the Ca^{++} conductance.

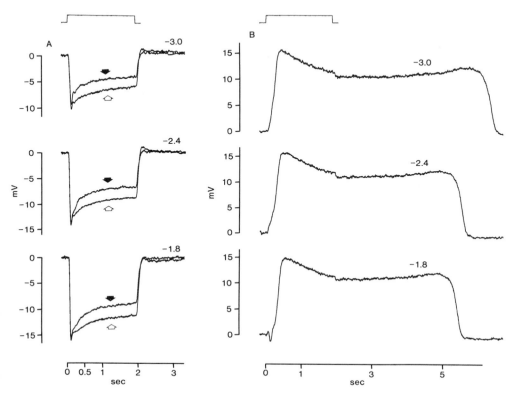

Fig. 4. Responses of a turtle cone to steps of light with the three light patterns used for Fig. 3, recorded intracellularly by means of an electrode filled with 3M-potassium chloride. Other experimental procedures as for Fig. 1. The relative light intensities are indicated in logarithmic units. A, responses to the small (open arrows) and large (filled arrows) circles. B, responses to the annulus. The series with the circles were obtained once to surround effect had stabilized, and the responses to the annulus were recorded afterwards. An additional series was subsequently recorded with each one of the stimulus patterns and the results reproduced those shown in this figure.

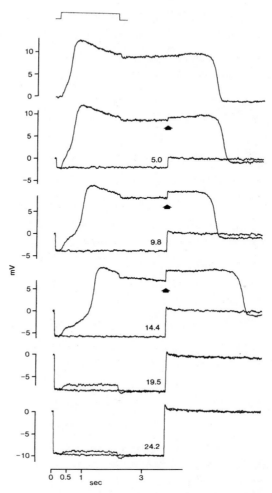

Fig. 5. Responses of a turtle cone to illumination with an annulus (O.D., 1100 μ; I.D., 240 μ) during hyperpolarization induced by extrinsic current. Relative light intensity −2.4 log units. The voltage drop across the microelectrode (filled with 3M potassium chloride) was canceled by means of the equivalent of a bridge circuit. Other experimental details as for Fig. 1. The top record is the response to the annulus in the absence of extrinsic current. Each one of the other records illustrates the response during a hyperpolarizing current pulse plus the same pulse in darkness (current in $A \times 10^{-11}$). The end of the pulse is marked by an arrow in those instances in which the surround response was still recorded. After the response is suppressed, a further increase in current evokes no significant change.

REFERENCES

Bader, C.R., Bertrand, D. and Schwartz, E.A. (1981). Voltage-activated and calcium-activated currents studied in solitary rod inner segments from the salamander retina, Abstr. Soc. Neurosci., 11th Meeting, p. 728.

Baylor, D.A., Fuortes, M.G.F. and O'Bryan, P.M. (1971). Receptive fields of cones in the retina of the turtle, J. Physiol.,214, 264-294.

Bennett, M.V.L. (1961). Modes of operation of electric organs, Ann. N.Y. Acad. Sci., 94, 458-509.

Fukuda, J. (1974). Chloride spike: A third type of action potential in tissue-cultured skeletal muscle cells from the chick, Science, 185, 76-78.

Fukuda, J., Henkart, M.P., Fischbach, G.D. and Smith, T.G., Jr. (1976). Physiological and structural properties of colchicine-treated chick skeletal muscle cells grown in tissue culture, Develop. Biol., 49, 395-411.

Fuortes, M.G.F., Schwartz, E.A. and Simon, E.J. (1973). Colour-dependence of cone responses in the turtle retina, J. Physiol., 234, 199-216.

Gaffey, G.T. and Mullins, L.J. (1958). Ion fluxes during the action potential in chara, J. Physiol., 144, 505-524.

Gerschenfeld, H.M. and Piccolino, M. (1980). Sustained feedback effects of L-horizontal cells on turtle cones, Proc. R. Soc. Lond B 206, 465-480.

Grundfest, H. (1971). The varieties of excitable membranes. In "Biophysics and Physiology of Excitable Membranes", W.J. Adelman, Jr., Ed., Van Nostrand Reinhold Co., N.Y. pp. 477-504.

Hartzell, H.C. (1981). Mechanisms of slow synaptic potentials, Nature, 291, 539-544.

Lasansky, A. (1981). Synaptic action mediating cone responses to annular illumination in the retina of the larval tiger salamander, J. Physiol. 310, 205-214.

O'Bryan, P.M. (1973). Properties of the depolarizing synaptic potential evoked by peripheral illumination in cones of the turtle retina, J. Physiol. 235, 207-223.

Piccolino, M. and Gerschenfeld, H.M. (1980). Characteristics and ionic processes involved in feedback spikes of turtle cones, Proc. R. Soc. Lond., B 206, 439-463.

MICROTUBULES IN VERTEBRATE PHOTORECEPTORS

M.A. Ali & M.A. Klyne

Département de Biologie, Université de Montréal, Canada

1. INTRODUCTION

Microtubules (MTs) are now recognised as being ubiquitous in eucaryotic cells. On the basis of their varied and wide occurrence, as well as the mode of action of specific inhibitors (e.g. colchicine, Vinca alkaloids) on cellular activies MTs, despite their simple and uniform structure, are postulated to have several functions. These include: direct or indirect participation in cell motility; intracellular transport of cytoplasmic particules or substances; and the formation and maintenance of asymmetrical cell shape as a sort of cytoskeleton. It is possible that the cytoplasmic MTs in retinas may participate in each of the above functions. Since many excellent reviews have appeared recently on the subject of MTs (Dustin, 1978; Gaskin & Shelanski, 1976; Goldman et al., 1976; Olmsted & Borisy, 1973; Roberts & Hyams, 1979; Sakai, 1980; Soifer, 1975; Stephens, 1975; Wilson & Bryan, 1974) only the essentials of MT structure and biochemistry required to understand the functions of the cytoplasmic MTs of the retina will be discussed in this chapter.

Ultrastructurally MTs appear as hollow cylinders with a cross-sectional (outer) diameter of 24±2 nm, and a wall which is approximately 5 nm thick. In length, MTs may range from less than 0.5 μm (viz. centrioles) to several millimetres (viz. flagella). The first report that MTs, in cross-section, are composed of 13 globular units (protofilaments) came from Ledbetter and Porter (1964) who employed the optical-reinforcement technique of Markham rotation (Markham and al., 1963). However, the subsequent introduction of Mizuhira's fixative (tanning acid and glutaraldehyde) which enabled MT-subunits to be seen without image reinforcement (Futaesuka et al., 1972; Tilney et al., 1973) showed the existence of special MTs with either 12 or 15 subunits (Burton et al., 1975; Nagano & Suzuki, 1975). Thus, there is evidence that some deviation in the number of protofilaments of MTs really exists. Subunit arrangement is similar in MTs from different sources (Tilney et al., 1973), nevertheless, these are composite microtubular structures (viz. flagella outer doublets, basal bodies, centrioles, etc.). An additional feature of MTs, especially those found in ordered arrays, is the bridge (lateral projection, junction, arm) (Mandelkow & Mandelkow, 1979; McIntosh, 1974). Although MT-bridges are generally seen between adjacent MTs and other cytoplasmic organelles have also been reported (Beckerle et al., 1979; Bikle et al., 1966; Heggenes et al., 1968; Murphy & Tilney, 1974; Schliwa & Bereiter-Hahn, 1973).

The structural units of MTs are equivalent to the tubulin monomer of molecular weight 55,000 (Mandelkow et al., 1977) but the chemical subunit (M.W. 100,000-120,000) is a heterodimer containing α - (M.W. 54,000 - 58,000) and β - (M.W. 46,000 - 54,000) tubulin in approximately equal amounts (Luduena et al., 1977; Mohri, 1976). Associated with tubulin is dynein, an ATPase protein, identified as the arms projecting out from MTs, which provides the generative force for sliding action (Afzelium, 1959; Gibbons, 1963; Summers & Gibbons, 1971). In addition, other proteins (MT-associated proteins or MAPs) associated with MTs render intrinsic properties to the tubules (c.f. Dustin, 1978; Roberts & Hyams, 1979).

This tubulin-dynein system (MT-system together with the actin-myosin system (microfilament-system) for the major means of motility in cells.

2. RETINA

The distribution and contribution of MTs in the pigment epithelium and photoreceptors of the retinas of lower vertebrates will be discussed in this chapter.

2.1. Retinal Pigment Epithelium (RPE)

The RPE, consisting of a single layer of cells, is not an integral part of the neural retina, however, it provides both metabolic and functional support for the retina (Bernstein, 1961; Cohen, 1963; Dowling & Gibbons, 1962; Lasansky & de Fisch, 1965; Moyer, 1969; Porter & Yamada, 1960).

One of the primary functions of the RPE is to phagocytose effete photoreceptor outer segments (Bairati & Orzalesi, 1963; Custer & Bok, 1969; Hollyfield & Ward, 1974 a,b; Young, 1971; Young & Bok, 1969). This involves the engulfment of the outer segments, their subsequent digestion and recycling and/or excretion of the by-products (Beauchemin & Leuenberg, 1977). Secondly, as the RPE forms the only "barrier" between the blood vessel and the neural retina in vertebrates not equipped with retinal circulation all metabolites to and from the retina must trasverse the RPE (Moyer, 1969). Thus, the RPE also functions as a selective barrier. Furthermore, in several lower vertebrates, melanin granules of the RPE migrate in response to light, thereby providing a variable shield for the light sensitive rod outer segments (Ali, 1971; Walls, 1942). These functions imply that elements of motility are required, and the cytoskeletal elements (microfilaments, 10-nm filaments, MTs) are thought to contribute to this; All three of these elements have been reported to occur in the RPE of vertebrates (microfilaments - Burnside, 1976; Murray & Dublin, 1975; 10-nm filaments - Klyne & Ali, 1981; Takeuchi & Takeuchi, 1979; MTs - Burnside, 1976; Klyne & Ali, 1981).

2.1.1. Phagocytosis

Phagocytosis entails a complex sequence of cellular phenomena: recognition, ingestion, fusion of ingested phagosomes with lysosomal granules and digestion (Edelman, 1976; c.f. Holtzman, 1976). Each of these processes, except digestion, depend on cellular motility. Although conflicting reports exist, it is generally accepted that recognition and attachment, and fusion of lysosomes with phagosomes is mediated by MTs (c.f. Berlin, 1975); while ingestion is mediated by microfilaments (Malawista, 1975; Simson & Spicer, 1973; Strossel, 1974; Weissmann et al., 1975). Evidence for this was shown by inhibitor studies. Cytochalasin B (a fungal metabolite which interferes with cytoplasmic microfilament) was found to block ingestion; the process of attachment and fusion being unaffected. Thus, in cytochalasin B treated cells lysosomes are observed to fuse with incomplete "phagosomes". On the order hand, in cells treated with MT-inhibitors (colchicine, _Vincia_ alkaloids) ingestion was not blocked, but the fusion of lysosomes and phagosomes was prevented. This interpretation is consistent with the numerous reports of MT-participation in the transport of cytoplasmic particles (c.f. Burnside, 1975).

The spatial disposition of MTs in teleost RPE cells, appropriate for taking part in phagocytosis, is illustrated in Fig. 1. MTs are

distributed throughout the RPE and even extend down the apical processes (Fig. 2). The presence of MTs within the apical processes may
function in recognition and attachment of effete photoreceptor outer
segments, while the close association of MTs with phagocytosed outer
segments and lysososomes suggest their contribution to the fusion
of these organelles.

2.1.2. Permeability Barrier

Retinas of vertebrates not provided with retinal circulation
must obtain their nourishment as well as excrete their metabolites
into the choroid capillary via the RPE. This may involve: 1) passive
transport along a concentration gradient from the neural retina to
the capillary, and vice versa, through the intracellular spaces
between the RPE cells; 2) engulfment of material (endocytosis) by
RPE, translocation of the vesicle to the site of requirement followed
by release (exocytosis) of the material; 3) diffusion (active or
passive) into the RPE cells, through the neural retina (or capillary)
and out of the RPE cells again. MT distribution in the RPE imply
that they may be involved in the first two of these processes.

Flow of material through intercellular space is regulated by
occluding junctions (tight junctions or zonulae occludents). These
junctions are present between adjacent cells of the RPE (Fig. 3).
Although the mechanism behind the formation of the junctional complex
is poorly understood, there is ultrastructural evidence to show that
microfilaments and MTs are closely associated with cellular junctions
(Farquhar & Palade, 1963; Goodenough & Revel, 1970; Wessells & Evans,
1968). However, inhibitor studies (colchicine, cytochalasin B)
showed that microfilament − and not MT-association with the plasma
membrane regulates the function of the junction (Meza et al., 1980).

Endocytosis and exocytosis imply that material, following engulfment, is translocated in membrane bound vesicles to the site to
requirement where the material is released. MTs have been shown to

                    Figures 1 to 3 ———————————————————————▶
Retinal pigment epithelium (RPE) of the common catfish (Fig. 1) and
the brook trout (Fig. 2, 3). Fig. 1 shows the close association of
microtubules (MT and the photoreceptor outer segment; Fig. 2, the
distribution of MTs and pigment granules (PG) within the apical process; Fig. 3, tight junction (TG) between adjacent RPE cells and the
presence of a coated-vesicle close to the plasma membrane.

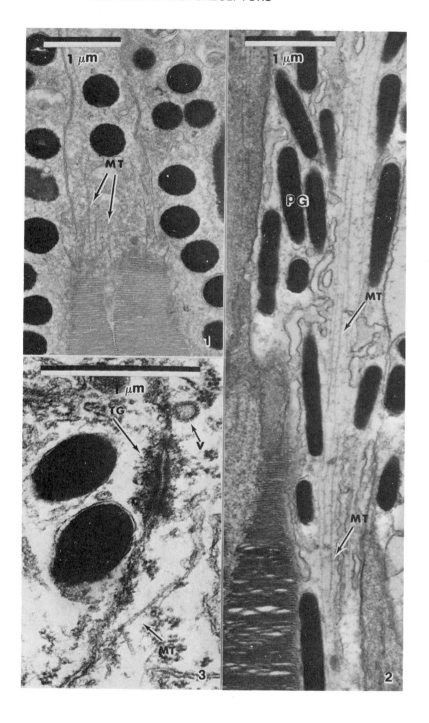

participate in this process (Edelman, 1976; Friend & Farquhar, 1967; Heiniger & Marshall, 1979; Matsusaka, 1967; Silverstein et al., 1977). (See also Section 2.3.2).

2.1.3. Retinomotor Responses

The eye of lower vertebrates responds to varying illumination, not by pupillary action, but rather by cellular movements within the retina itself. These so-called photomechanical or retinomotor responses include, in some instances, the extension of the apical processes of the RPE and the migration of pigment granules within these processes during light-adaptation (Ali, 1971; Walls, 1942). Cytoskeletal elements (microfilaments, MTs) have been reported to operate in this mechanism.

Murray and Dublin (1975), in a study on the RPE of the frog, reported the absence of MTs within the apical projections of the RPE and suggested that the microfilament system is responsible for pigment migration. However, subsequent studies (Burnside, 1976; Klyne & Ali, 1981) on the retinas of fishes showed that MTs of the RPE may participate in pigment migration in a manner similar to that found in dermal melanophores of various species. In these retinas MTs were seen alongside the elongated pigment granules of the light-adapted retina (Fig. 2). MTs may affect pigment migration by direct association (Murphy & Tilney, 1974) or indirectly through the micro-trabecular lattice (Luby & Porter, 1980; c.f. Section 2.3.2).

2.2. Photoreceptors

The retinas of vertebrate (except the strictly nocturnal or diurnal species) generally contain 2 types of photoreceptors: 1) the scotopic rods, which function at low light intensities; and 2) the photopic cones, which operate at higher light intensities. As mentioned in the preceeding section (Sect on 2.1.3) the eye of lower vertebrates responds to light also by retinal movements. In addition to movements of the RPE, one or both of the photoreceptor types may also undergo contraction and elongation.

2.2.1. Rods

The visual pigments of the scotopic photoreceptors would be bleached if exposed to light intensities. The amount of light reaching the photo-sensitive outer segments may be mediated through pupillary or photomechanical action of the retinal cells (Ali, 1971;

Walls, 1942). In the latter instance, rods respond to light by
elongation, thereby pushing their sensitive outer segments between
the processes of the RPE. In darkness or low light intensities,
rods contract, thus exposing their outer segments to the incoming
radiation. Most of the elongation and contraction occur within the
myoid - that region of the photoreceptor cell between the ellipsoid
and nucleus. Both MTs and microfilaments are reported (Ferrero et
al., 1979; Klyne & Ali, 1981; O'Connor & Burnside, 1981) to be present in this region; and have been implicated in these rod responses,
however, the actual mechanism involved have not been resolved.
Couillard (1975) may function in the same way as they do in unicellular organisms.

Current investigations (Anctil et al., 1980; O'Connor & Burnside,
1981), employing the use of inhibitors (colchicine, cytochalasin B),
noted that colchine (MT-inhibitor) prevented rod contraction while
cytochalasin B (microfilament-inhibitor) prevented rod contraction.
From these studies they postulated that, in rods, contraction is
mediated by MTs and elongation by microfilaments. Ultrastructural
evidence advanced in support of the above includes the complete
absence of microfilaments in the myoids of rods (brown trout -c.f.
Anctil et al., 1980) and the absence of microfilaments in contracted
dark-adapted rod myoids while MTs were present both in the light-
and dark-adapted states (the cichlid, Sarotherodon mossambicus) -
c.f. O'Connor & Burnside, 1981). Although the preceeding mechanism
may be operating in these teleosts there is evidence that differences
exist. Contrary to the above observations prominent microfilament
bundles were observed only in the contracted, dark-adapted rods of
the brook trout, while both light- and dark-adapted rod contained
MTs (Fig. 4, 5, 6, 7; Klyne & Ali, 1980). Furthermore, MT-inhibitors
(colchicine, vinblastine) were found to disrupt the organised struc-

---

Figures 4 to 9 (on following page).
Photoreceptors of charrs in the light- (Fig. 4, 5, 8, 9) and dark-
adapted (Fig. 6, 7) states. Fig. 4, rod myoid of a light-adapted
Arctic charr showing the distribution of microtubules (MT). Fig. 5,
high magnification of MTs of Fig. 4. Fig. 6, rod inner segment of
a dark-adapted brook trout; note the reduction in the amount of MTs
and the presence of microfilament bundles (MF). Fig. 7, high
magnification of MTs and MF of Fig. 6. Fig. 8, cone inner segment
of light-adapted brook trout showing the distribution of MTs and MF
bundles. Fig. 9, high magnification of Fig. 8 to show MTs and MF.
(C - cone; R - rod)

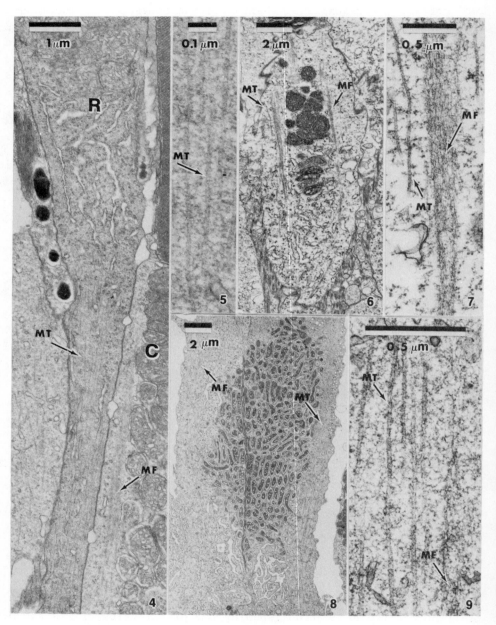

Figures 4 to 9

ture of both light- and dark-adpted retinas (Klyne & Ali, 1980) and
hence the precise location of the rods. Thus indicating that the
interpretation of inhibitor effects should consider all the cells
of the photoreceptor layer (RPE, rods, cones) rather than an isolated
cell within a heterogenous tissue where the cellular components react
different to the radiation stimulus.

2.2.2. Cones

Cones, the photopic photoreceptors, contribute to vision during
periods of higher light intensities than do the rods. Thus, in
vertebrates exhibiting photomechanical changes, cones contract in
light and elongate in darkness. The elongation and contraction of
cones, as in rods, is via the neck-like myoid, and all three cytoskeletal elements (MTs, intermediate (10-nm)- and micro-filaments)
have been observed in cones (Fig. 7, 8; Burnside, 1976 a, 1978;
Ferrero et al., 1979; Klyne & Ali, 1980; Warren & Burnside, 1978).

The basis of the photomechanical response of cones has been
studied in greater detail than that of the rods. Inhibitor studies
colchicine, cytochalasin B) have shown that in cones, contrary to
rods, microfilaments mediate contraction (Burnside, 1976 a) while
MTs mediate elongation (Adomian & Sj strand, 1973; Anctil et al.,
1980; Burnside, 1976 a, 1978; Klyne & Ali, 1980; Warren and Burnside,
1978). The mechanisms whereby these cytoskeletal elements affect
motility is still not quite resolved. Myosin binding studies by
Burnside (1978) showed that cones contain actin filaments of opposite
polarity and suggested that contraction was due to the sliding of
two sets of oppositely directed actin filaments. The elongation
process is less clearly understood, and both the assembly/dissassembly
of MTs (Adomian & Sjöstrand) and sliding interactions between MTs
close enough to overlap (Anctil et al., 1980; Klyne & Ali, 1980;
Warren & Burnside, 1978) have been suggested as possible mechanisms.
However, the solution of these mechanisms still rests on the localization of MT organising centres (for the first proposal) and MT bridges
(for the second proposal).

Figures 10 to 13 (on following page).
Retinas of the eel (Fig. 10, 11) and the common catfish (Fig. 12,
13). Fig. 10, eel photoreceptors showing the tiered rods. Fig. 11,
high magnification of the rod myoid to show microtubules (MT). Fig.
12, Cone (C) of the common catfish. Fig. 13, high magnification of
the cone myoid to show MTs.
(C-cone; R - rod)

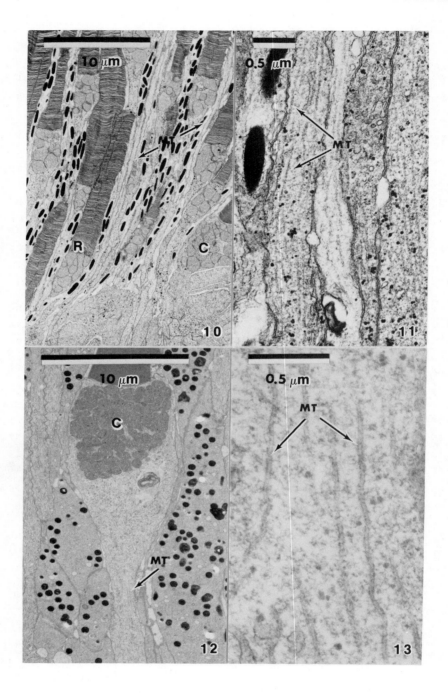

Figures 10 to 13

2.3. Other Retinal Functions Associated with MTs

Current interest in the motility aspects of the cytoskeletal elements of retinas started when Couillard (1975) suggested that the responses of photoreceptor myoids of teleost could be the result of interplay between microfilament-mediated contraction, and MT-mediated elongation; nevertheless, microfilaments and MTs may also function in support (viz. cytoskeleton) and translocation (viz. neural impulse, cytoplasmic particles, etc.).

2.3.1. Cytoskeletal Role

Il MTs functioned solely as contractile elements in photo-receptors which do not exhibit photomechanical movements, however, MTs have also been reported in these photoreceptors. The tiered rods of the eel apparently do not migrate with different light in-tensities yet MTs, in abundance, are observed within their myoids (Fig. 10, 11); likewise MTs are also present within the static cones of the walleye and the common catfish (Fig. 12, 13). It is easy to comprehend the need for support, if not in the cones then in the slender myoids of the rods. Furthermore cytoskeletal elements, including the MTs of the inner segments of photoreceptors, have been cited as contributing to the maintenance of orientation of the photo-receptor unit (Laties & Burnside, 1979).

2.3.2. Cytoplasmic Transport

An integral function of many cellular functions is the directed transport of specific components from one site within a cell to another. In many instances the presence of MTs has been associated with the movement of these components. Directed transport is not only of prime importance in the RPE, which provides metabolic support for the neural retina (Bernstein, 1961; Cohen, 1963; Dowling &

Figures 14 to 18 (on following page).
Retinal pigment epithelium of the Arctic charr (Fig. 14, 15) showing the presence of dense bodies (DB), microtubules (MT), Golgi (G) and vesicle, most likely of Golgi origin (V). Fig. 15, high magnifica-tion of Fig. 14. Fig. 16 shows the presence of coated-vesicles (V) close to the plasma membrane of the pigment epithelium cell; while Fig. 17 shows the presence of microtubule bridges (arrows-heads) between adjacent microtubules (MT) and pigment granule (PG). Fig. 18 shows the 9 + 0 doublets of the centrioles (C) of walleye photo-receptors. (TG - tight junction; BM - Bruch's membrane).

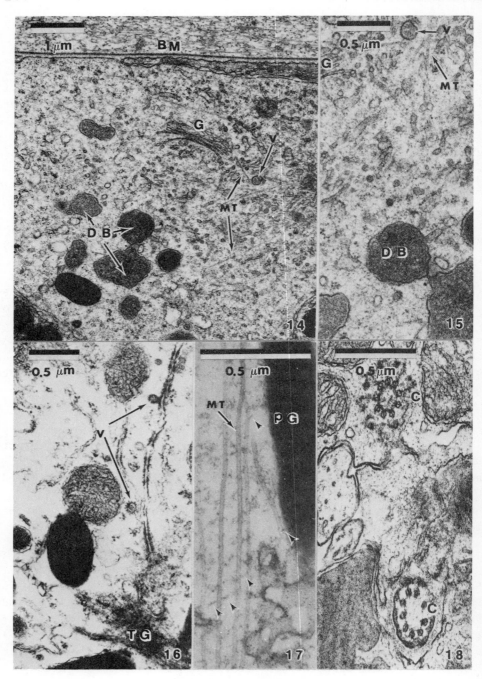

Figures 14 to 18

Gibbons, 1962; Lasansky & de Fish, 1965), but, also in the photoreceptors where sensory transduction takes place. The mechanism(s)
which MTs participate in cytoplasmic flow is complex and multifaceted;
and several theories have been advanced to explain the role of MTs
(c.f. Porter, 1966; Tucker, 1979; Weatherbee, 1981; Wuerker &
Kirkpatrick, 1972).

Schmitt (1968) proposed the "sliding vesicle theory" - a mechanism for the interaction between MTs and particles passing through
the cell; where the MT acts as a conveyor belt, as well as providing
the motive force (ATP). The discovery of dynein arms (an ATPase
protein) on the outer doublets of cilia (Gibbons & Rowe, 1965) led
to the suggestion that the function of the tubulin-dynein system
may be analogous to the actin-myosin system. Although MT-arms
(bridges) had been reported initially to be present in systems with
organized arrays of MTs (e.g. flagella, cilia) they are also present
in other cytoplasmic MTs. The exact nature of the bridges is still
unknown, however, they are thought to convey the particles along
the MTs. Particulates and organelles reported to be coupled to MTs
in this manner include: adjacent MTs (c.f. Haimo et al., 1979;
McIntosh, 1974), endoplasmic reticulum (Franke 1971), membrane-bound
vesicles (Allen, 1974, 1975), vesicle-enclosed transmitters (Schmidt,
1968; Smith, 1971; Smith et al., 1975), mitochondria (Smith et al.,
1975, 1977), 10-nm filaments (Rice et al., 1980), food vacuole membranes (c.f. Lynn, 1981). Membrane-bound vesicles located in the
RPE (Fig. 14, 15, 16) have been implicated in the metabolic functions
of the retina while in the photoreceptors they are thought to be
the means by which membranes are transported (c.f. Holtzman & Mercurio, 1980). The presence of bridge-like structures on retinal MTs
was mentioned briefly (Klyne & Ali, 1981), however, there is no
evidence against the possibility of retinal MTs transporting cytoplasmic organelles and particulates via the sliding hypothesis.
Bridge-like structures of retinal MTs of the brook trout are shown
in Fig. 17.

In additional to the above mechanism, MTs may aid in the
translocation of particulates by exerting the motive force as well
as by defining the channels through which the particles move; pigment
granules are postulated to be transported in this manner (Bikle et
al., 1966; Green, 1968; Malawista, 1971).

MTs are also thought to be implicated in sensory transduction
(Schafer & Reagan, 1981; Wueker & Kirkpatrick, 1972) because cilia

1956; Sjöstrand, 1953) and cones (De Robertis & Lasansky, 1958; Sjöstrand, 1953) have been shown to possess the 9 outer doublets; the central pair, however, is absent (Fig. 18). Here again it is not clear how MTs contribute to sensory transduction, but transduction failed to occur following treatments of colchine and vinblastine (MT poisons) (Moran & Varela, 1970, 1971). It is suggested that perhaps MTs support the plasmalemma so that deformation can occur – deformation is a basic mechanism for action potential generation (Loewenstein, 1960) –; or whether cilia themselves have an inherent potential generating capacity. Nevertheless, it is clear that MTs and tubulin are associated with the plasma membrane of cells where neuronal transmission occurs e.g. desmosomes, pre-and post-synaptic densities of membranes in synaptic junctions (c.f. Weatherbee, 1981).

3. CONCLUDING REMARKS

Due to the nature of this subject and the information presently available it would be inappropriate to make any generalisations on the roles and mechanisms of MTs in the retina. Ultrastructural and inhibitor studies clearly demonstrate that MTs are an intrisic part of the retina and necessary for its proper functioning, however the manner in which the MTs function still remains speculative. Data and ideas presented as to the properties, mode of assembly, associated enzymes, role in motility and other physiological phenomena are often conflicting; even the structure of MTs has not been explicitly resolved. Furthermore, there is often a tendency to explain cell motility on the basis of information and hypotheses emerging from the biochemistry and biology of muscle. MTs, which are often seen in intimate contact with cellular organelles, may contribute in other way(s) in addition to the sliding mechanism. For example, the polymerization-depolymerization of MTs influences the ionic concentration of the cytoplasm which can then alter the gel-sol state of the cytoplasm and hence affect motion. Thus, much more work (biochemical, morphological) still needs to be done before the role of MTs can be resolved.

It is quite clear at present that MTs are involved in the cytoskeletal (e.g. photoreceptor orientation) and motility (e.g. phagocytosis, sensory transduction, retinomotor responses) aspects of the retina. However, the exact manner in which MTs mediate these functions as yet to be resolved.

4. REFERENCES

Adomian, G.E. & Sjöstrand, F.S. (1973) Morphology of myoid elongation and shortening, J. Cell Biol., 59, 2A.

Afzelius, B.A. (1959) Electron microscopy of the sperm tail: Results obtained with a new fixative, J. Biophys. Biochem. Cytol., 5, 269-278.

Ali, M.A. (1971) Les responses retinomotrices: Caracteres et mechanismes, Vision Res., 11, 1225-1288.

Allen, R.D. (1974) Food vacuole membrane growth with microtubule-associated membrane transport in Paramecium, J. Cell Biol., 63, 904-922.

Allen, R.D. (1975) Evidence for firm linkages between microtubules and membrane-bounded vesicles, J. Cell Biol., 64, 497-503.

Anctil, M. Ali, M.A. & Couillard, P. (1980) Cone myoid elongation and rod contraction are inhibited by colchicine in trout retina, Experientia, 36, 574-575.

Baraiti, A., Jr. & Orzalesi, N. (1963) The ultrastructure of the pigment epithelium and of the photoreceptor-pigment ephitelium junction in the human retina, J.Ultrastruct. Res., 9, 484-496.

Beauchemin, M.L. & Leuenberger, P.M. (1977) Effects of cholchicine on phagosome-lysosome interaction in retinal pigment ephitelium, A. Graefes Arch. Klin. Exp. Ophthal., 203, 237-251.

Beckerle, M.C., Byers, R.H., Fujiwara, K. & Porter, K.R. (1979) Indirect immunofluorescent and stero high voltage electron microscopic evidence for microtubule-associated migration of pigment granules in erythrophores, J. Cell Biol., 83, 352a.

Berlin, R.D. (1975) Microtubules and the fluidity of the cell surface, Ann. N.Y. Acad. Sci, 253, 445-454.

Bernstein, M.H. (1961) Functional architecture of the retinal epithelium. in: "Structure of the Eye, G.K. Smelser, ed. , p. 139-150. Academic Press, New York.

Bikle, D., Tilney, L.G. & Porter, K.R. (1966) Microtubules and pigment migration in the melanophores of Fundulus heteroclitus L., Protoplasma, 61, 322-345.

Burnside, B. (1975) The form and arrangement of microtubules; an historical, primarily morphological, review, Ann. N.Y. Acad. 253, 14-16.

Burnside, B. (1976a) Microtubules and actin filaments in teleost visual cone elongation and contraction, J. Supramol Struct., 5, 257-275.

Burnside, B. (1976b) Possible roles of microtubules and actin filaments in retinal pigmented epithelium, Exp. Eye Res., 23, 257-275.

Burnside, B. (1978) Thin (actin) and (myosinlike) filaments in cone
    contraction in the teleost retina, J. Cell Biol., 78, 227-246.
Burnside, B. & Laties, A.M. (1979) Pigment migration and cellular
    contractility in the retinal pigment epithelium. in: "The
    Retinal Pigment Epithelium", K.M. Zinn & M.F. Marmor, eds.,
    Harvard University Press, Cambridge, Mass.
Burton, P.R., Hinkley, R.E. & Pierson, G.B. (1975) Tannic acid-
    -stained microtubules with 12, 13, and 15 protofilaments, J.
    Cell. Biol., 65, 227-233.
Cohen, A.I. (1963) Vertebrate retinal cells and their organization,
    Biol. Rev., 38, 427-459.
Couillard, P. (1975) Approaches to the study of contractility in
    rods and cones, in: "Vision in Fishes", M.A. Ali, ed., p.
    357-368, Plenum Press, New York.
Custer, N.V. & Bok, D. (1975) Pigment epithelium-photoreceptor in
    the normal and dystrophic rat retina, Exp. Eye Res., 21, 153-166.
De Robertis, E. (1956) Electron microscope observations on the sub-
    microscopic organization of the retinal rods, J. Biophys.
    Biochem. Cytol., 2, 319-330.
De Robertis, E. & Lasansky, A (1958) Submicroscopic organization of
    retinal cones of the rabbit, J. Biophys. Biochem. Cytol., 4,
    743-746.
Dowling, J.E. & Gibbons, I.R. (1962) The fine structure of the pig-
    ment epithelium in the albino rat, J. Cell Biol., 14, 459-474.
Dustin, P. (1978) "Microtubules". Springer-Verlag, Berlin,
    Heidelberg, New York. 452 pp.
Edelman, G. (1976) Surface modulation in cell recognition and cell
    growth, Science, 192, 218-226.
Farquhar, M. & Palade, G. (1963) Junctional complexes in various
    epithelia, J. Cell Biol., 17, 375-412.
Ferrero, E., Anctil, M. & Ali, M.A. (1979) Ultrastructural correlates
    of retinomotor responses in inner segments of vertebrate photo-
    receptors, Rev. Can. Biol., 38, 249-264.
Franke, W.W. (1971) Cytoplasmic microtubules linked to endoplasmic
    reticulum with cross-bridges, Exp. Eye Res., 66, 486-489.
Friend, D.S. & Farquhar, M.G. (1967) Functions of coated vescicles
    during protein absorption in the rat vas deferens, J. Cell Biol.,
    35, 357-376.
Futaesaku, Y., Mizuhira, V. & Nakamura, H. (1972) A new fixation
    method using tannic acid for electron microscopy and some
    observations of biological specimens, in: "Histochemistry
    and Cytochemistry", T. Takeuchi, K. Ogawa & S. Fujita, eds., p.
    155-165, Nakanishi Printing Co., Tokyo.

Gaskin, F. & Shelanski, M.L. (1976) Microtubules and intermediate filaments, Essays Biochem., 12, 115–146.

Gibbons, I.R. (1963) Studies on the protein components from cilia Tetrahymena pyriformis, Proc. Natl. Acad. Sci., 50, 1002–1010.

Gibbons, I.R. (1965) Chemical dissection of cilia, Arch. Biol., 76, 317–352.

Gibbons, I.R. & Rowe, A.J. (1965) Dynein: A protein with adenosine triphosphates activity from cilia. Science 149: 424–426.

Goldman, R.D., Pollard, T. & Rosenbaum, J. (Eds) (1976) "Cell Motility", Cold Spring Harbor, New York.

Goodenough, D.A. & Revel, J.P. (1970) A fine structural analysis of intercellular junctions in the mouse liver, J. Cell Biol., 45, 272–290.

Green, L. (1968) Mechanism of movements of granules in melanocytes of Fundulus heteroclitus, Proc. Natl. Acad. Sci., 59, 1179–1186.

Haimo, L.T., Telzer, B.R. & Rosenbaum, J.L. (1979) Dynein binds to and cross-bridges cytoplasmic microtubules, Proc. Natl. Acad. sci., 76, 5759–5763.

Heggeness, M., Simon, M. & Singer, S.J. (1968) Association of mitochondria with microtubules in cultured cells, Proc. Natl. Acad. Sci., 75, 3863–3866.

Heiniger, H.J. & Marshall, J.D. (1979) Pinocytosis in L cells: Its dependence on membrane sterol and the cytoskeleton, Biol. Int. Rev., 3, 409–420.

Hollyfield, J.G. & Ward, A. (1974a) Phagocytic activity in the retinal pigment epithelium of the frog Rana pipiens. I. Uptake of polystyrene spheres, J. Ultrastruct. Res., 46, 327–338.

Hollyfield, J.G. & Ward, A. (1974b) Phagocytic activity in the retinal pigment epithelium of the frog Rana pipiens. II. Exclusion of Saraner subflava, J. Ultrastruct. Res., 46, 339–350.

Holtzman, E. (1976) Lysosomes: A survey. Cell Biology Monographs, Vol. 3, 298 pp., Springer-Verlag, Wein, New York.

Holtzman, E. & Mercurio, A.M. (1980) Membrane circulation in neurons and photoreceptors: Some unresolved issues, Int. Rev. Cytol., 67, 1–67.

Klyne, M.A. & Ali, M.A. (1980) Retinomotor responses: Role of microtubules, Mikroskopie, 36, 199–210.

Klyne, M.A. & Ali, M.A. (1981) Microtubules and 10 nm-filaments in the retinal pigment epithelium during the diurnal light-dark cycle, Cell Tissue Res., 214, 397–405.

Lasansky, A. & de Fisch, F.W. (1965) Studies on the function of the pigment epithelium in relation to ionic movement between retina and choroid, in: "The structure of the Eye", II Symposium, J.W.

Rhoen, ed., p. 139-144, Schattauer, Stuttgart.

Laties, A.M. & Burnside, B. (1979) The maintenance of photoreceptor orientation, in: "Motility in Cell Function", Proceedings of the First John M. Marshall Symposium in Cell Biology. F.A. Pepe, J.W. Sanger & V.T. Nachmias, eds., p. 285-298.

Ledbetter, M.C. & Porter, K.R. (1964) Morphology of microtubules of plant cells, Science, 144, 872-874.

Loewenstein, W.R. (1960) Biological transducers. Sci. Am. 203 (2): 98-108.

Luby, K.J. & Porter, K.R. (1980) The control of pigment migration in isolated erythrophores of Holocentus ascensionis (Osbeck). I. Energy requirements, Cell, 21, 13-23.

Luduena, R.E., Shooter, R.M. & Wilson, L. (1977) Structure of the tubulin dimers, J. Cell Biol., 252, 7006-7014.

Lynn, D.H. (1981) The organization and evolution of microtubular organelles in ciliated protozoa, Biol. Rev., 56, 243-292.

Malawista, S.E. (1971) The melanocyte model, J. Cell Biol., 49, 848-855.

Malawista, S.E. (1975) Microtubules and the mobilization of lysosomes in phagocytizing human leukocytes, Ann. N.Y. Acad. Sci., 253, 738-749.

Mandelkow, E.M. & Mandelkow, E. (1979) Junctions between microtubule walls, J. Mol. Biol., 129, 135-148.

Mandelkow, E., Thomas, J & Cohen, C. (1977) Microtubule structure at low resolution by X-ray diffraction, Proc. Natl. Acad. Sci., 74, 3370-3374.

Markham, R., Frey, S. & Hills, G.J. (1963) Methods for the enhancement of image detail and accentuation of structure in electron microscopy, Virol., 20, 88-102.

Matsusaka, T. (1967) The intracytoplasmic channel in pigment epithelial cells of the chick retina, Z. Zellforsch., 81, 100-113.

Meza, I., Ibarra, G., Sabanero, M., Martinez-Palomo, A. & Cereijido, M. (1980) Occluding junctions and cytoskeleton components in a cultured transporting epithelium, J. Cell Biol., 87, 746-754.

McIntosh, J.R. (1974) Bridges between microtubules, J. Cell Biol., 61, 166-187.

Mohri, H. (1976) The function of tubulin in motile systems, Biochim., Biophys. Acta, 456, 85-127.

Moran, D.T. & Varela, F.G. (1970) Microtubules and sensory transduction, J. Cell Biol., 47, 145a.

Moran, D.T. & Varela, F.G. (1971) Microtubules and sensory transduction, Proc. Natl. Acad. Sci., 68, 757-760.

Moyer, F.H. (1969) Development structure, and function of the retinal pigmented epithelium, in: "The Retina: Morphology, Function and

Clinical Characteristics", B.R. Straatsma, M.O. Hall, R.A. Allen & F. Crescitelli, eds. p. 1-30, Univ. Calif. Press, Berkley and Los Angeles.

Murphy, D.B. & Tilney, L.B. (1974) The role of microtubules in the movement of pigment granules in teleost melanphores, J. Cell Biol., 61, 757-779.

Murray, R.L. & Dubin, M.W. (1975) The occurrence of actinlike filaments in association with migrating pigment in frog retinal pigment epithelium, J. Cell Biol., 64, 705-710.

Nagano, T. & Suzuki, F. (1975) Microtubules with 15 subunits in cockroach epidermal cells, J. Cell Biol., 64, 242-245.

O'Connor, P. & Burnside, B.(1981). Actin dependent cell elongation in teleost retinal rods: Requirement for actin filament assembly, J. Cell Biol., 89, 517-524.

Olmsted, J.B. & Borisy, G.G. (1973) Microtubules, Ann. Rev. Biochem., 42, 507-540.

Porter, K.R. (1966) Cytoplasmic microtubules and their functions, in: "Principles of Bimolecular Organization", Ciba Found Symp. 1965, G.E.W. Wolstenholme & M. O'Connor, eds., p. 306-336, J. & A. Churchill Ltd., London.

Porter, K.R. & Yamada, E. (1960) Studies on the endoplasmic reticulum. V. Its form and differentiation in pigment epithelial cells of the frog retina, J. Biophys. Biochem. Cytol., 8, 181-205.

Rice, R.V., Roslansky, P.F., Pascoe, N. & Houghton, S.M. (1980) Bridges between microtubules and neurofilaments visualized by stereoelectron microscopy, J. Ultrastruct. Res., 71, 303-310.

Roberts, K & Hyams, J.S. (Eds.) (1979) Microtubules, Academic Press, London, Toronto, 595 pp.

Sakai, H. (1980) Regulation of microtubule assembly in vitro, Biomed. Res., 1, 359-375.

Schafer, R. & Reagan, P.D. (1981) Colchicine reversibly inhibits electrical activity in Arthropod mechanoreceptors, J. Neurobiol., 12, 155-166.

Schliwa, M. & Bereiter-Hahn, J. (1973) Pigment movements in fish melanophores: morphological and physiological studies. III. The effect of colchicine and vinblastine, Z. Zellforsch., 147, 127-148.

Schmitt, F.O. (1968) Fibrous proteins - neuronal organelles, Proc. Natl. Acad. Sci., 60, 1092-1101.

Silverstein, S.C., Steinman, R.M. & Cohn, Z.A. (1977) Endocytosis, Ann. Rev. Biochem., 46, 669-722.

Simson, J.V. & Spicer, S.S. (1970) Activities of specific cell constituents in phagocytosis (endocytosis), Int. Rev. Exp. Pathol., 12, 79-118.

Sjöstrand F.S. (1953). The ultrastructure of the inner segments of the retinal rods of the guinea pig eye as revealed by electon microscopy, J. Cell Comp. Physiol., 42, 45-70.

Smith D.S. (1971). On the significance of cross bridges between microtubules and synaptic vesicles. Philos. Trans. RI Soc. Lond. Ser. B Biol Sci., 261, 395-405.

Smith D.S., Jarlfors U. & Cameron B.F. (1975). Morphological evidence for the participation of microtubules in axonal transport, Ann. N.Y. Acad. Sci., 253, 472-506.

Smith D.S., Jarlfors U., Cayer M. & Cameron B.F. (1977). Structural cross-bridges between microtubules and mitochondria in central axons of an insect (Periplaneta americana), J. Cell Sci, 27, 255-272.

Soifer D. (Ed.) (1975). The Biology of Cytoplasmic Microtubules, Ann. N.Y. Acad. Sci., New York. Vol. 253, 848 pp.

Stephens R.E. (1975). Structural chemistry of the axoneme: Evidence for chemically and functionally unique tubulin dimers in outer fibers, in: "Molecules and Cell Movement", S. Inoué & R.E. Stephens eds., pp. 181-206, Raven Press, New York.

Strossel T.P. (1974). Phagocytosis. Part II, N. Eng. J. Med., 290, 774-780.

Summers, K.E. & Gibbons, I.R.(1971). Adenosine triphosphate-induced sliding of tubules in trypsin-treated flagella of sea urchin sperm, Proc. Natl. Acad. Sci., 68, 3092-3096.

Takeuchi I.K. & Takeuchi Y.K. (1979). Intermediate filaments in the retinal pigment epithelial cells of the goldfish, J. Electron. Microsc., 28, 134-137.

Tilney L.G., Bryan J., Bush D.J., Fujiwara K., Mooseker M.S., Murphy D.B. & Snyder D.H. (1973). Microtubules: Evidence for 13 protofilaments, J. Cell Biol., 59, 267-275.

Tucker J.B. (1979). Spatial organization of microtubules, in: Microtubules. K. Roberts & J.S. Hyams eds., pp. 315-357, Academic Press, London.

Walls G.L. (1942). The Vertebrate Eye. Hafner Publishing Co., New York.

Warren R.H. & Burnside B. (1978). Microtubules in cone myoid elongation in the teleost retina, J. Cell Biol., 78, 247-259.

Weatherbee J.A. (1981). Membranes and cell movement: Interactions of membranes with proteins of the cytoskeleton, Int. Rev. Cytol. Suppl., 12, 113-176.

Weissman G., Goldstein I., Hoffstein S. & Tsung P. (1975). Reciprocal effects of cAMP and cGMP on microtubule-dependent release of lysosomal enzymes, Ann. N.Y. Acad. Sci., 253, 750-762.

Wessells N.K. & Evans J. (1968). Bundles of microfilaments encircling the cell apex have been found in association with junctions in developing pancreatic cells, Dev. Biol., 17, 413-446.

Wilson L. & Bryan J. (1974). Biochemical and pharmacological properties of microtubules, Adv. Cell Mol. Biol., 3, 21-72.

Wuerker R.B. & Kirkpatrick J.B. (1972). Neuronal microtubules, neurofilaments, and microfilaments, Int. Rev. Cytol., 33, 45-75.

Young R.W. (1971). Shedding of discs from rod outer segments in the Rheseus monkey, J. Ultrastruct. Res., 34, 190-213.

Younk R.W. & Bok D. (1969). Participation of the retinal pigment epithelium in the rod outer segment renewal process., J. Cell Biol., 42, 392-403.

A QUANTITATIVE STUDY ON SYNAPTIC RIBBONS IN THE PHOTORECEPTORS OF TURTLE AND FROG

R.L. Pierantoni[*] and G.D. McCann

California Institute of Technology, Bio-Information
System 286-80 Pasadena 91125 California U.S.A.

Since their discovery and correct description Siøstrand (1953 a, 1953 b), Carasso (1957) synaptic ribbons have been found ubiquitously in the vertebrate nervous system. They are present in the outer plexiform layer of the retina at the junctions between the photo-receptors and the second order neurons: Siøstrand (1953 a, 1953 b), Carasso (1957), Siøstrand (1958), Ladman (1958), Lanzavecchia (1960), Cohen (1960), Fine (1962), Kidd (1962), Cohen (1963), Evans (1966), Matsusaka (1957), Foos (1969), Gray (1971), Fisher (1974), Gray (1976), Siøstrand (1974). In the inner plexiform layer of the retina at the junctions between the bipolar cells and the third order neurons: Kidd (1962), Goodland (1966), Witkowsky (1973), Wong-Riley (1974). In the organs of the lateral line of fishes: Bartes (1962), Flock (1965), Derbin (1969), Mullinger (1969), Hama (1977). In the lateral line of the salamander: Jorghensen (1973). In the inner ear hair cells: Smith (1961). In the pineal gland at the pynealocyte synapse: Hopsu (1964), Kelly (1965), Wollrath (1973), Nulty (1980). Ribbon-like structures have been described in the chick ciliary ganglion: De Lorenzo (1960), the visual system of the fly: Burkardt (1976) and in the giant synapse of the squid: Martin (1975).

Some characteristics of the synaptic ribbons (SRs) may be taken as specific of these intracellular organelles: the proximity to a pre-synaptic membrane, the association with synaptic vesicles

---

*Permanent address: Istituto di Cibernetica e Biofisica del C.N.R.
16032 Camogli, Genova - Italy.

(SVs), the biochemical affinity for osmium and permanganate, the digestion with proteolytic enzymes.

The present study will concern only the SRs located in the outer plexiform layer of the retina of the frog and the turtle. The rod-like aspect of the SR, as it appears on the ultra-thin sections, had initially deceived the observer (Siøstrand, 1953 a) but soon their lamellar structure was recognized Siøstrand, 1953 b; Carasso, 1957). The actual shape of the SR can be reconstructed only using serial sections encompassing the whole object and taking in consideration that the image on the micrograph is the geometrical projection on the section plane of an object contained in the section itself. Siøstrand (1958) was the first to measure both the surface area and the thickness of the SRs. Table I summarized the available information on Srs dimensions and shape.

The classic study in three-dimensional reconstruction of the photoreceptor synaptic terminal in the rabbit (Siøstrand, 1974) does not provide quantitative data on SRs morphology.

An interesting point is the inner structure of the ribbon itself. Matsusaka (1967) describes a penta-laminar structure: two external layers (dark 20-25 A°), two internal lines (light 70 A°) and a central line (dark 20 A°). Cohen (1963) has shown the dependance of the laminar structure from the fixation-staining procedure. With lead stain the SRs exhibit two external dark profiles and a central light region. Permanganate fixation produces a pentalaminar structure, however. Furthermore, the ribbon thickness seems to be affected by the fixation procedure as well: osmium fixation gives a value of 250-300 A° whilst permanganate raises this value to 450 A°.

A not yet settled problem concerns the cytological site of origin of the SRs within the photoreceptor. They have been followed during the pre-natal and embryological stages in many animals. Table II gives some information on this subject.

From the above observations summarized in Table II it should be inferred a non-membranal origin of the Srs. This has been challenged by Spadaro et al. (1978) who maintain a membranal origin of the ribbon, at least in the albino rat. These authors suggest that the SRs will take origin from an unfolding of the plasmalemma. Grün (1980), on the other hand, maintains a cytoplasmic origin of the SRs in Xaenopus and Tilapia. According to this author the SRs appear very early in the cytoplasm with a characteristic "drop-

Table I

Surface area of completely reconstructed synaptic ribbons

Animal	Organ	Dimensions (in micron)	Thickness	Author
Guinea Pig	O.P.L.	2.3 x 0.2	350 A°	Siøstrand (1958)
Cat	I.P.L.	0.1 x 0.2	200/400 A°	Kidd (1962)
Human	O.P.L.	max length 1.4	270/290 A°	Foos (1969)
Salamander	Lateral. line	Diameter 0.7		Jorghenses (1973)

Table II

Early appearence and cytological locations of synaptic ribbons during embryogenesis

Animal	Early appearance	Cytological location	Organ	Author
Chick	15/17 days after fec.	Near the triadic compl.	Retina	McLaughlin (1976)
Chick	16 days after fecund.	Terminal cytoplasm	Retina	Meller (1977)
Chick	17 days after fecund.	Terminal cytoplasm	Retina	
	18 days after fecund.	Contact with plasmalemma	Retina	Meller (1964)
Mouse	2nd post natal day	Perinuclear region (morphological precursors)	O.P.L.	
	7th post natal day	association with the plasmalemma	O.P.L.	
	10th post natal day	Ribbon synapse	I.P.L.	Olney (1968)
Rat	6th post natal day	Perinuclear region (morphological precursor)	O.P.L.	
	7th post natal day	Triadic complex	O.P.L.	
	8th post natal day	Triadic complex completed	I.P.L.	Weidman (1969)
Mouse	4th post natal day	Terminal cytoplasm	O.P.L.	Blancks (1974)
Rabbit	0 day (birth)	Perinuclear region	Retina	
	3rd day	Contact with the plasmal.	O.P.L.	
	9th day	Ribbon synapse complete	I.P.L.	McArdle (1977)
Primate	76th day of gestation	Perinuclear region (morphological precursors)	O.P.L.	
	80th day of gestation	Intermediate position between the nucleus and the plasmalemma	O.P.L.	Smealser (1974)

shaped" appearance and with an occasional tendency to branch. We
have observed, in the turtle after 48 hrs of continuous illumination a very similar morphology and, in the inner plexiform layer,
cases of abortive branches in bipolar ribbons.

The function of the SRs is still controversial. Almost simultaneously Gray and Pease (1971) and Bunt (1971) put forward an
hypothesis on the SRs function. Their hypothesis may be named the
"conveyor belt" hypothesis. According to this suggestion the SRs
convey the SVs to the plasmalemma in "an orderly fashion". Gray
and Pease enriched their hypothesis with an interpretation of the
arciphorm density (a densely stained portion of the plasmalemma
facing the synaptic edge of the ribbon). According to Gray and
Pease this arciphorm density will detach the SVs away from the SR
surface. In fact, the SVs closer to the arciphorm density appear
in a different geometrical relatioship with the SR and this was
interpreted as an intermediate stage of the detachment from the SR
surface. On the order hand Bunt added to her hypothesis the valua-
ble information that SRs are digested by the enzymes of the pronase
family. The "conveyor-belt hypothesis" was not shared by Osborne
and Thornhill (1972) who observed how the reserprine and the gua-
netidine, both known to deplete the mono-amine reservoires, reduce
the staining properties of the SRs in the inner ear of the bullfrog.
These authors interpret their results as an evidence that SRs (more
precisely synaptic bars) are actually mono-amine reservoires. The
SVs, according to this hypothesis, will crowd around the SR to load
themselves with the transmitter accumulated into the SR.

Another series of observations on ribbon modifications under
different illumination conditions has been published recently:
Wagner (1973), Wagner and Ali (1977). According to these authors,
in the trout, the dimensions and the number of the SRs decrease
dramatically during the dark adaptation state. Spadaro (1978) has
shown a similar chronobiological pattern in the SRs populations of
the albino rats. Other observations on this line concern the fate
of the SRs during hibernation in the ground squirrel. The ribbon
morphology, under these conditions, is very close to the image
obtained from immature animals and sometimes the SRs appear decom-
posed in thin parallel sub-units (Remé and Young, 1977). In reti-
nitis pigmentosa in man, Szamier and Bersen (1977) have shown SRs
strongly reduced both in dimension and in number and freely floating
in the perinuclear region.

Another point of interest concerns the spatial relationships between SRs and SVs. Since the early observations SRs were described as surrounded by an "halo" of synaptic vesicles. This association between SRs and SVs establishes itself quite early in the embryogenesis. Measurements on SVs concentration in the peri-ribbon regions are already available: Pierantoni (1978, 1979, 1980). These finding will be discussed later in detail. The actual site of contact between the SR surface and the SVs of the "first row" has been studied using the EPTA-staining by McLaughlin and Bodkins 1977). These authors have been able to show some "cup-like" projections covering the ribbon lateral surface. These elements may play an important role in establishing the relative positions between the vesicles and the ribbon surface. Finally, it must be remembered that in the receptor terminal is always present a complex network of neuro-filaments. Gray (1976), using his fixation method involving the albumin has been able to evidentiate clearly this network. The filaments are clearly associated with the SVs but their points of contact with the SRs remain problematic. Similar networks have been described by Glees and Spoerri (1977) and Loves (1971), but in these cases as well the ribbon-filaments relationships are not clear. In general, the common belief is that the neuro-filaments network helps the SVs to find their way to the SRs.

From the above reviewed material it results very clearly the need for new quantitative information on SRs structure, dimensions, location and their relationships with SVs and the post-synaptic thickening (PST).

In particular this study will provide information on these subjects: "Complete tri-dimensional reconstruction of SRs in frog and turtle", "Analysis of two extreme dark-light adaptation conditions on SR morphology", "Quantitative analysis of the SVs population in close contact with the ribbon and in regions remote from it", "A qualitative model explaining the basic morphology of the concentration gradients of the SVs around the SR", "An interpretation of the SRs function related to the analysis of the synaptic noise power spectrum".

MATERIAL AND METHODS

Eyes of the turtle (Emis scripta) and frog (Rana catesbeiana) were enucleated, their retinae isolated and processed routinery for electron microscopy (3% gluaralehyde in phosphate buffer, post-fixation in 1% osmium, stain in block, cut in serial sections). The

explored area was in the region of the central disk. Only cone
pedicles were studied.

The electronmicrographs were digitalised using the image processing program developed in our laboratory. The image processing
involved basically the following steps:
1) Tracing the micrographs with a Tektronik magnetic tablet.
2) Digitalization of selected profiles: plasmalemma, post-synaptic
   thickenings, ribbons and synaptic vesicles coordinates.
3) Building of a set of polygonal surfaces connecting one section
   with the next one.
4) Visualization at a Comptal Color-TV terminal of the reconstructed
   objects.

This step was accomplished through and interactive program
setting the positions of the viewer, the object and the source of
"light". Other variables were elaborated at this stage of the image
processing: the reflectance qualities of the built surface, the
position of the primary and secondary shadows and the colours of
the surfaces.

5) Quantitative evaluation of geometrical parameters associated with
   the reconstructed objects: surface area, perimeter, volume,
   radium of curvature of profiles and similar data.

RESULTS

The ribbon geometry and the vesicles of the "first row"

It is convenient, at beginning, to study the ribbon geometry
independently from its relationships with other elements. In frog
and turtle the SRs are never contained in a single section as a
consequence of their twisting and turning according to the local
geometry of plasmalemma. In the cases in which the whole SR has
been reconstructed the following statements may be made.

A) Ribbons never branch. This quite obvious statement reflects the
   yet unknown dynamics of the SR growth which takes place on a
   plane without branchings.
B) Ribbons have sharp edges. In many instances, in fact, the whole
   ribbon disappears in a single section. Considering that the
   largest dimension of a SR may attain 2 microns in length this
   is a clear indication of a very sharp ribbon edge. This structure suggests a crystal-like structure of the ribbon inner matrix.

C) Ribbons have a constant thickness. In our case the SRs have a constant thickness of 350 A°. The SR surface, when seen in tangential sections, does not reveal fine details about its inner structure, but an indirect information on ribbon surface geometry may come from a close analysis of the SVs distribution on the SR face. In a good tangential section they appear to be distributed according to an exagonal lattice (see Fig. 1 and Fig. 2). This geometrical distribution may be passive consequence of spherical particles on a surface but, in another instance, may depend from an inner regularity of the surface itself housing the vesicles only at given places. A classical arrangement of this kind is the so called "presynaptic grid" (Akert, 1969).

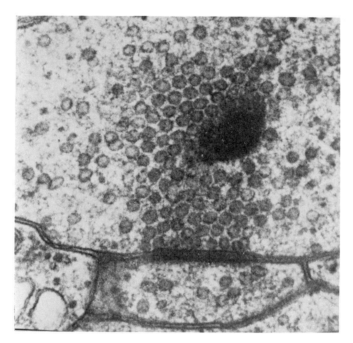

Fig. 1.   Synaptic ribbon in a bipolar terminal (turtle). The quasi-tangential section allows to see the exagonal lattice of the synaptic vesicles. Note the non-tangential contact between adjacent vesicles. The dark area is the portion of the synaptic ribbon present in the section.

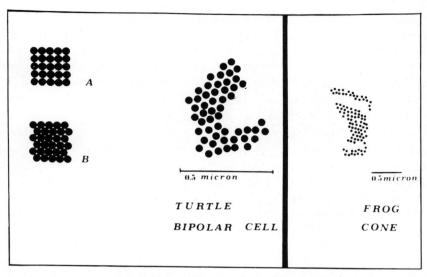

Fig. 2.   In A and B are represented two possible lattices. The two
          drawings on the right represent the actual distribution of
          the synaptic vesicles in two cases: a bipolar cell (turtle)
          and a cone (frog). The exagonal lattice is present in both
          cases.

D) Synaptic ribbons, in turtle and frog, tend to have rectangular
   shapes. We call A the surface area, a, the longer side and b
   the shorter one. Some measurements of A, a and b are listed
   below. Frog, cone, light condition non controllated:
   A = 1.048 micron^2 ± 0.26   a, b, values not available N=6
   Turtle, cone, 48 hrs continuous illumination:
   A = 0.542 micron^2 ± 0.19   a = 1.16 micron ± 0.6
                                        b = 0.44 micron ± 0.03   N=22
   Turtle, cone, 48 hrs continuous darkness:
   A = 0.264 micron^2 ± 0.09   a = 0.80 micron ± 0.7
                                        b = 0.27 micron ± 0.03   N=17
   a/b = 2.99 in the dark - a/b = 2.89 in the light.
   The above data on ribbon geometry show the effect on the SRs di-
   mensions by the light conditions.
E) Dark adaptation reduces the average surface area of the SR to an
   half of the value measured after 48 hrs of continuously illumination. The ribbon geometry is not affected, however. In fact,
   the a/b ratio is identical in the two states of adaptation (see
   Fig. 3). An interesting point is the statistical distribution

of the lengths of the short and the long side of the rectangle.
The distribution of the length of the short sides (b) is much
more uniform than the length of the long ones (a). The standard
deviation on b measurement gives: in the dark 0.7 and in the light
0.6. While for the long side a the standard deviation is much
lower and identical under the two conditions 0.03. This suggests
a quite different growth strategy for the two sides.

F) Side a (the longer one) attains a wider spectrum of values than
side b. It may be remembered that side b is the shorter distance
travelled by a synaptic vesicle on the SR surface and which is
bound to the synaptic edge. The large difference in scattering
of the data between the a and b population indicates that the
growth along the b direction is under the strict control of a
limiting factor which, apparently, does not influence the growth
along the a direction.

G) The SVs closer to the synaptic edge of the SR are in tangential
contact with its surface, the other ones are separated from the

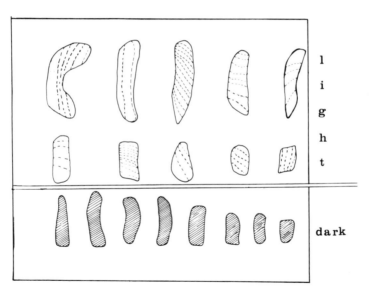

Fig. 3.   This figure shows 10 synaptic ribbons after 48 hrs of light
          (turtle). The smaller dimensions of the dark-adapted rib-
          bons is obvious. The dotted lines crossing the light-
          adapted ribbons indicate the shape assumed by each ribbon
          after section, e.g. the first light-adapted ribbon has been
          reconstructed from 7 consecutive sections, the second one
          was contained, instead, in only three sections.

ribbon surface by a claireance of about 400 A°. From the early
observations, an "halo" of synaptic vesicles has been observed
flanking the ribbon on both sides. Fig. 4 gives a conventional
representation of the ribbon/vesicle system. A more detailed
representation of the system may be observed in Fig. 5. Here
the distance between the SVs of the first row and the SR surface
is plotted against the SR length. The distance, or claireance,
between the two association modes is quite sharp. It may be
suggested that a supra-molecular substrate, not stainable with
our procedure, keeps the SVs away from the SR surface. The
absence of this "supra-molecular structure" at the synaptic edge
of the SR may be accounted for the tangential contact between
SVs and SR at this site. The "cup-like" projections stained by
McLaughlin (1977) with the EPTA staining may be the hypothised
structure which keeps away the SVs from the SR surface. When,
instead, the SR is seen "en face", it is possible to locate with

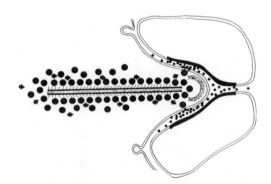

Fig. 4.   A conventional representation of a ribbon synapse. The
           small arrows indicate the probable direction of motion of
           the synaptic vesicles associated with the ribbon. The
           short segments attached to the ribbon are nothing else but
           a visual metaphor of a possible transport mechanisms
           associated with the ribbon. The smaller dots into the
           synaptic cleft suggest the diffusional area of the trans-
           mitter. Please note the tangential contact between the
           ribbon and the synaptic vesicles closer to the ribbon
           synaptic edge.

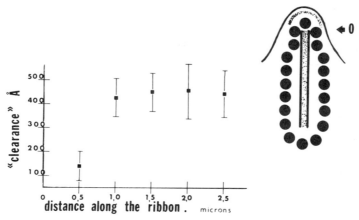

Fig. 5. The diagram shows the distance (in A°) of the synaptic
         vesicles from the synaptic ribbon surface plotted in func-
         tion of the ribbon length. The origin of the ribbon is
         the synaptic edge (see the insert on the right). Note the
         sudden change in the value of the distance at about 0.75
         microns from the synaptic edge (frog, cone).

great precision each SV on its surface. Fig. 2 gives two examples
of such a distribution, but an important point has to be made now.

H) The SVs are not in tangential contact one with another but each
   one is surrounded by an empty space. In few words: the overall
   geometry is an exagonal array of spheres separated from their
   neighbours by a distance greater than their diameter. Assuming
   for the SV a radium of about 400 A° it is possible to calculate
   the maximum number of SVs arranged in an exagonal and in a
   tangential rectangular pattern on a plane. Exagonal simmetry
   = 1297 vesicles/micron^2 (calc.), rectangular simmetry = 1190
   vesicles/micron^2 turtle, cone, 48 hrs light = 657 vesicles/micron^2
   (measur.), turtle, cone 48 hrs dark = 1060 vesicles/micron^2
   (measur.). It is possible to see that, under both experimental
   conditions, the SV concentration is far below the maximum. This
   finding suggests that the SVs are repelling each other at some
   extent or that the SR houses them at certain evenly distributed
   sites. It is impossible, on our data alone, to give an answer
   to this question but may be remembered here the results of Ohsawa
   et al. (1981). These authors have shown that the SVs, in the
   rat superior cervical ganglion, are associated with a coloumbian
   repulsive field and all the SVs are negatively charged.

I) Synaptic vesicle concentration on the SR surface is greater in
the dark and attains an higher degree of order. In only few
cases the quite cumbersome procedure of the reconstruction of
the SR together with its associated first row of vesicles has
been accomplished. Fig. 6 shows one of such reconstructions.
The SR (turtle, cone, 48 hrs of continuos illumination) has been
represented on both sides to show the distribution of the SVs on
the two "faces". The whole ribbon was contained in seven consecutive sections. The SVs are distributed, on the SR surface,
in a very irregular fashion with extensive empty spaces and
occasional clusters. Furthermore, there is a visible difference
in SV concentration on the two faces: face "b", which is the
richer one in SV, is the one which "looks" at cytoplasm, whilst
the face "a", closer to the plasmalemma, is poorer in SV density.
The SV concentration changes under different illumination con-

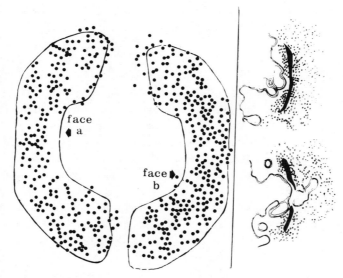

Fig. 6. The insert on the right shows two drawings of two consec-
         utive sections of the same ribbon. On the left the complete
         ribbon, together with the population of the synaptic vesi-
         cles of the first row. Face a looks at the plasmalemma
         whilst face b looks at the cytoplasm. The synaptic edge
         is the concave one. Note the irregular distribution of
         the synaptic vesicles on the ribbon faces (turtle, cone,
         light-adapted).

ditions. Fig. 7 shows three cases for each state of adaptation.
It is obvious the greater order of the vesicle distribution in
the dark adapted state. After 48 hrs of continuous illumination,
on the order hand, the SV distribution appears coarser and much
less orderly.

Spatial distribution of synaptic vesicles around the ribbon

We will deal here with the vesicle population immediately
surrounding the ribbon but not in direct contact with it. The high
vesicle concentration at the SR surface has attracted the attention
more than the study of spatial structure of the population at greater
distances. We have studied such distribution calculating the local
vesicle concentration (number of vesicles/micron^2). The results
are shown in Fig. 8. It is evident that the concentration reaches
its maximum at the SR surface, but, if we move away from it along
a direction normal to the surface we encounter a clear minimum at
0.3 microns of distance from the SR. At distances greater than
0.3 microns the value of concentration rises again to level off
eventually to an intermediate value. These data have been obtained

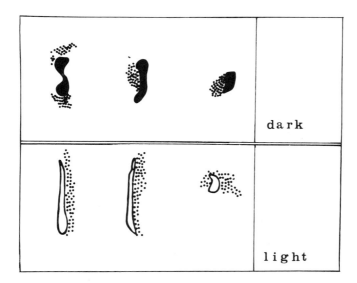

dark

light

Fig. 7. The figure shows six cases of synaptic vesicles distribution in the two adaptation states. These are not complete
reconstructions of synaptic ribbons but just drawings of
single sections. The higher density and order of the
synaptic vesicles in the dark adaptation is evident.

from 70 fully reconstructed SRs in the frog cones. It should be
noted, however, that the depletion belt is immediately recognizable
after a coarse inspection of the micrographs. The spatial distribution of the SVs has been calculated along a direction parallel to
the cytoplasmic edge of the SR (turtle, cone, light and dark adaptation states).

In all the cases the maximum of the concentration is attained
along the ribbon edge and falls outside its boundaries. The values
of the SVs concentration are very different in the two adapting
states: 16 SV/O. 1 $micron^2$ in the dark and only 6 SV/O. 1 $micron^2$
in the dark and only 6 SV/O. 1 $micron^2$ in the light (see Fig. 9).

Spatial vesicles distribution away from the ribbon

In region far away from the "ribbon field" the SVs show a more
homogeneous distribution. In three cases in which the whole pedicle
has been reconstructed we have observed a marked belt of reduced
SV concentration along the plasmalemma border and, in the more
central portion of the terminal, the SV population shows also very
interesting clusters and depletion zones. See Fig. 10 to have an
idea of the spatial distribution of the SVs in a terminal. The local
concentration of the SVs is represented by isoclynes whose density
is proportional to the local SV density. Fig. 11, instead, shows
the same area but according to a different visual rendering of the
data: a pseudo-perspective view. The total count of the SVs contained in the whole pedicle is 250.000.

Plasmalemma modifications in different adaptation states

Schaeffer and Raviola (1976, 1977) have noted a dramatic
"response" of the plasmalemma to dark adaptation state. According
to these authors, dark induces an invagination of the SR into the
plasmalemma foldings and, on the contrary, light causes a general
flattening of the membrane with consequent "extrusion" of the SR.
The Schaeffer and Raviola data did not receive an adequate morpho-
metric treatment and they do not appear to come from the analysis
of serial reconstructions. We tried to fill this little gap using
our material. We measured, section by section, the total length
of the plasmalemma of a pedicle and the length of a straight line
connecting the two extremes of the plasmalemma profile. The two
extremes A and B of the straight line (which are of course also the
extremes of the plasmalemma portions measured) have been established
in a quite standard way as the two points, where, in that section,

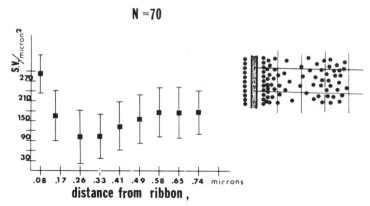

Fig. 8.   The figure represents the relationships between the synaptic
          vesicles concentration (number of synaptic vesicles/micron^2)
          and the distance from the ribbon. The insert on the right
          shows the graphical procedure. The data have been obtained
          from 70 completely reconstructed ribbons (frog, cone).

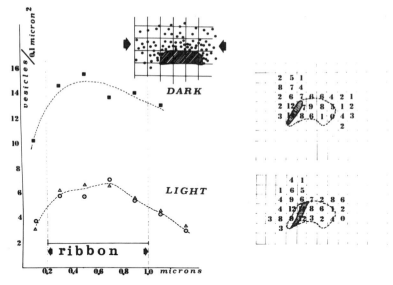

Fig. 9.   Synaptic vesicles concentration measured along a direction
          parallel to the cytoplasmic edge of ribbon under the two
          adaptation states. See the inserts above and on the right
          which show the procedure. In particular the insert on the
          right shows two consecutive sections of the same ribbon:
          the figures give the number of synaptic vesicles present
          into the squares (turtle, cone, dark and light adaptation).

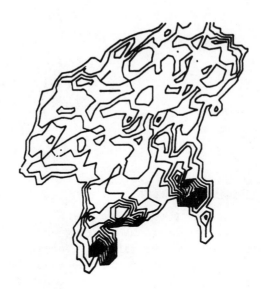

Fig. 10. Computer hard copy showing the synaptic vesicles concentra-
         tion over a section of a cone pedicle (turtle). The iso-
         clynes density gives the local concentration of synaptic
         vesicles. The two "ribbon fields" are immediately recogniz-
         able at the bottom of the pedicle profile.

the pedicle "touches" the adjacent Müller cells. Fig. 12 shows the
procedure. This method allows to measure the relative value of the
folding of the plasmalemma under the two extreme experimental conditions. A sensible parameter is the ratio between the total plasmalemma length and the A-B distance along the straight line. The
average value for this ratio gives 3.67 for the dark and 2.10 for
the light. The difference in value between the two ratios gives a
convincing evidence about the correct interpretation given by
Schaeffer and Raviola.

Geometrical relationships between ribbon and the post-synaptic
thickning

     A morphological characteristic of the second-order post-synaptic
dendritic terminal is the presence of the post-synaptic thickening
(PST). This modification of the dendritic terminal appears as a
thicker line bordering, from the inside, the profile for a portion
of this lenght (Pfenninger, 1978). In the case of the ribbon synapse this structure is readily recognizable and shows a kind of
proportionality with the dimensions of the SR itself. In some cases

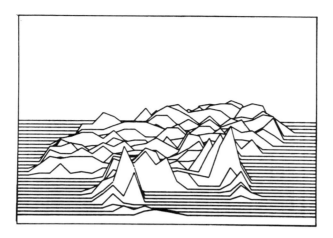

Fig. 11. The same data as Fig. 10 but displayed according to a
"bird-view" perspective. Again, the two mountains in the
foreground are two "ribbon field". The "sea" represents
the extracellular space where the synaptic vesicle concentration is zero. Note how low in concentration is the
cytoplasmic belt immediately bordering the plasmalemma.

we have reconstructed, together with the SR, the two PSTs bordering
the second-order neuron profiles. The following table, Table III,
gives the values of the surface areas of the SRs and its associated
PSTs (turtle, cone 48 hrs light). The values are in microns^2.

According to these measures we can say that the ratio between
the SR surface and the PSTs flanking it, in the light adapted state,
is close to 1. Geometrically speaking the PSTs may be considered
a sort of projection of the SR on the post-synaptic membrane of

Table III
Surface area of synaptic ribbons and related post-synaptic thickness

Ribbon	PST 1	PST 2
0.472	0.45	0.65
0.239	0.41	0.27
0.317	0.36	0.07
0.143	0.11	0.08

(the values are given in micron^2)

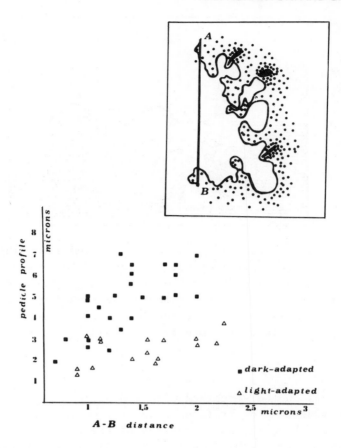

Fig. 12. The figure shows the relationships between the plasmalemma
         and the length of a straight line connecting two points on
         the plasmalemma. The insert on the right shows the graphi-
         cal procedure. From the coarse inspection of the plot it
         is possible to observe, at a given value of the A-B dis-
         tance (e.g. 1.5) two different values of the plasmalemma
         lenght.

the second-order neuron. In reality this is an overt over-simplifica-
tion because it is necessary to take into consideration the different degree of invagination of the SR into the plasmalemma fold.
In general the "duller" is the synaptic wedge, the shorter is the
PST, the "sharper" is the wedge the longer is the PST, at a given
value of the ribbon dimensions. Owing to the complex shape of the
plasmalemma at the synaptic region it is not easy to figure out a
simple law relating the two geometrical parameters one with another.

DISCUSSION

Although the function of the SRs is still unknown, it is possible to follow a series of logical steps leading to a tentative of interpretation of the functional meaning of these pre-synaptic structures. In short: the SRs are located always near a synapse, are surrounded by a dense population of SVs, a large part of this population is in tangential contact with the SR surface, their dimensions are modifiable under different light-dark adaptation states. As a logical consequence of the above the SRs study should follow two main lines of scientific thought: the "vesicle hypothesis" and the "Trifonov hypothesis". The first one does not need any comment here. According to this hypothesis the transmitter substance might be contained in SVs which, by secretory mechanisms, release their content into their synaptic cleft (Zimmermann, 1979; Ceccarelli and Hurlbut, 1980). The "Trifonov hypothesis" is specific for the synaptic transmission between photoreceptors and second-order neurons and it has been nicely summarized by Cervetto: "Trifonov (1968) formulated the hypothesis that the transmission of signals from photoreceptors may be mediated by a depolarizing transmitter released in the darkness. Accordingly, the hyperpolarization of the receptor membrane would reduce the liberation of the transmitter and hyperpolarize the horizontal cells". (Cervetto, 1976, Trifonov, 1968). The logical link between these two hypotheses may be represented by the Gray-Bunt suggestion according to which the SR acts as a "conveyor belt" and brings the SVs in an "orderly fashion" at their release sites on the plasmalemma (Bunt, 1971).

Both hypotheses, the "vesicle" and the "Trifonov", have received a large body of experimental evidence and may be taken as the best intellectual framework coping with the experimental data. The "Trifonov hypothesis" has received confirmation both from the electrophysiology than from morphology. One of the most impressive evidence based only on morphological ground came from the contribution of Schaecher et al. (1973, 1974, 1976). According to these authors horse-radish peroxidase (HRP) present in the extra cellular space is taken up by endocytic SVs into frog cone terminals. In the light-adapted state the SVs loaded with HRP and present into the terminal are very few, if not absent at all. On the contrary, dark adaptation, brings about an high number of loaded SVs. Furthermore, the amount of the SVs associated with the SR and loaded with HRP reflects the amount of loaded vesicles present into the terminal.

A basic difficulty with the Gray-Bunt hypothesis concerns the reduction in surface area of the SRs the dark adaptation state (Raynauld, 1978; Wagner and Ali, 1977; Spadaro, 1978). Our observations tend to confirm, in general, these findings. The contradiction in the conveyor-belt idea may be stated as follows: why the SRs reach their maximum surface area when the tansmitter release is inhibited and tend to disappear, or at least to reduce its surface area, when the transmitter is actively released? If the SRs act as a conveyor-belt should it not be other way round?

A possible solution of this may be found looking at the problem along a different line. SRs may have the basic function to block the SVs when the photo-receptor is illuminated and allow them to reach for the release site when the photo-receptor is in the dark. It is perhaps worth to analyse in some detail this suggestion underlining its advantages in explaining some finding and its drawbacks when compared with other data. Let us remember now the "depletion zone" surrounding the SR and characterized by a low concentration of SVs. The general shape of this area is elliptical and the SR is always in contact with some SVs of the surrounding population along its protoplasmic edge, whilst is kept separated by them all along the remaining surface by the quasi-constant value of 0.3 micron. As pointed out above it has been given evidence that the SVs are associated with a coloumbian field because they are all negatively charged (Ohsawa et al., 1981). On the other hand, from the enzymatic analysis carried out by Bunt (1971), we know that the SRs are digested by the enzymes of the pronase family. These enzymes have a strong affinity for the lysine and arginine residuals which are associated to positive charges. In first approximation we may think of a SR in the cytoplasm a positive charged object immersed in an acqueous solution of different ions (Na^+, K^+, Ca^{++}, and Cl^-). In the same solution an high number of negatively charged spherules are free to move. Below a certain distance from the SR surface the free-moving vesicles will be attrached by the positive coloumbian field associated with the SR. In consequence of this a large number of SVs will cover the SR surface. We know from the embryogenesis that the SV/SR system establishes itself very early during the photo-receptor morphogenesis.

The SV/SR complex will appear as a strongly negative-charged object. A free moving SV will be, henceforth, repelled by such a field, the repulsive force being at its maximum if the SV "try" to reach the SR along a direction normal to its face and pointing at

its geometrical center. The repulsive force will be at its minimum
if the SV will "try" to reach the SR along a direction parallel to
its surface, in few words if it reaches the SR in a way to land on
it at its protoplasmic edge. The immediate consequence of this
simplified electrostatic model will be: a) around the SR, and mainly
along its sides, there will be a "no man land" for vesicles.
b) The only landing site for the SV will be the cytoplasmic edge
of the SR.
c) The overall geometry of the "no man land" will be elliptical.

According to these suggestions, the SVs, once on the SR surface,
will be free to move on it with a minimum of enery expenditure because
they are moving along an isopotential surface. The only way to leave
the SR is to "roll" or "slite" on the SR surface pushed by the other
SVs on the SR in direction of the synaptic edge. This should be the
condition in the dark when the only link between the SVs and the SR
is the electrostatic mutual attraction. The situation will be different when the photoreceptor is illuminated. Under this condition
it may be suggested that a stronger interaction will develop itself
between SVs and SR. It is a well established fact that SVs exhibit
the so called "Ca-spot" (Politoff, 1975). It has been suggested
also that SVs, in order to become "active" must align themselves
in relation to the membrane at the accepting site (Ceccarelli,
Hurlbut, 1980). It may be possible that, in the illuminated photoreceptor, the SVs bind themselves to the SR though an unknown mechanism: under this condition they will be not allowed to reach for the
plasmalemma. It has been demonstrated that intra-cellular injection
of Ca^{++} mimic the hyperpolarizing effect of light. A Ca-dependent
mechanism able to hold the SVs on the surface may explain the halt
of the synaptic transmitter at the ribbon synapses. This suggestion
encounters a major difficulty when is confronted with the fact that
Ca^{++}, in general, acts a mobilizing agent for the transmitter release
(Rahamimoff, 1976; Alanes & Rahamimoff, 1975). Another difficulty
resides in the fact that intracellular concentration of Ca^{++} does
not increase significantly during illumination (Hubbel & Bownds,
1979).

It may be noted however that the data on Ca^{++} mobilizing action
have been obtained from synapses rich in mitochondria. Mitochondrial
Ca^{++} sequestred and then released in the crystae plays a critical
role in the mobilizing effect. During the complete reconstruction
of the cone pedicles in turtle and frog, we have not encountered a
single mitochondrion. The working mode of a mitochondria-free
synapse may present unknown variables. Although the intracellular
Ca^{++} concentration during illumination does not show a significant

increase, very little is known about the biochemical events taking place in the inner segment of the photoreceptor away from the well known studied region of the outer segment.

Another interesting point concerns the function of the Srs in the dark. We have seen how reduced in surface area they appear under this condition: on the other hand the SV concentration at the SR surface increases significantly. Fig. 6 gives the distribution of SVs in case of light adaptation and Fig. 7 (upper row) shows three examples of dark adaptation. Under the latter condition the SVs are clustered at higher density and, henceforth, with higher order. The quite high order of the SV distribution on the SR surface should introduce an high level of temporal order in the transmitter release time-course. This order must be significantly different from the statistical distribution of the quantal release at the flat synapse. It has been demonstrated, in fact, that photoreceptors establish synaptic contacts, at least with bipolar cells, at two different synaptic locations: the ribbon synapes and the flat (or superficial) synapses (Lasansky, 1969-1971).

The transmitter release at the two sites should follow different statistical structures. The "conveyor belt" should introduce an high order in the release whilst the absence of the SVs around the site of release, i.e. henceforth their statistical of arrival. The SVs may be considered, under this point of view, as data buffer whose action is to transform a random arrival of a signal (the landing of a vesicle at the sytoplasmic edge) in an orderly output (the leaving of a vesicle at the synaptic edge). It may be useful to remember now the quasi-constant value of the short side $\underline{b}$. This constant value may be the minimum lenght which is necessary to introduce a sufficient order in the SVs population on the ribbon surface.

As a logical consequence of the above the main function of the SRs in the dark is to keep the membrane of the second-order neuron under a constant depolarization. An irregular flow of transmitter could be "read" at lower levels of the image processing chain in the retina as short flashes of light. We should not forget that the hyperpolarization of a second-order neuron in the "retina-language" means simply: light.

This hypothetical interpretation of the SRs as data buffers should receive some indirect confirmation from the synaptic noise statistical structure. It may be pertinent to remember here the findings published by Ashmore and Falck (1977 a,b). According to these authors the synaptic noise recorded in a bipolar cell of the dog-fish retina exhibits two components when its laurentian curve is plotted. Tho two components have two distinct plateau levels of the power and two distinct roll-off frequencies. The two components are present in the dark only, however. When dim flashes illuminate the retina, the higher frequency component disappears leaving only the lower component, which has an higher power level. The data have been interpreted by Ashmore and Falck as an indication of the presence of a synaptic component which interferes with the "dark noise". According to our suggestion in the dark both synapses, the ribbon and the flat, work in bringing the SVs to the plasmalemma. The ribbon synapse will work, presumably, at higher release rate of the flat synapse and furthermore its release time course should be more regular. This will explain the first and the second noise component. When light is shone on the retina, the ribbon synapse will be blocked because of the development of the molecular interaction between SR and SVs. Only the flat synapse will be able to work. This could explain the disappearance of the higher frequency/lower power component. Anatomical data are required to account for such a result: the same bipolar cell must entertain both ribbon and flat synapses with the photo-receptor. In the turtle Dacheux (1980) has shown, through a complete tridimensional reconstruction, that the same bipolar cell entertains both kind of synapse with the same cone pedicle.

ACKNOWLEDGEMENTS

    The authors wish to thank Ms. Devra Spurr whose skill in serial cutting at the ultramicrotome allowed them to count on long, un-interrupted, serial sections. Mr. Ron Fargasson is kindly acknowledged for having taken care of the Computer Image Processing. Prof. Jean Paul Ravel (Caltech, Division of Biology) allowed one of us to use the facilities of his laboratory with great generosity.

REFERENCES

Akert K., Moor H., Pfenninger K., Sandri C. (1969). Contribution of new impregnation methods and freeze etching to the problem of synaptic fine structure, Akert & Waser eds., Elsevier - Amsterdam, vol. 31 p. 223-240.

Alanes E. & Rahamimoff R. (1975). The role of the mitochondria in transmitter release from motor nerve terminals, J. Physiol., 248, 285-297.

Ashmore J.F. & Falk G. (1977). Fluctuations in retinal bipolar cell responses to dim light flashes, J. Physiol. 269, 27-28P.

Ashmore J.F. & Falk G. (1977). Dark noise in retinal bipolar cells and stability of rhodopsin in rods, Nature, 270, 69-71.

Barets A., Szabo T. (1962). Appareil synaptique des cellules sensorielles de l'ampoule de Lorenzioni chez la Torpille: Torpedo marmorata, J. Micr., 1, 47-54.

Blanks J.C., Adinolfi A.M., Lolley R.N. (1974). Synaptogenesis in the photoreceptors terminal of the mouse retina, J. Comp. Neur., 156, 81-94.

Bunt A.H. (1971). Enzymatic digestion of synaptic ribbons in amphibians retinal receptors, Brain Res., 25, 571-577.

Burkardt W., Braitenberg V. (1976). Some peculiar synaptic complexes in the first visual ganglion of the fly, Cell Tiss. Res., 173, 287-308.

Carasso N. (1957). Etude au microscope electronique des synapses des cellules visuelles chez le tetaud d'Alyster obstetrician, C.R. Acad. Sci. Paris, 245, 216-219.

Ceccarelli B., Hurlbut W.P. (1980). Vesicle hypothesis of the release of quanta of acetylcholine, Physiol. Rev., 60, 396-441.

Cervetto L. (1976). Interaction between cones and second-order neurons in the turtle retina, in Neural Principles in Vision Zettler, Weiler, eds., p. 131-142, Springer-Verlag Heidelberg.

Cohen A.I. (1963). The fine structure of the visual receptors of the pigeon, Exp. Eye res., 2, 88-113.

Dacheux R.F. (1980). Connections between small bipolar cells and photoreceptors in the turtle retina, Suppl. Invest. Ophtal. Vis. Sci., 70.

De Lorenzo A.J. (1960). The fine structure of the synapses in the ciliary ganglion of the chick, J. Biophys. Biochem. Cytol., 7, 31-36.

Derbin, C., Denizot J.P., Szabo T. (1969). Ultrastructure of the type B sense organ of the specific line system of Gymnarchus niloticus, Zellforsch., 98, 262-276.

Evans E.M. (1966). On the ultrastructure of the synaptic region of visual receptors in certain vertebrates, Zellforsch., 71, 499-516.

Fine B.S. (1962). Synaptic lamellae in the human retina: an electron microscope study, J. Neuropath. exp. Neurol., 22, 255-262.

Fisher L.J. (1972). Changes during maturation and metamorphosis in the synaptic organisation of the tadpole inner plexiform layer, Nature, 235, 391-393.

Flock A. (1965). Electronmicroscopic and electrophysiological
    studies on the lateral line canal organ, Acta Oto-Laring.
    (Stockholm). Suppl., 199, 1-90.

Foos R.Y., Miyamamasu E., Yamada Y. (1969). Tridimensional study
    of an anomalus synaptic ribbon in the human retina, J. Ultr.
    Res., 26, 391-398.

Glees P., Spoerri P.E. (1977). Microtubule-vesicle-ribbon associa-
    tions in the monkey retina, J. Neurocytol., 6, 353-354.

Goodland H. (1966). The ultrastructure of the inner plexiform layer
    of the retina of the cat., Exp. Eye Res., 5, 198-200.

Gray E.G. (1976). Microtubules in synapses of the retina, J. Neuro-
    cytol., 5, 361-370.

Gray E.G., Pease H.L. (1971). On understanding the organization of
    the retinal receptor synapses, Brain Res., 35, 1-15.

Grün G. (1980). Developmental dynamic in synaptic ribbons of retinal
    receptor cells (Tilapia Xenopus), Cell Tissue Res., 207, 331-
    339.

Hama K., Saito K. (1977). Fine structure of the efferent synapse
    of the hair cells in the saccular macula of the gold-fish:
    with special reference to the anastomising tubules, J. Neuro-
    cytol., 6, 361-373.

Hopsu V.K., Arstilla A.V. (1964). An apparent somato-somatic syn-
    aptic structure in the pineal gland of the rat, Exp. Cell Res.,
    37, 484-487.

Hubbell W.L. & Bownds M.D. (1979). Visual transduction in vertebrate
    photoreceptor, Ann. Rev. Neurosci, 2, 17-34.

Jorghensen J.M., Flock A. (1973). The ultrastructure of the lateral
    line sense organs in the adult salamander Amblystoma mexicana,
    J. Neurocytol., 2, 133-142.

Kelly D. (1965). Ultrastructure and development of amphibian pienal
    organ, in "Structure and Function of the Ephysis Cerebri",
    Brain Research, vol. 10, Ariens Kappers J., Schade J.P., eds.,
    p. 270-285, Elsevier.

Kidd M. (1962). Electron microscopy of the inner plexiform layer
    of the retina of the cat and pigeon, J. Anat., 96, 179-187.

Ladman A.J. (1958). The fine structure of the rod-bipolar cell
    synapse in the retina of the Albino rat, J. Biophys. Cytol.,
    4, 459-466.

Lasansky A. (1969). Basal junctions at synaptic endings of turtle
    visual cells, J. Cell. Biol., 40, 577-592.

Lasansky A. (1971). Synaptic organization of the cone cells in
    the turtle retina, Phil. Trans. Roy. Soc. London B, 262, 365-
    385.
Lanzavecchia G. (1960). Ultrastruttura dei coni e dei bastoncelli
    della retina di Xenopus laevis, Arch. Ital. Anat. Embr., 65,
    417-435.
Loves B. (1971). Tubular networks in the terminal endings of the
    visual receptor cells in the humans, the monkey, the cat and
    the dog, Zellforsch., 121, 341-357.
Martin R., Miledi R. (1975). A pre-synaptic complex in the giant
    synapse of the squid, J. Neurocytol., 4, 121-129.
Matsusaka T. (1967). Lamellar bodies in the synaptic cytoplasm of
    the accessory cone from the chick retina as revealed by the
    electron microscope, J. Ultr. Res., 18, 55-70.
Meller K. (1964). Elektromicroscopische befunde sur Differenzierung
    der Rezeptor Zellen und Bipolarzellen der Retina und ihr syn-
    aptischen Verbindungen, Zellforsch., 64, 733-750.
Meller K., Tetloff W. (1977). The development of membrane special-
    ization in the receptor-bipolar-horizontal cell synapses in
    the chick embryo retina, Cell Tiss. Res., 181, 319-326.
Mullinger A.M. (1969). The organization of ampullar sense organs
    in the electric fish: Gymnarchus niloticus, Tissue and Cell,
    1, 31-52.
McArdle C.B., Dowling J.E., Masland R.H. (1977). Development of
    outer segments and synapses in the rabbit retina, J. Comp.
    Neur., 175, 253-274.
McLaughlin B.J. (1976). A fine structural and E-PTA study of photo-
    receptor synaptogenesis in the chick retina, J. Comp. Neur.,
    170, 347-364.
McLaughlin B.J., Bogkins L. (1977). Ultrastructure of E-PTA stained
    synaptic ribbons in the chick retina, J. Neurocytol., 8, 91-96.
Nulty J.A. (1980). Ultrastructural observations on synaptic ribbons
    in the pineal organ of the goldfish, Cell Tissue Res., 210,
    249-256.
Ohsawa K., Ohshima S., Ohki K. (1981). Surface potential and sur-
    face charge density of the cerebral-cortex synaptic vesicle
    and stability of vesicle suspension, Biochim. Biophys. Acta,
    648, 206-214.
Olney J.W. (1968). An electron microscope study of synapse forma-
    tion, receptor outer segment development and other aspects of
    developping mouse retina, Invest. Opht. Vis. Sci., 7, 250-268.

Osborne M.P., Thornhill R.A. (1972). The effect of monoamine depleting drugs upon the synaptic bars in the inner ear of the bullfrog, Zellforsch., 127, 347-355.

Pfnninger K.H. (1978). Organization of neuronal membranes, Ann. Rev. Neurosci., 1, 445-471.

Pierantoni R.L., Citron M.C., McCann G.D. (1978). Spatial relationships between synaptic vesicles and synaptic ribbons in the rods of frog retina, Suppl. Invest. Opht. Vis. Sci. April 1978, 116.

Pierantoni R.L., Citron M.C., McCann G.D. (1979). A computer-assisted tridimensional reconstruction of the photoreceptor synapses in the frog retina, Atti V Congresso Nazionale di Cibernetica e Biofisica del C.N.R., 81-86.

Pierantoni R.L., Citron M.C. (1980). Ribbons as perturbators of synaptic vesicles population, Suppl. Invest. Opht. Vis. Sci. April 1980, 163.

Politoff A.L., Rose S., Pappas G.D. (1974). The calcium binding sites of synaptic vesicles of the frog sartorius neuromuscolar junction, J. Cell Biol., 61, 818-823.

Rahamimoff R., Erulkar S.D., Alnaes E., Meiri H., Rotschenker S., Rahamimoff H. (1976). Modulation of transmitter release by calcium ions and nerve impulses, in Cold Spring Harbor Symposia on Quantitative Biology Vol. XL "The synapse". Cold Spring Harbor Laboratory, 107-116.

Raynauld J.P., Wagner H.J. (1978). Goldfish retina synaptic ribbon cycles and single unit activity, Suppl. Invest. Opht. Vis. Sci. April 1978, 261.

Remé Ch. E., Young R.W. (1977). The effects of hibernation on cone visual cells in the ground squirrel, Invest. Opht. Vis. Sci., 16, 815-840.

Schacher S.E., Holtzmann E., Ebragz T. (1973). Cytochemical studies of peroxidase uptake and other features of frog terminal photoreceptor cells, J. Histochem. Cytochemistry, 21, 410-427.

Schaecher S., Holtzmann E., Hood D. (1974). Uptake of HRP by frog photoreceptor synapse in the dark and in the light, Nature, 249, 261-263.

Schaecher S., Holtzmann E., Hood D.C. (1976). Synaptic activity of frog retinal photoreceptor. A peroxidase uptake study, J. Cell Biol., 70, 178-192.

Schaeffer S.F., Raviola E. (1976). Ultrastructural analysis of
    functional changes in the synaptic endings of turtle cone
    cells, in Cold Spring Harbor Symposia on Quantitative Biology
    Vol. XL "The synapse". Cold Spring Harbor Laboratory, 521-
    528.
Schaeffer S.F., Raviola E. (1977). Membrane recycling in the cone
    endings of the turtle retina, J. Cell Biol, 79, 802-825.
Siøstrand F.S. (1953 a). The ultrastructure of the retinal rod
    synapse of the guinea pig, J. Appl. Physics, 24, 1422.
Siøstrand F.S. (1953 b). The ultrastructure of the outer segments
    of the rods and cones of the eye as revealed by the electron
    microscope, J. Cell Comp. Physiol., 42, 15-44.
Siøstrand F.S. (1958). Ultrastructure of retinal synapses of the
    guinea pig eye as revealed by three-dimensional reconstruction
    from serial sections, J. Ultr. Res., 2, 122-170.
Siøstrand F.S. (1974). A search for the circuitry of directional
    selectivity and neural adaptation through three-dimensional
    analysis of the outer plexiform layer of the rabbit retina,
    J. Ultr. Res., 49, 60-156.
Smealser G.K., Ozamics V., Rayborn M., Segun D. (1974). Retinal
    synaptogenesis in the primate, Invest. Opht., 13, 340-361.
Smith C.A., Siøstrand F.S. (1961). A synaptic structure in the
    hair cells of the guinea pig cochlea, J. Ultr. Res., 5, 184-
    192.
Spadaro A., De Simone I., Puzzolo D. (1978). Ultrastructural data
    and chronobiological patterns of the synaptic ribbons in the
    outer plexiform layer in the retina of albino rats, Acta Anat.,
    102, 365-373.
Szamier P.B., Bergsen E.L. (1977). Retinal ultrastructure in ad-
    vanced retinitis pigmentosa, Inv. Opht. Vis. Sci., 16, 947-
    961.
Trifonov Yu. A. (1968). Study of synaptic transmission between
    photoreceptors and horizontal cells by means of the electrical
    stimulation of the retina, Biophysica, 13, 809-817.
Wagner H.J. (1973). Darkness-induced reduction of the number of
    synaptic ribbons in the fish retina, Nature New Biol., 246,
    53-55.
Wagner H.J., Ali M.A. (1977). Cone synaptic ribbons and retinomotor
    changes in the brook trout, Salvelinus fontinalis, under various
    experimental conditions, Can J. Zool., 55, 1684-1691.
Weidman T.A., Kuwabara T. (1969). Development of the rat retina,
    Invest. Opht. Vis. Sci., 8, 60-69.

Witkowsky P., Stell W.K. (1973). Retinal structure in the smooth
     dogfish Musteles canis: electron microscopy of serially sectioned
     bipolar cell synaptic terminals, J. Comp. Neur., 150, 147-168.
Wollrath L., Huss H. (1973). The synaptic ribbons of the guinea pig
     pineal gland under normal and experimental conditions,
     Zellforsch., 139, 417-426.
Wong-Riley M.T. (1974). Synaptic organization of the inner plexiform
     layer in the retina of the tiger salamander, J. Neurocytol., 3,
     1-33.
Zimmermann H. (1979). Vesicle recycling and transmitter release.
     Neuroscience Vol. 1773 to 1804 Pergamon Press Ltd.

A NOTE ON THE SYNAPTIC EVENTS IN HYPERPOLARIZING BIPOLAR CELLS OF THE TURTLE'S RETINA[*]

P.B. Detwiler, A.L. Hodgkin and T.D. Lamb

The Physiological Laboratory, University of Cambridge and the Department of Physiology and Biophysics, Schools of Medicine, University of Washington, Seattle, USA

Several authors have shown that hyperpolarizing bipolar cells are electrically noisy in the dark and that most of this noise is suppressed by a patch of light centred on the cell (Simon, Lamb & Hodgkin, 1976; Ashmore & Falk, 1980; Ashmore and Copenhagen, 1980). This fits with the suggestion by Trifonov (1968) that vertebrate rods and cones release transmitter continuously in the dark and that the effect of light is to reduce this release by making the inside of the photoreceptor more negative. According to Trifonov's hypothesis the noise of a hyperpolarizing bipolar cell in darkness should be composed of a random sequence of depolarizing synaptic potentials each having a time course that is consistent with the frequency spectrum of the dark noise.

The present note contains a brief account of experiments carried out in 1976 which provided tentative information about the polarity and time course of the synaptic potentials in a hyperpolarizing bipolar cell. In one type of analysis we depended on a single experiment in which there was clear evidence of positive going unitary

---

[*]This article is based on a talk given by one of us at the conference on Noise in Biological Membranes held at Erice in March 1977. This was the last occasion on which we met Mike Fuortes; he was already suffering from his final illness, but with characteristic courage took an active part in the proceedings of the conference. Two of the present authors (A.L.H. and P.B.D.) were introduced to visual physiology by Fuortes.

synaptic potentials that appeared in a random sequence as the effects of a sustained bright light wore off. In the other we relied
on interrupting a bright light for a brief time in the hope that
this would give an approximately synchronous volley of synaptic
potentials.

METHODS

    All experiments were done on the peripheral-dorsal retina of
the red-eared swamp turtle, Pseudemys scripta elegans. The apparatus
and methods were the same as those described by Detwiler and Hodgkin
(1979). The posterior half of an enucleated eye was drained of
vitreous and placed in a chamber aerated with moist 95% O_2, 5% CO_2
at room temperature. Microelectrodes filled with 4 M potassium
acetate and having resistances of 200 to 500 MΩ, were advanced into
the retina from the vitreal surface. Bipolar cells were penetrated
most frequently just distal to the horizontal cell layer. Stimuli
centred on the impaled cell were formed by an optical bench of the
Baylor & Hodgkin (1973) design. Hyperpolarizing bipolar cells gave
a hyperpolarizing response to a spot of light and a depolarizing
response to annular illumination. The unattenuated intensity of
the light after passing through a narrow-band 650 nm interference
filter was 1.55×10^3 erg cm^{-2} sec^1 (5.1×10^6 photon μm^{-2} sec^{-1}).
Data were recorded on an FM tape recorded with a bandwidth of d.c.
to 12350 Hz. Selected regions of the tape were digitized and noise
analysis was performed according to the procedure described by Lamb
& Simon (1976).

RESULTS

Bipolar cell noise and miniature synaptic potentials

    Figure 1 illustrates one rather complete experiment in which
there was clear evidence of potential changes resembling discrete
miniature synaptic potentials. The figure shows the response of
the cell to three different intensities of steady 650 nm light.
In darkness the cell voltage fluctuated randomly at low frequencies
over a range of 4 to 5 mV peak to peak. The response to a step
of light consisted of a negative peak followed by a slow decline
to a plateau. A positive-going peak and a slow positive phase was
seen in B when a light of moderate intensity was turned off. The
absence of brief depolarizing transients on switching off the strong
lights used in A and C is probably explained by the fact that lights

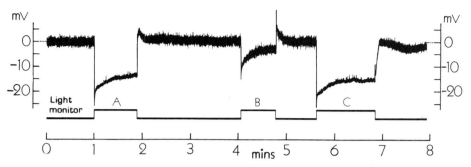

Fig. 1.   Reduction of bipolar cell noise by steady illumination.
          Intracellular voltage was recorded d.c. coupled. Step
          intensities expressed as photon μm^{-2} sec^{-1} at 650 nm were
          from left to right: 1.2×10^6, 9.0×10^3, and 5.1×10^6.
          Here the stimulus was a spot 1.76 mm in diameter, but
          smaller spots (0.1 to 0.2 mm) were usually employed.
          Temperature 22° C.

of this intensity and duration may leave the cone depolarized for
many seconds (Baylor, Hodgkin & Lamb 1974). The electrical noise
was greatly reduced by light and returned at the end of the period
of illumination. All this is essentially similar to the description
given by Simon et al. (1975). The new feature of the experiment is
that during the relatively quiet plateau, when most of the noise
had been suppressed, the base line was disturbed by the random
occurrence of relatively brief positive going potentials. These
are most clearly illustraded by Fig. 2 which is an oscilloscope
recording, taken at 25 times the speed of Fig. 1, from the third
exposure to light. The records were selected to show all those
cases in which the amplitude of a spontaneous potential change exceeded 2 mV. When these waves were normalised and superposed we
obtained the mean potential change in Fig. 2B. This is a biphasic
wave consisting of an initial depolarizing phase lasting 30 msec
and a subsequent hyperpolarizing phase of about the same duration.
The possibility that events with this time course and shape might
give rise to the dark noise was tested by comparing the power
spectrum of the noise suppressed by light with the square of the
modulus of the Fourier transform of the average spontaneous wave.
As can be seen from Fig. 3 the spectrum of the measured noise peaks
at a lower frequency than the spectrum predicted from the discrete
waves, suggesting that the average unit event underlying the noise
must be slower than that shown in Fig. 2B.

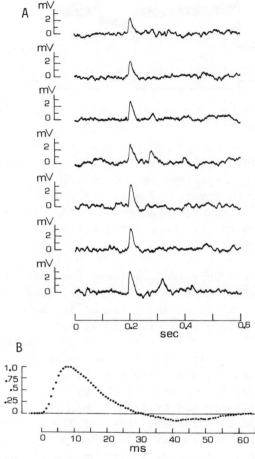

Fig. 2.   Discrete spontaneous potential changes during steady il-
          lumination.   A. Selected traces showing 7 spontaneous
          potential changes with amplitudes greater than 2 mV, from
          the same cell as Figure 1 during the brightest light.
          The peak amplitudes of the 7 events were normalized and
          their rising phases superimposed to obtain the mean spon-
          taneous potential change shown in B.   The largest event
          was 3.3 mV and the mean amplitude 2.8 mV.
          In order to reduce baseline drifts the records shown in
          this figure were taken from an a.c. coupled channel with
          a 1-sec time constant which should have little effect on
          the event shape.

The magnitude of the unit event underlying the noise was also smaller than the spontaneous potentials. Its approximate magnitude, estimated by dividing the change in voltage variance by mean voltage change, was 60 μV whereas the seven spontaneous changes in Fig. 2 had an average amplitude of 2.8 mV. The size of the unit event calculated from noise in 10 hyperpolarizing bipolar cells varied between 60 and 300 μV with a mean of 160 μV.

If the discrete spontaneous potentials in Fig. 2 were responsible for the noise in the dark we must explain why they were larger and faster than the unit synaptic event inferred from the analysis of the dark noise. One possibility is that the spontaneous waves arose close to the soma and were much less affected by electronic spread along the dendrites than the majority of synaptic events contributing to the dark noise. This seems quite plausible as the bipolar cell illustrated in Figs. 1-3 had an unusually large receptive field (c. 100 μm) and the cable properties of its dendrites would be expected to reduce amplitude and prolong time course.

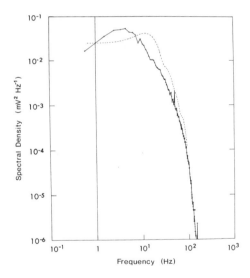

Fig. 3. Comparison of the power spectrum of light sensitive noise with the power spectrum predicted from the mean spontaneous potential change. The solid line shows the difference between the noise spectrum in darkness and the sum of the spectra during the two brightest lights in Figure 1. The dashed line is the square of the modulus of the Fourier transform of the mean spontaneous potential shown in Figure 2B, vertical position arbitrary.

Another explanation for the discrepancy between the two spectra in Fig. 3 is that low-frequency components are added to the noise spectrum by the effect of cone voltage noise in modulating the release of transmitter. This would be consistent with the experiments and analyses of Ashmore & Copenhagen (1980).

The biphasic shape of the spontaneous events in Fig. 2 fits with the finding that the spectral frequency of the dark noise had a maximum at about 4 Hz and declined at lower frequencies (Fig. 3). Similar results were obtained in other experiments; the frequency of the peak averaged 2.9 Hz (7 cells, 21-23°C).

Flashes of darkness

A different way of estimating the shape of the synaptic potentials is to apply a steady light which suppresses most of the dark noise and then interrupt it for a brief period with a 'flash

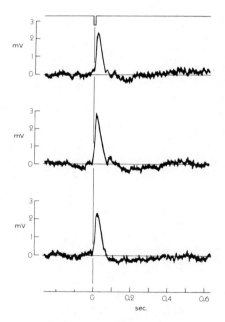

Fig. 4.   Response of another bipolar cell to flashes of darkness. A steady white light which delivered the equivalent of 2.3×10^5 photon μm^{-2} sec^{-1} at 644 nm was turned off for 12 ms at 2 second intervals. The light covered a circle 0.55 mm in diameter. Temperature 23°C.

of darkness'. As can be seen from Fig. 4 this gave a biphasic potential change consisting of an initial positive phase followed by
a slower and smaller negative phase. The biphasic wave resembles
the spontaneous potentials in Fig. 2 but is slower. Figure 5 shows
that its power spectrum is similar to that of the dark noise in the
same cell. This type of analysis was performed on five bipolar
cells and the agreement between the two spectra was always reasonably
good. However, exact agreement would not be expected because the
finite duration of the cone response may prolong the bipolar cells
response and there is no reason why the low frequencies introduced
in this way should correspond exactly to those produced by the
interaction of cone and bipolar cells intrinsic noise (see Ashmore
& Copenhagen 1980).

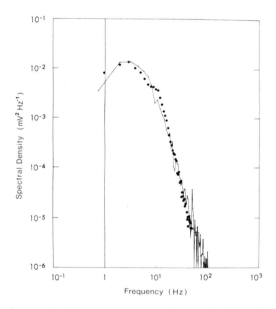

Fig. 5. Comparison of the power spectrum of the light sensitive
         noise with the power spectrum predicted from the cell's
         response to a flash of darkness. The spectrum of the
         light suppressed noise (solid line) is the spectrum of the
         noise in darkness minus the spectrum in steady light equiv-
         alent to 2.3×10^5 photons μm^{-2} sec^{-1} at 644 nm. The
         solid circles plot the power spectrum of the mean of 25
         responses to flashes of darkness from the series from which
         the 3 samples in Figure 4 were taken, vertical position
         arbitrary.

DISCUSSION

The tentative conclusion of this note is that the dark noise
of hyperpolarizing bipolar cells is generated by the continuous release of packets of cone transmitter which generate unitary synaptic
potentials in the processes of the bipolar cell. These synaptic
potentials consist of an initial depolarization followed by a slower
and smaller hyperpolarization. A step of light hyperpolarizes the
cell and reduces its noise by shutting off the release of cone
transmitter and reducing the frequency of the depolarizing miniatures.
The biphasic shape of the synaptic potentials is supported by the
shape of the noise spectrum of the cell's dark noise, by the biphasic
response to a flash of darkness and in one experiment by the presence of discrete biphasic waves resembling miniature synaptic potentials. It also agrees with the more recent observations that
the response of both hyperpolarizing and depolarizing bipolars to
weak flashes is biphasic (Ashmore & Copenhagen 1980).

The experiments of Baylor & Fettiplace (1977) on the transfer
of information between turtle photoreceptors and ganglion cells show
that the transmission pathway acts like an electrical band-pass
filter containing delay and differentiating stages. It is clear
from experiments such as that in our Fig. 1 that some of the differentiation has already occurred by the time information about
ligth intensity has been converted into bipolar cell voltage. Thus
Baylor & Fettiplace's theoretical plot of synaptic excitation in
an off-centre ganglion cell in response to a brief depolarization
of the cone is similar in shape and time scale to the voltage response of a hyperpolarizing bipolar to a flash of darkness, as may
be seen by comparing Fig. 4 of the present note with Fig. 4C of
Baylor & Fettiplace 1977. In both cases the wave is biphasic with
the first depolarizing phase occupying about 70 msec and the second
hyperpolarizing phase roughly 200 msec. It should be said that this
type of signal is consistent with the spikes seen when a moderate
light is turned on and off, and that the slow decline of potential
during or after the light which occurs with a time constant of
several seconds is clearly a separate phenomenon that probably would
not have been noticed in the experiments of Baylor & Fettiplace who
used relatively brief exposures to light.

Generating biphasic miniature synaptic potentials would seem
to be a neat method of differentiating signals in the nervous system.
This would not be difficult in bipolar cells where the dark potential
of -35 mV is some 40 mV less negative than the probable value of the

potassium equilibrium potential. In that case a biphasic wave like that in Fig. 4 would be expected if the depolarization produced by the cone transmitter caused a delayed increase in potassium conductance which subsequently relaxed with a time constant of about 50 msec.

REFERENCES

Ashmore J.F. & Copenhagen D.R. (1980). Different postsynaptic events in two types of retinal bipolar cell, Nature, 288, 84–86.

Ashmore J.F. & Falk G. (1980). Responses of rod bipolar cells in the dark-adapted retina of the dogfish Scyliorhinus canicula, J. Physiol. Lond., 300, 115–150.

Baylor D.A. & Fettiplace R. (1977). Transmission from photoreceptors to ganglion cells in the retina of the turtle, J. Physiol. Lond., 271, 391–424.

Baylor D.A. & Hodgkin A.L. (1973). Detection and resolution of visual stimuli by turtle photoreceptors, J. Physiol. Lond., 234, 163–198.

Baylor D.A., Hodgkin A.L. & Lamb T.D. (1974). The electrical response of turtle cone to flashes and steps of light, J. Physiol. Lond., 242, 685–727.

Detwiler P.B. & Hodgkin A.L. (1979). Electrical coupling between cones in turtle retina, J. Physiol. Lond., 291, 75–100.

Lamb T.D. & Simon E.J. (1976). The relation between intracellular coupling and electrical noise in turtle photoreceptors, J. Physiol. Lond., 263, 257–286.

Simon E.J., Lamb T.D. & Hodgkin A.L. (1975). Spontaneous voltage fluctuations in retinal cones and bipolar cells, Nature, 256, 661–662.

Trifonov Yu.A. (1968). Study of synaptic transmission between the photoreceptor and the horizontal cell using electrical stimulation of the retina, Biofizika, 13, 809–817 (in Russian); Biophysics, 13, 948–957 (in English).

QUANTITATIVE MORPHOLOGY OF AMACRINE CELLS IN TELEOST RETINA

*S. Deplano and S. Vallerga

Istituto di Cibernetica e Biofisica del C.N.R.

Camogli

INTRODUCTION

Amacrine cells in the vertebrate retina mediate the processing of visual information in the inner plexiform layer (IPL) from bipolar cells to ganglion cells, and between neighbouring amacrine cells. Although the synaptic circuitry of the IPL of teleostean retinae has been extensively investigated (Witkowsky and Dowling, 1969; Kaneko, 1973; Toyoda et al., 1973; Famiglietti et al., 1977), and we know that amacrine cells can be presynaptic and postsynaptic to bipolar and to other amacrine cells, as well as presynaptic to ganglion cells, up to now there has been no comprehensive morphological description of amacrine cells in fish retinae since the work of Cajal (1972) in the Cyprinidae and Percidae retinae. Cajal classified amacrine cells into two main groups according to the organization of their dendritic tree within the IPL: the diffuse and stratified amacrine cells. He observed a pentalamination of the IPL and therefore subdivided the stratified units into cells of the first, second, third, fourth and fifth sublayer, as well as bilayered and multilayered cells. The number of sublayers differs among different species; Scholes (1975) found six layers in the rudd, and as many as seven sublayers were observed in the Nannacara (Wagner, 1976). With the aid of flat mounted Golgi preparations the extension of

---

*Permanent address: Istituto di Anatomia Comparata dell-Università di Genova.

the dendritic field has been added as a second descriptive criterion
used to classify amacrine cells. Famiglietti and Siegfried (1980)
classified amacrine cells in the rabbit retina into three groups
according to the spread of their dendrites: narrow-, medium-wide,
and wide-field units. An exhaustive morphological description of
amacrine cells of the cat retina has been recently given by Kolb
et al. (1981). They divided amacrine cells into four broad classes
narrow-, small-, medium- and wide-field, and recognized 22 types of
cells on the basis of both dendritic spread and stratification at
the IPL.

The morphological variety has been, at least partly, related
to the physiological diversity of amacrine cells. Broadly stratified and multistratified cells found their physiological correlate
in units giving transient responses, narrowly stratified cells are
linked to sustained responses (Murakami and Shimoda). A correspon-
dance has been established between the polarity of the response and
the level of layering at the IPL for certain amacrine cells in the
cat (Famiglietti and Kolb, 1976) and in Cyprinid fishes (Famiglietti
et al. 1977). Recent immunocytochemical and autoradiographic studies
indicate that the level of stratification and dendritic morphology
may be related to the transmitter(s) present in an amacrine cell (Lam
et al., 1979; Marc et al., 1978, Masland and Mills, 1979; Hayden et
al., 1980; Pourcho, 1981; Ball and Dickson, 1981; Famiglietti and
Vaughn, 1981; Yazulla, 1981).

An accurate morphological description is therefore required in
the search for unequivocal correlation between functional and morphological characteristics, with the goal of a single classification
scheme of amacrine cells, and possibly the recognition of an unique
functional role for each morphological type.

The purpose of our study is to give a comprehensive morphological classification of amacrine cells in a teleost retina, considering
as the most descriptive criteria the shape, extension and organization
within the IPL of their denditic fields. With this aim we also attempted to define quantitatively the five-tier sublayering of the IPL
and establish the pattern and level of branching of the different
types of amacrine cells responsible for such pentalamination.

METHODS

All the experiments were performed with retinae of adult bogues,
Boops boops, a shallow water fish of the Sparidae family, quite common
in the northern Mediterranean and on the eastern Atlantic shores. The

isolated retinae were stained according to the rapid Golgi method
described by Cajal (1972). The impregnated retinae were than embed-
ed in Epon and cut in tangential or cross sections 50-70 μm thick,
by a rotary microtome using a modification of West's (1972) technique. Golgi impregnated cells were studied by light microscopy
(see Fig. 1) and drawn with the aid of a camera lucida.

NOMENCLATURE

    A simple code is used to define the cells observed in cross
or in tangential sections. We name a cell X_1 X_2 X_3 where: X is
either a number, which e.g., X_1 X_2 X_3 defines the sublayer(s) of the
N (narrow), S (small), M (medium), and W (wide). The last key, X_3,
denotes the shape of the dendrites: K (knotty), R (radiate), W
(webbed), S (semithick) and T (thick). Displaced units are sig-
nalled by a bar over the code. The details for each type are given
in the Results section.

RESULTS

    In this study we classify amacrine cells in a three dimensional
scheme according to:
a) branching pattern in the inner plexiform layer
b) extension of dendritic field
c) dendritic morphology

a) Branching pattern in the IPL

    Amacrine cells are separated into two broad groups according
to the localization of their terminal ramifications in the IPL:
stratified units have processes segregated in specific sublayers,
diffuse units ramify through the entire IPL (Cajal, 1972). We
evaluated the average width of individual sublayers by measuring the
bands drawn by dendrites of amacrine, bipolar and ganglion cells.
Figure 2 shows the five-tier organization of the inner plexiform
layer and the types of bipolar cells sending axon terminals into
each sunlayer; and the thickness of each sublayer relative to the
whole IPL. Depths in the IPL are given as % of the distance from
the inner border (0) to the outer border (100) of IPL. The
first sublayer, S1, lies at the outer boundary of the inner plexiform layer, its mean level is at 13+5% of the IPL. S2 is at 33+6%
of the depth of the IPL. The third sublayer is the thinnest one,

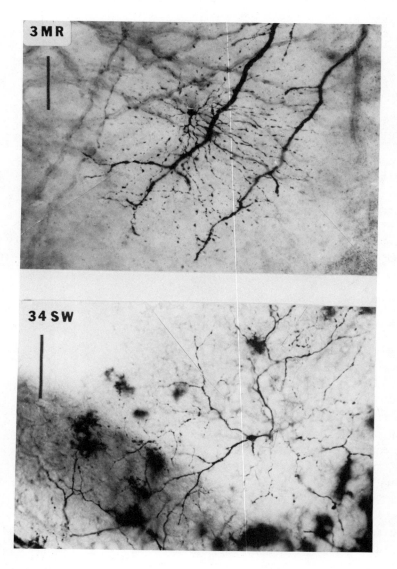

Fig. 1   (a) Light-micrographs of Golgi-impregnated amacrine cells
in the bogue retina as seen in flat-mounted preparations.
3MR: medium-field radiate unit of the third sublayer.
345WS: multistratified wide-field amacrine cell with semithick type dendrites, found in the same region as 3MR.

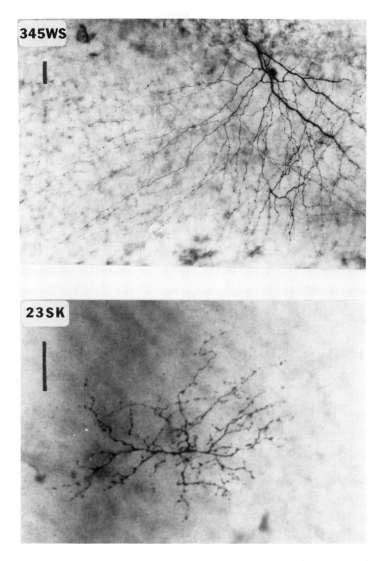

Fig. 1   (b) 34SW: bistratified small-field unit with net-like W
type dendrites.
23SK: bistratified small-field cell with knotty type dendrites.   Bar=50 µm.

accounting for less than 10% of the IPL; its mean level is 48+3%.
The proximal half of the IPL is divided into two sublayers of roughly
the same thickness, S4 (at 61+7%) and S5 (at 93+10%).

Cone bipolar cells with spread axon terminals and in sublayers
1, 2 and 3 ; while cone bipolar cells with globular terminals form
a regular band at about the level of 67% of the IPL depth, (S4);
rod bipolar cells send conical footpieces at two levels, both in the
fifth sublayer at about 82% of the IPL, and just above the ganglion
cell somata (Vallerga and Deplano, manuscript in preparation). Using
the terminology of Cajal (1972) we call cone bipolars the units with
small soma and flat dendritic terminals at the level of cone pedicles
and rod bipolars the cells with large soma and long dendrites reaching the rod spherules. However, both types of bipolars may be functionally connected to both types of photoreceptors.

According to the pattern of the terminal branching of bipolar
cells, the IPL can be divided into two parts whose nomeclature we
adopt after the functional bisublamination proposed by Famiglietti
and Kolb (1976), and we call sublayer 1 to 3 (where spread terminals
are found) sublamina a, and sublayers 4 and 5 (the region of bulbous
terminals) sublamina b. The functional correlation for such a two-
part division of the IPL has yet to be demonstrated in the Sparidae
retina, but the assumption is supported by findings in other fish
families (Famiglietti et al., 1977).

b) Extension of the dendritic field

Amacrine cell dendrites may reach as far as 2 mm from the soma
or remain as close as 20 μm. Since the dendritic field is often
elliptical or asymmetrical we chose as a criterion to evaluate the
dendritic spread the maximum distance D between soma and dendritic
terminals.

Narrow-field cells (class N) are units with D<50 μm (Fig. 3,
SNW), small-field cells (class S) have a dendritic range of 50<D<150
μm, (Fig. 3 1SR), medium-field cells (class M) have a dendritic
span of 150<D<250 μm (Fig. 3, 2KM), and wide-field amacrine cells
class W) have a maximum D exceeding 250 μm (Fig. 3, 5WR). The
measured mean values and standard deviations of D are: 30±5 μm for
narrow-field, 100±300 μm for small field, 190±20 μm for medium-field,
and 400±200 μm for wide-field. The elements of classes N, S and M
are well grouped around the mean value and thus form significant
classes, while cells of class W are scattered over a wide range.

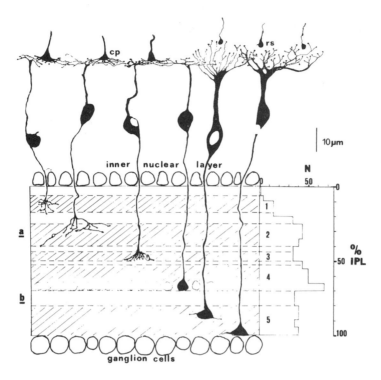

Fig. 2.   Five-tier sublayering of the inner plexiform layer. Sub-
          layers 1, 2 and 3 (sublamina a) receive the spread axon
          terminals of small soma bipolar cells with dendrites at
          the level of cone pedicles (cp). Sublayer 4 is character-
          ized by small bipolar cells contacting cone pedicles. At
          two levels in sublayer 5 are the conical footpieces of large
          soma bipolar cells with long dendrites reaching rod spher-
          ules (rs). N represents the observed number of bipolar,
          amacrine and ganglion cells ramifying at a given level of
          the IPL.

     We did not oberve any systematic variation in the size of
dendritic field with increasing distance from the optic disc as
observed in mammals (Boycott and Wässle, 1974), possibly because
in lower vertebrates the reason for the variation of eccentricity
is missing, since they lack the visual cortex (Braccini et al.,
1982).

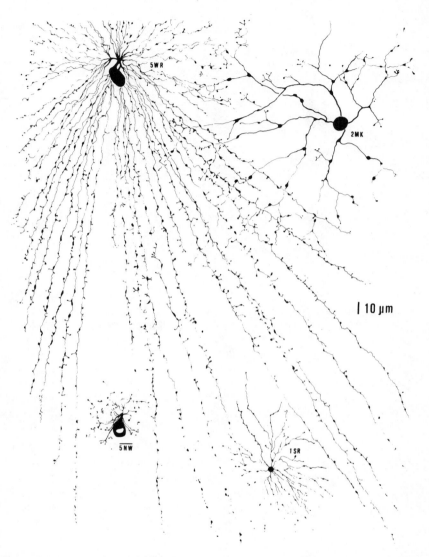

Fig. 3.   Camera lucida drawings of flat mounted Golgi-impregnated
          amacrine cells. Examples of different types of dendritic
          field size. Narrow-field (N): SNW, displaced amacrine
          cell of the fifth sublayer, with webbed dendrites. Small-
          field (S): 1SR, radiate unit of the first sublayer. Medium-
          field (M): 2KM, knotty unit branching in the second sub-
          layer. Wide-field (W): SWR, partly drawn radiate amacrine
          cell with many spines protrunding from the fine beaded
          dendrites.

c) Dendritic morphology

Amacrine cell dendrites are markedly diversified: their diameter may vary from 0.1 to 4 µm, they may or may not exhibit small or large regularly spaced swellings, may or may not divide and may be straight or billowy. To take into account the differences in dendritic configuration we grouped amacrine cells into five classes (Fig. 4):
1) Knotty (class K), cells with sparse dendrites (∿1 µm diameter) containing regularly spaced bulbous swellings (3÷4 µm). The mean value of the soma size is 8.5x14 µm (Fig. 4 2MK).
2) Radiate (class R), cells with many fine dendrites that depart radially from the soma of from a single apical stem and stratify narrowly. The dendrites bear small beads (∿1 µm diameter) and on occasion spines, and divide only in the terminal part of their field. Soma 8x12.5 µm (Fig. 4, 3MR).
3) Webbed (class W), cells with many fine spiny and wavy dendrites which intertwine continuously, and are either diffuse or broadly stratified. Many small beads are present along their length. Soma 8x12 µm (Fig. 4, 34MW).
4) Semithick (class S), cells whose dendrites are coarse (∿4 µm) close to the soma and tapered toward the periphery of dendritic field. Soma 8x13 µm (Fig. 4 345WS).
5) Thick (class T), cell with few large caliber (∿4 µm) smooth and straight dendrites whose diameter remains constant for distances in some cases up to 400 µm (Fig. 5, 5WT), and then end abruptly in a burst of fine processes. Soma 9x14 µm (Fig. 4, 3MT).

The different types of dendrites seem to have a peculiar organisation, in each sublayer the sequence most frequently observed is distally to proximally: type knotty (K), radiate (R), webbed (W), semithick (S), and thick (T). Over these bands are scattered the net-like dendrites of the diffuse amacrine cells.

Cells of the first sublayer

We observed in S1 five morphological types of monolayered units: one narrow-field (1NW), three small-field. (1SK, 1SR and 1ST), and one medium-field (1MT). The maximum D for these units does not exceed 200 µM.

The narrow-field units (1NW) have an ovoid cell body (8x10 µm) and broadly stratified, fine wavy dendrites that form a cobwed like tree within the first sublayer (Fig. 5, 1NW). 1SR type cells have very fine beads interlaced with fine dendrites, typical of

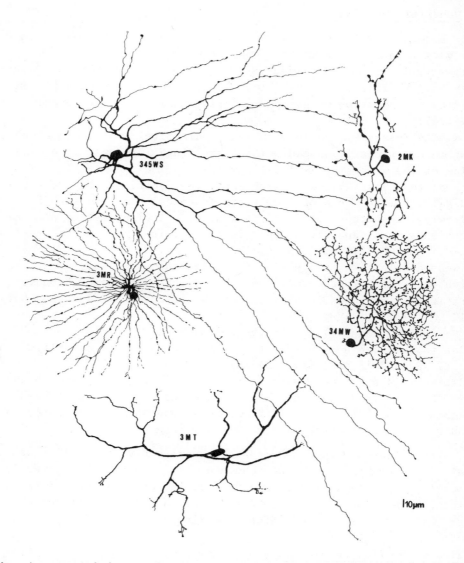

Fig. 4.   Dendritic morphology. Knotty (K): 2MK, large beads are
           interlaced with the sparse dendrites. Radiate (R): 3MR,
           the fine dendrites spread virtually undivided from the
           cell body. Webbed (W): 34MW, the filamentous dendrites
           are thickly intertwined to form a cobwed-like tree.
           Semithick (S): 345WS, coarse primary dendrites are contin-
           uously tapered toward the periphery. Thick (T): 3MT,
           smooth cylindrical processes end in a tuft of fine branches.

the R (radiate) class, and a miniature soma, 4x4 μm (Fig. 3, 1SR).
1SK, 1ST and 1MT have large somata (11x14 μm), pyriform (1SK) or
hemispherical (1ST and 1MT). The two latter cells resemble the
units described by Cajal (Pl i Fig. 5B, 1972) in the Percidae and
Cyprinidae fishes.

Cells of the second sublayers

There are six types of stratified amacrine cells that branch
in the second sublayer: three small-field (2SR, 2SW and 2ST) and
three medium-field (2MK, 2MR and 2MW).

2SR has a large pyriform soma (8x15 μm) and its very fine,
undivided dendrites branch in a single plane at about the 28% level
(Fig. 5), it recalls the monostratified cell of the second sublayer
described by Cajal (Pl 1 Fig. 5C, 1972). Small beads are regularly
spaced at intervals of about 10 μm. 2SW has a small soma (5x6 μm)
and fine wavy dendrites that end with small swellings. 2ST is a
typical type T cell, with smooth thick dendrites which on occasion
bear bulbous appendages. 2MK (Fig. 4 2MK) has sparse dendrites with
large swellings; the size of somata for this cell type is about
10x10 μm. 2MR closely resembles 1SR in soma size (4x4 μm) and
dendritic morphology (fine, beaded, radiating). 2MW has medium
calibre branches bifurcating several times and terminating in
delicate tufts. The soma is round (10x10 μm) and crested with short
apical processes.

Cells of the third sublayer

The units we observed branching at this sublayer are one small-
field (3ST) and two medium-field (3MR and 3MT). 3ST has large
caliber dendrites bearing bulbous appendages and a large, ovoid
soma (10x16 μm). 3MR (Fig. 4 and 5) has a symmetrical dendritic
tree with very fine-grained, beaded dendrites departing radially
from several coarse main branches. 3MT has a markedly pyriform
soma (9x20 μm) and large dendrites bearing many short processes
($\sim$5 μm) ending with knobs (Fig. 4).

Cells of the fourth sublayer

A peculiarity of the fourth sublayer is the regular row of
globular bipolar axon terminals narrowly packed at level 67%; this
line is an accumulation point for amacrine cells, and many types

branch close to this level we have seen two small-field (4SR and
4ST), three medium-field (4MR, 4MS and 4MT) and one wide field
(4WR).

4SR has an elongated soma (7x13 µm) and an elegant spread of
fine spiny processes radiating from a thick main dendrite at about
level 56%. 4ST bifurcates into dendrites as thick as the descending
trunk (∿4 µm) at level 70%. At the same level as 4RS are found the
branches of the medium-field units of the R class, the 4MRs. The
cells with semithick dendrites (4MS) have small pyriform somata
(6x11 µm) and sparse dendrites with many knobby appendages. The
soma of the 4MT type resembles a bulbous expansion of the principal
stem, from which depart thick dendrites with many drumsticks and
terminating with fine processes. The 4WR units have giant somata
(14x30 µm). The 4WR units have giant somata and long spiny dendrites confined in a narrow region around level 60% (Fig. 5).

Cells of the fifth sublayer

The conical axon terminals of rod bipolar cells end both at
level 80% and directly above ganglion cell somata. Within these
two levels branch several types of amacrine cells: one narrow-field
(5NW), a displaced unit, one small-field (5SK), two medium-field
(5MK and 5MS) and three wide-field (5WS and 5WT).

5SK and 5MK, the cells with type K dendrites, have large somata
(10x18 µm) independent of the extension of their dendritic field.
The straight, primary dendrite divides several times within sublamina b, branching within S5 with typical fine processes interlaced
with large swellings. 5MS and 5WS also present a descending trunk
that divides into several branches, but their dendrites are coarse,
with many varicosities. 5WR are commonly found in our Golgi impregnated retinae; they have large ovoid somata (∿10x17 µm) and
their long undivided dendrites bear many spines (Fig. 3 5WR). 5WT
is an elegant unit with a bat-shaped soma, smooth, thick dendrites
bearing knobby pedicles, and ending in a tuft of small processes
(Fig. 5 5WT).

Diffuse Cells

The amacrine cells with dendrites diffusing throughout the
entire IPL account for only 5% of the cells completely stained in
our Golgi preparation. We observed two types, DNW (Fig. 5) and
DMW, whose common feature is the dendritic type. All of them have,

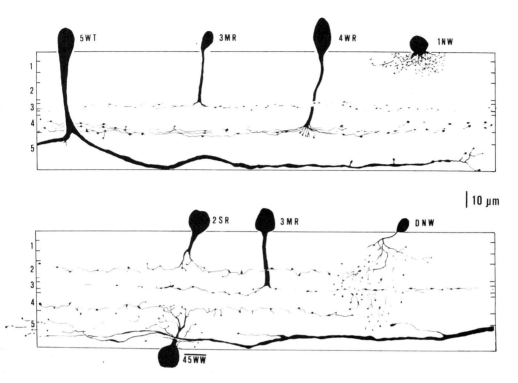

Fig. 5. Camera lucida drawings of cross sections of Golgi impreg-
ated retinae. Top: 5WT, wide-field cell with thick dendrites branching in the fifth sublayer. 3MR: medium-field
radiate unit of the third sublayer. 4WR, wide-field radiate
cell of the fourth sublayer. 1NW, narrow-field amacrine
spreading with net-like dendrites in the first sublayer.
Bottom: 2SR, small-field radiate cell of the second sublayer. 3MR: large soma subtype of medium-field cell with
radiating dendrites. DNW, diffuse unit with narrow-field
and webbed type dendrites. 45WW, wide-field displaced
amacrine cell bistratified within sublamina b.

in fact, W webbed (W) type processes, with a high degree of dichoto-
my, and many small beads. The somata of diffuse units are pyriform
and range from 4x7 to 7x13 μm, according to the extension of the
dendritic tree, which ranges from narrow to medium. The lower and
upper limits of the observed maximum radius D were 25 and 180 μm,
respectively. This finding agrees with the observations that in
rabbit and cat retina most wide-field amacrine cells are unistrati-
fied (Famiglietti and Siegfried, 1980; Kolb et al., 1981).

Asymmetric cells

        A peculiar type of amacrine cell frequently observed in our
Golgi preparations, has dendrites directed centrifugally from the
cell body, spreading through the whole IPL except S1. The extremely
fine (0.1 μm), billowy dendrited of these units bear many small
beads and can be ascribed to the W type (Fig. 6), but they are less
intertwined than the typical W dendrites. The extension of the
dendritic tree varies from 160 to 450 μm, and therefore these cells
are confined to the medium and wide-field classes. The somata of
asymmetric cells range from 6x8.5 μm for medium-field cells (AMW)
to 7x13 μm for wide-field units (AWW), and are located preferentially
close to the embryonic fissure.

Displaced cells

        Amacrine cells whose cell bodies are displaced to the ganglion
cell layer can be easily distinguished from ganglion cells, firstly
because they lack an axon, and secondly because the soma is small
and pyriform and the nucleus is often cupped, giving the cell the
coronate look described by Hughes and Vaney (1980), and Vaney (1980)
in the rabbit retina. Their dendritic type is webbed, and we observed two varieties; one narrow-field monostratified (5NW) (Fig. 3),
and one wide-field bistratified (45WW) (Fig. 5).   The latter unit
has a narrow dendritic field in S5, and long processes extending
horizontally into S4 at the 67% level. The somata are 8x8 μm for
45WW. We did not find that, the somata of displaced amacrine cells
were, on the average, larger than those of amacrine cells of the
inner nuclear layer as observed in the rabbit (Hughes and Vaney,
1980). Like displaced cells in other species, amacrine cells of the
bogue ramify only in the sublamina close to their soma, namely
sublamina b.

Multilayered Cells

        Amacrine cells may send dendrites to more than one sublayer,
we observed two bistratified units within sublamina a (23SK and
23MK), and three bistratified (15WS, 34SW and 34MW) and two tri-
stratified (124MS and 345WS) cells bracking in both sublamina a
and b.

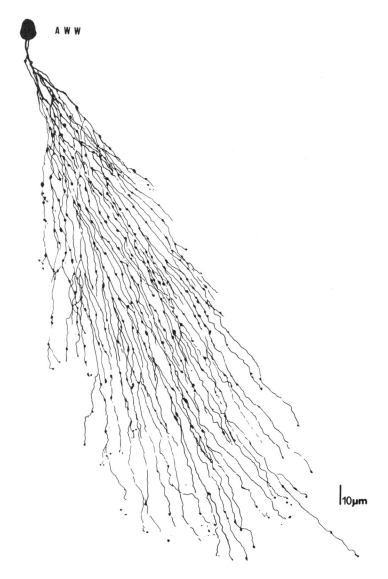

Fig. 6. Flat-mounted asymmetric amacrine cell. The soma of this peculiar type of cell is located close to the embryonic fissure and the very fine beaded dendrites are directed centrifugally.

23SK (Fig. 7) has coarse dendrites in the small-field range branching at level 33% and fine processes terminating at level 50%, at the boundary between the two sublaminae. 23MK, a medium-field unit, has two levels of branching, at 21% and 46%, in both levels the cell ramifies with knotty dendrites. The dendritic tree is less extensive in S3 than in S2. 15WS has a small soma (6x8 μm) and long, coarse dendrites with few branches. 34SW and 34MK have round somata (10x10 μm), and wavy, spiny dendrites extending across the border between sublamina a and b (Fig. 4 34MW). 124MS is a typical bistratified cell with ramification in non-contiguous sublayer; the soma is pyriform (10x15 μm), and the coarse, primary dendrites are tapered toward the periphery, as usual in type S dendrites. 345WS has a large hemilunar cell body (12x15 μm) from which depart two thick branches that ramify repeatedly in S3, S4 and S5 (Fig. 4 345WS). Coarse and short (∿150 μm) dendrites terminate just above the ganglion cell somata, while fine and long (∿1 mm) processes remain within S4. This cell closely resembles the transient unit stained by Kaneko (1970) in the goldfish retina.

DISCUSSION

We observed thirty-nine different types of amacrine cells in the retina of the bogue, classified according to three morphological parameters: spatial organization of their dendrites at the inner plexiform layer, extension of the dendritic tree and dendritic morphology (Fig. 8). Nineteen morphological types were previously described in teleost retina on the basis of branching pattern and cell body size (Cajal, 1972). We did not consider the size of the soma as an index for classification because the slight variations observed seem to be related mostly to the extension of dendritic field. The only significant diversity we found is that the somata of diffuse units are on the average 20% smaller than those strati-fied cells. More types may be suspected because of the capricious-ness of the Golgi staining technique, which is extremely powerful but completely unpredictable. The reason for the large observed variety as compared with mammals (Kolb et al., 1981) may be found in the original observation of Boycott and Dowling (1969) that the retinas of lower vertebrates with less developed cortical visual area contain a large morphological diversity of neuronal units and a distinctly laminated inner plexiform layer, possibly because much of the visual information is processed within the retina.

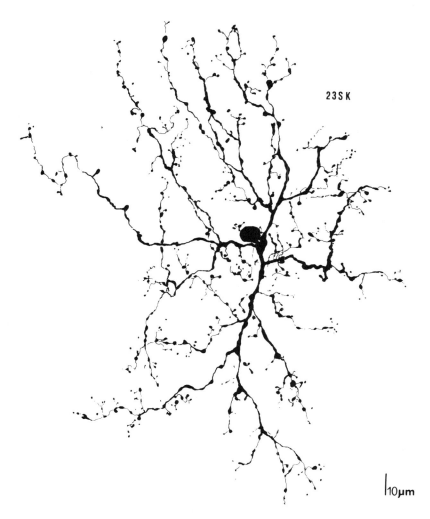

23S K

10μm

Fig. 7.　Bistratified amacrine cell of sublamina a.　The coarse
dendrites are layered in sublayer 2, and the fine ones
invade S3.　The large beads interlaced with dendrites
ascribe this cell to the knotty dendride type.

LEVEL OF LAYERING		DENDRITIC FIELD			
SUB LAYER	MEAN % IPL	NARROW <50 μ	SMALL 50÷150	MEDIUM 150÷250	WIDE >250μ
1	13±5	1NW	1SK 1SR 1ST	1MT	
2	33±6		2SR 2SW 2ST	2MK 2MR 2MW	
3	48±3		3ST	3MR 3MT	
4	61±7		4SR 4ST	4MR 4MS 4MT	4WR
5	93±10		5SK 5MS	5MK	5WR 5WS 5WT
DIFFUSE		DNW		DMW	
ASYMMETRIC				AMW	AWW
DISPLACED		5 NW			45WW
MULTI– LAYERED		23SK 34SW	23MK 34MW 124MS		15WS 345WS

(Left vertical label: STRATIFIED)
(Right vertical labels: K=KNOTTY R=RADIATE W=WEBBED S=SEMITHICK T=THICK DENDRITIC TYPES)

Fig. 8.   Diagram of the observed amacrine cell types in the bogue
           retina. The first symbol of the code represents the
           sublayer of branching for stratified cells, or whether
           the cell is diffuse uniformly (D) or asymmetrically (A).
           The second letter gives the size of dendritic field, and
           the third letter the dendritic type.

    In this study on Boops boops retina we have chosen parameters for
classification which have some basis in function. Patterns of
branching are probably associated with the waveform of the responses,
even if the relation is different for different animal species. Thus
it has been noted in the carp retina (Murakami and Shimoda, 1977)
that broadly stratified of diffuse amacrine cells produce transient
responses, while narrowly stratified cells are associated with
sustained responses. In contrast, diffuse amacrine cells give
sustained responses in the cat (Kolb and Nelson, 1981) and in the
turtle (Marchiafava and Weiler, 1982), where narrowly stratified
amacrine cells produce sharp transient responses, and broadly
stratified units are associated with slow transient responses. Level
of stratification of dendrites within the inner plexiform layer is
known to be related to the polarity of ganglion cell responses

(Famiglietti and Kolb, 1976; Nelson et al., 1978). Thus OFF-centre
ganglion cells branch in sublamina a, while sublamina b contains
the dendrities of ON-centre units. This same relation holds for the
ganglion cells in the salamander retina (Vallerga and Deplano, 1980),
and for certain amacrine cells in the cyprinid fish retina (Famiglietti et al., 1977).

We observed a two-part structural subdivision of the IPL according to the shape of bipolar endings; the three distal sublayer (S1,
S2 and S3 contain the branched axon terminals of cone bipolar cells,
while in S4 and S5 are found round and compact terminals of both
cone and rod bipolars (Fig. 2). We assume that sublayers S1 to S3
form sublamina a, where the "OFF" pathway is confined, and S4 and S5
are sublamina b where terminate the cells of the "ON" pathway of
the visual information. The functional correlation of the structural
bisublamination of the IPL has to be proved in the Sparidae retina,
but it is supported by the study on cyprinid fish retina (Famiglietti et al., 1977).

The criterion we used to define the extension of the dendritic
field differ slightly from other authors (Famiglietti and Siegfried,
1980; Kolb et al., 1981). They chose the maximum diameter of the
dendritic tree, while we have measured the maximum distance from
the soma to the dendritic terminals (D) because we assume that this
is more representative of the actual maximum distance a signal
travels. Since the dendritic field of amacrine cells is often
elliptical or asymmetric. The values of D are from 20 μm to 1 mm,
and these values are grouped rather naturally into three classes:
narrow-field (class N) for D<50 μm, small-field (S) for 50<D<150
μm, medium-field (M) for 150<D<250 μm. In the wide-field class D
ranges from 250 μm to 1 mm, and there is no accumulation point around
the mean value.

We did not observe any systematic variation in the size of
dendritic field with increasing distance from the optic disc as
observed in the cat (Boycott and Wässle, 1974; Kolb et al., 1981).
A recent paper gives a reason for this finding, Braccini et al.
(1982) suggest that in mammals the dendritic fields of amacrine
and ganglion cells increase with eccentricity to satisfy constraints
due to the logarithmic mapping on the visual cortex. In fishes the
lack of visual cortex removes the requirement for geometrical
variation of dendritic field.

Dendritic morphology is known to affect the electrotonic properties of neurons. The large diversification of the dendritic shapes
of amacrine cells in fish retina suggests a specific functional role
for each dendritic type in the visual circuitry. A functional
meaning for a specific morphological type of dendrite has been
provided by Kolb and Nelson (1981) in the cat retina. They observed
that the small beads of large-field amacrine cells with fine dendrites branching in sublamina b, are the sites of reciprocal synaptic
interactions with rod bipolar cells. Our 4WR could be the counter-
part of such a unit in the fish retina.

The need to identify amacrine cells by the level of branching
and dendritic morphology has recently been stressed by immunocytochemical and pharmacological studies which suggest that different
neurotransmitters can be found within different morphological types
of amacrine cells. Indications are provided that in the mammalian
retina dopamine and GABA are released by units of the K class
(Pourcho, 1981; Famiglietti and Vaughn, 1981). Cholinergic amacrine
cells can be recognized as units of the R class branching in sub
lamina a, or in sublamina b when their somata are displaced to the
ganglion cell layer (Hayden et al., 1980; Masland and Mills 1979;
Massey et al., 1981). In the newt retina displaced amacrine cells
with W type dendrites have been reported to be GABA-ergic and
taurinergic (Ball and Dickson, 1981). In goldfish, GABA-ergic units
are confined to sublamina b, and are pyriform amacrine cells of the
T class (Lam et al., 1979; Marc et al., 1978; Yazulla, 1981); our
4MT and 5WT (Fig. 5) closely recall the morphology of GABA-ergic cells
cells. Glycine is accumulated by narrow-field, weakly bistratified
cells in the human retina (Frederick et al., 1981). Indoleamine
has been found in amacrine cells of sublamina a which are pre- and
post-synaptic to other amacrine cells, and in amacrines of sublamina
b which contact bipolar cells (Holmgren, 1981).

The low morphological resolution of neurochemical and electrophysiological technique emphasize the need for a detailed morphological desctiption of each cell type to serve as a reference standard. The Golgi study may act as trait d'union to link pharmacological and physiological units, with the aim of depicting in its en-
tirety the functional role of each amacrine cell type.

REFERENCES

Ball A.K. and Dickson D.H. (1981). Taurinergic and GABA-ergic
    amacrine cells in the ganglion cell layer of the newt retina,
    Invest. Ophthal. Visual Sci. ARVO Suppl., p. 204.
Boycott B.B. and Dowling J.E. (1969). Organization of the primate
    retina: light microscopy, Phil. Trans. R. Soc. B., 255, 109-
    184.
Boycott B.B. and Wässle H. (1974). The morphological types of
    ganglion cells of the domestic cat's retina, J. Physiol. Lond.,
    240, 397-419.
Braccini C, Gambardella G., Sandini G. and Tagliasco V. (1982). A
    model of the early stages of the human visual system: func-
    tional and topological transformations performed in the
    peripheral visual field, Biol. Cybern, (in press).
Cajal Ramon Y.S. (1972). "The Structure of the Retina" (trans.
    Thorpe S.A. and Glickstein M.), p. 17-38, Thomas C.A.,
    Springfield, Illinois.
Famiglietti E.V. (1981). Starburst amacrines: 2 mirror-symmetric
    retinal networks, Invest. Ophthal. Visual Sci. ARVO Suppl.,
    p. 204.
Famiglietti E.V., Kaneko A. and Tachibana M. (1977). Neuronal
    architecture of on and off pathways to ganglion cells in carp,
    Science, 198, 1267-1269.
Famiglietti E.V. and Kolb H. (1976). Structural basis for 'ON' and
    'OFF'-center responses in retinal ganglion cells, Science, 194,
    193-195.
Famiglietti E.V. and Siegfried E.C. (1980). The amacrine cells of
    rabbit retina, Invest. Ophthal. Visual Sci. ARVO Suppl., p. 70.
Famiglietti E.V. and Vaughn J.L. (1981). Golgi impregnated amacrine
    cells and GABA-ergic retinal neurons: a comparison of dendritic
    immuno-cytochemical, and histochemical stratification in the
    inner plexiform layer of rat retina, J. Comp. Neurol., 197,
    129-139.
Frederick J.M., Lam Dominic M.K., Rayborn M.E. and Hollyfield J.G.
    1981). Identification of neurotransmitters in the human retina.
    Invest. Ophthal. Visual Sci. ARVO Suppl., p. 203.
Hayden S.A., Mills J.W., Masland R.M. (1980). Acetylcholine
    synthesis by displaced amacrine cells, Science, 210, 435-437.
Holmgren I.T., Ehringer B. and Dowling J.E. (1981). Synaptic
    organization of the indoleamine- accumulating neurons in the
    cat retina, Invest. Ophthal. Visual Sci. ARVO Suppl., 203.

Hughes A. and Vaney D.I. (1980). Coronate cells: displaced amacrines of the rabbit retina, J. Comp. Neurol., 189, 169-189.

Kaneko A. (1970). Physiological and morphological identification of horizontal, bipolar and amacrine cells in goldfish retina, J. Physiol., 270, 623-633.

Kaneko A. (1973). Receptive field organization of bipolar and amacrine cells in the goldfish retina, J. Physiol., 235, 133-153.

Kolb H. and Nelson R. (1981). Three amacrine cells of the cat retina: morphology and intracellular responses, Invest. Ophthal. Visual Sci. ARVO Suppl., p. 184.

Kolb H., Nelson R. and Mariani A. (1981). Amacrine cells, bipolar cells and ganglion cells of the cat retina: a Golgi study, Vision Res., 21, 1081-1114.

Lam D.M.K., Su Y.Y.T., Swain L., Marc R.E., Brandon C. and Wu J.Y. (1979). Immunocytochemical localization of L-glutamic and decarboxylase in the goldfish retina, Nature, 278, 565-567.

Marc R.E., Stell W.K., Bok D. and Lam D.M.K. (1978). GABA-ergic pathways in the goldfish retina, J. Comp. Neurol., 172, 221-246.

Marchiafava P.L. and Weiler R. (1982). The photoresponses of structurally identified amacrine cells in the turtle retina, Proc. R. Soc. Lond. B, 214, 403-415.

Masland R.H. and Mills J.W. (1979). Autoradiographic identification of acetylcholine in the rabbit retina, J. Cell Biol., 83, 159-178.

Massey S.C., Crawford M.L.J. and Redburn D.A. (1981). Many cholinergic amacrine cells in rabbit retina receive ON input, Invest. Ophthal. Visual Sci. ARVO Suppl., p. 44.

Murakami M. and Shimoda Y. (1977). Identification of amacrine and ganglion cells in the carp retina, J. Physiol., 264, 801-818.

Nelson R., Famiglietti E.V. and Kolb H. (1978). Intracellular staining reveals different levels of stratification for ON and OFF-center ganglion cells in cat retina, J. Neurophysiol., 41, 472-483.

Pourcho R.G. (1981). Dopaminergic amacrine cells in the cat retina, Invest. Ophthal. Visual Sci. ARVO Suppl., p. 203.

Scholes J.H. (1975). Colour receptors and their synaptic connexions, in the retina of a cyprinid fish, Proc. R. Soc. Lond B, 270, 61-118.

Toyoda J.I., Hashimoto H., Ohtsu K. (1973). Bipolar-amacrine transmission in the carp retina, Vision Res., 13, 295-307.

Vallerga S. (1981). Physiological and morphological identification of amacrine cells in tiger salamander retina, Vision Res., 21, 1307-1317.

Vallerga S. and Deplano S. (1980). Structural basis for amacrine and ganglion cell responses, Invest. Ophthal. Visual Sci. ARVO Suppl., p. 285.

Vaney D.I. (1980). A quantitative comparison between the ganglion cell populations and axonal outflows of the visual streak and periphery of the rabbit retina, J. Comp. Neurol., 189, 215-233.

Wagner J. -H. (1976). Patterns of Golgi impregnated neurons in a predator type fish retina, in "Neural Principles in Vision" F. Zettler and R. Weiler, eds., p. 7-26 Springer-Verlag, Berlin.

West R.W. (1972). Superficial warming of epoxy blocks for cutting 25-150 μm sections to be sectioned in the 40-90 nm range, Stain Technol., 47, 201-204.

Witkowsky P. and Dowling J.E. (1969). Synaptic relationships in the plexiform layers of carp retina, Z. Zellforsch. Mikrosk. Anat., 100, 60-82.

Yazulla S. (1981). GABA-ergic synapses in the goldfish retina: an autoradiographic study of 3H-Muscimol and 3H-GABA binding, Invest. Ophthal. Visual Sci. ARVO Suppl., p. 184.

CHROMATIC ORGANIZATION AND SEXUAL DIMORPHISM

OF THE FLY RETINAL MOSAIC

Nicolas Franceschini

Institut de Neurophysiologie et Psychophysiologie
CNRS, 31, Chemin Joseph-Aiguier
13277 Marseille Cedex 9, France

·INTRODUCTION

Whether in vertebrates or in invertebrates, mapping the spectral organization of a retinal mosaic with single cell resolution often remains an insuperable task, for which microspectrophotometry and intracellular recordings appear as cumbersome tools. The need for methods capable of revealing at a glimpse the mosaic pattern of the individual spectral types across a large receptor array has led to many ingenious techniques, some of which are listed in Table 1.

This account presents the knowledge we have gained over the last few years about the spectral properties of individual receptor cells and their topographic distribution across the fly retinal mosaic. Several methods used for analyzing the properties of single cells (microspectrophotometry, intracellular recordings, intracellular dye injections and electron microscopy) have been associated with a technique of "ommatidial fundus fluoroscopy". This technique reveals individual spectral types of receptors in the live insect from their characteristic autofluorescence colour (Fig. 2).

Like many vertebrates, flies possess a duplex retina. The chromatic organization of the retinal mosaic now appears amazingly complex with a number of spectral types that is reminiscent of the highly differentiated avian retina (Bowmaker and Knowles, 1977; Mariani and Leurre du Pree, 1978).

319

Table 1. Some methods which have been used to reveal the topographic
          distribution of the various spectral types of retinal re-
          ceptors with single cell resolution. The methods of group
          (I) merely provides a way of labelling various receptor
          types. The possible presence of screening or sensitizing
          pigments in some photoreceptor cells calls for caution in
          inferring the spectral sensitivity from transmission meas-
          urements. The methods of group (II) offer a more direct
          insight into the spectral sensitivity of the revealed pho-
          toreceptor cells.

Method	Authors	
Spectral absorbance	Denton and Wyllie	(1955)
	Scholes	(1975)
	Kirschfeld et al.	(1978)
Receptor autofluorescence	Liebman and Leigh	(1969)
	Franceschini et al.	(1981)
Use of oil droplets	Brown	(1969)
	Granda and Haden	(1981 a, b)
	Meyer and May	(1969)
	Bowmaker and Knoles	(1970)
	Mariani and Leure	
	Du Pree	(1978)
	Kolb and Jones	(1982)
Slective uptake of dyes	De Monastrio et al.	(1981)
Activity staining	Gribakin	(1969)
	Marc and Sperling	(1976)
	Levine et al.	(1979)
	Basinger et al.	(1979)
	Fernald	(1981)
Selective induction of pigment migration	Butler	(1971)
	Menzel	(1972)

I (brackets group spanning from "Brown (1969)" through "De Monastrio et al. (1981)")

II (brackets group spanning from "Gribakin (1969)" through "Menzel (1972)")

As regards the neural processing of visual information, an interesting aspect of insects and in particular flies, is the possibility to correlate physiological and behavioural data. Hence the two last chapters concern a characteristic sexual dimorphism of the receptor mosaic which is likely to play a role in the sexual pursuit of the female by the male. The emerging message is of ethoneurological nature, which states that looking at the behaviour of an animal may help understand even the post peripheral part of a neurosensory circuitry.

STRUCTURE AND AXONAL PROJECTIONS OF THE PHOTORECEPTOR CELLS

Two compound eyes containing a total of $\sim$ 50 000 receptor cells confer upon the housefly a panoramic vision (Fig. 9a). In each of the 3000 ommatidia of an eye, the receptor cells are arranged in groups of 8, according to a characteristic, asymmetrical pattern (Fig. 1a, b, c). The light-sensitive part of a cell is called a rhabdomere (hatched in Fig. 1a, b, c), which is a slender rod (diameter $\sim$ 1 μm) acting as an absorbing waveguide. Six peripheral cells (R 1-6) encircle two smaller cells (R 7-8) whose rhabdomeres curiously lie on top of each other and build a continuous light-guide (Fig. 1c). As a consequence, R7 inevitably acts as a screen for the underlying R8.

Both peripheral (R1-6) and central (R7-8) cells respond to light with a depolarizing receptor potential (Järcilehto, 1971; Smola and Meffert, 1975; Eckert et al., 1976; Hardie, 1977) having a peak level of $\sim$ 50 mV and a time-to-peak of $\sim$10-50 ms (Scholes, 1969; Hardie, 1977).

Due to the neat separation of the 7 rhabdomere endings in the focal plane of the corneal lenslet, each ommatidium samples the few degrees of its visual field along seven eigen-direction (Kirschfeld, 1967; Kirschfeld and Franceschini, 1968). But the projection of the receptor axons onto the first optic ganglion (the lamina or outer plexiform layer) takes advantage of this situation not for improving the angular resolution of the eye but rather for improving its quantum catch. Each cartridge of the lamina receives axons from six receptor cells (of type 1-6) which belong each to a different ommatidium but which look all in the same direction of space. This is the remarkable connectivity principle of the "neural superposition eye" of flies (Vigier, 1909; Braitenberg, 1967; Kirschfeld, 1967; Reviews in Kirschfeld, 1972; Braitenberg and Strausfeld, 1973; Shaw, 1981). In view of the photon noise affecting each receptor channel, a ben-

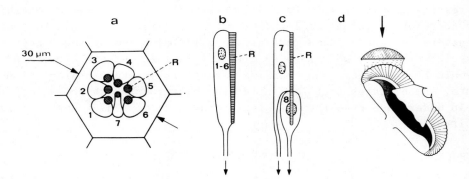

Fig. 1.   (a-c) Sensory outfit of a housefly ommatidium (after Trujil-
          lo-Cenoz and Melamed, 1966; Boschek, 1971).   (a) six recep-
          tor cells R1-6 whose longitudinal section is shown in (b)
          surround two smaller, central cells R7 and R8 which lie on
          top of each other as shown in (c).   The hatched part of each
          cell is the rhabdomere, which houses the visual pigment(s).
          (d) method used for visualizing the rhabdomeres in vivo in
          a large number of ommatidia (see Fig. 2).   "Ommatidial fundus
          fluoroscopy" is achieved by optically neutralizing the cor-
          neal surface with a drop of water and observing the distal
          receptor endings with epi-fluorescence microscopy (blue ex-
          citation).   (from Franceshini et al., 1981 b).

eficial effect of the signal summation which takes place within a
cartridge (Scholes, 1969) appears to be an improvement (by factor
√6) in the signal-to-noise ratio, a parameter which sets limits to
both absolute and contrast sensitivity.

     A slight variant of this scheme is encountered at the equator
of the eye, on each side of which the rhabdomere patterns exhibit a
mirror-image symmetry (Dietrich, 1909).   Here 7 to 8 receptor cells
of type 1-6 looking in the same direction of space (Kirschfeld, 1967)
and it has been shown that the lamina cartridges correspondingly receive 7 to 8 axons instead of the usual 6 (Horridge and Meinertzhagen,
1970; Boschek, 1971).   This provides a kind of "visual streak" with
improved quantum catch that could help the fly navigate in low light
level environments (Franceschini, 1975).

     For each sampling direction, vision is brought about by two vis-
ual subsystems having co-axial receptive fields.   The one is mediated
by the second order neurons leaving each cartridge and projecting to

various sublaminae of the medulla, the other is mediated by the two central cells R7 and R8 whose axons bypass the underlying cartridge and project directly to the medulla (Cajal and Sanchez, 1915; Trujillo-Cenoz and Melamed, 1966; Campos-Ortega and Strausfeld, 1972). An optical phenomenon which we have called the "reduced corneal pseudopupil" provides direct evidence for the strict coaxiality of the elementary receptive fields of these two integrated visual subsystems (Franceschini and Kirschfeld, 1971b; and Franceschini, 1975).

The present review summarizes our knowledge about the spectral properties of these two visual subsystems and about a conspicuous departure from the general connectivity pattern outlined above which affects a strategic region of the male eye.

NATURAL FLUORESCENT LABEL ON EACH SINGLE CELL

Early intracellular recordings made by Burkhardt (1962) have revealed that the compound eye of flies is equipped with receptor cells of various spectral sensitivities. The recent discovery of rhabdomere autofluorescence has shed a new light upon the precise chromatic organization of the retinal mosaic.

The convex corneal lenslets of the fly's eye can be optically neutralized if one applies a clear medium of appropriate refractive index (~ 1.5) onto the corneal surface (Franceschini and Kirschfeld, 1971a). Under such conditions (Fig. 1d) each lenslet (diameter $\sim$ 30 μ m, see Fig. 1a) becomes a kind of tiny flat window through which one can discover the intimacy of the retinula. Recent association of this technique of "optical neutralization of the cornea" with epifluorescence microscopy has revealed that most rhabdomeres of the eye of flies are fluorescent under various excitations (Franceschini, 1977; Franceschini et al., 1981b). The most colourful palette is observed under blue excitation (e.g. 436 nm Hg-line) which simultaneously reveals a homogeneous population of red-emitting R 1-6 rhabdomeres and a mixed population of green- and non-fluorescing R7's (Fig. 2).

These fluorescence phenomena are interesting in three respects. Firstly, they allow visual pigment properties to be studied in individual, living cells by using in vivo microspectrofluorimetry (review in Franceschini, 1982). Secondly, they confer upon each individual cell a characteristic color label which allows detailed mapping of the retinal mosaic to be carried out with single cell resolution (sections 7-8). Thirdly, they can be used for attributing to a given cell the results of an intracellular electrical recording (section 5).

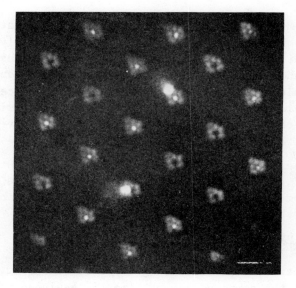

Fig. 2.   In vivo epifluorescence observation of the individual photo-
          receptor cells in the eye of a female housefly (mutant
          white). The whole retina is more than 100 times larger than
          the retinal patch viewed here. Calibration bar: 10 μm.
          The method of "ommatidial fundus fluoroscopy" schematically
          described in Fig. 1d was used here (neutralizing agent:
          water; objective: 25x water, numerical aperture 0,65; blue
          excitation: mercury arc 100 Watts with interference filter
          436 nm; barrier filter: 510 nm; aperture filtering as de-
          scribed in Franceschini, 1982). On this black-and-white
          print of the original colour slide (Ektachrome 400 Asa),
          the colour-code is the following: grey spots = red-fluor-
          escing R1-6 rhabdomeres; bright central spots = green-fluor-
          escing R7 rhabdomeres (R7y); dark central spots = non-fluor-
          escing R7 rhabdomeres (R7p). The two bright and large spots
          reveal the yellow fluorescence of the two cells which have
          been impaled by the microelectrode and stained by iontopho-
          retic injection of procion yellow (see Section 5). (From
          Franceschini and Hardie, in preparation).

     So far our analysis of the fluorescence colours observed under
blue excitation can be summarized as follows. The red emission stems
from a related form, M' of metarhodopsin, which is created under
intense blue irradiation (Franceschini et al., 1981b; Stavenga et
al., in prep.). The green emission belongs to a peculiar class of
central rhabdomeres (R7y) which contain, in addition to their rhodop-

sin, a blue-absorbing accessory-pigment (probably β-carotene according to the three-fingered absorption spectrum measured with microspectro-photometry: Kirschfeld et al., 1978; Mac Intyre and Kirschfeld, 1981). Evidence that the green emission stems from this accessory pigment (rather than from the specific rhodopsin of this cell: Kirschfeld, 1979) is provided by recent fluorescence observations done under polarized blue excitation (Franceschini, unpublished). By contrast to the red emission from R 1-6 which is maximal when the E-vector of the exciting light is parallel to their microvilli (hatched in Fig. 1a) the green emission is maximal when the E-vector is perpendicular to the R7 microvilli. This is precisely what is expected if the e-mission stems from the accessory pigment because the latter confers upon the cell an unusual dichroism such that maximal absorption in the blue occurs when the E-vector is perpendicular to the microvilli (Kirschfeld and Franceschini, 1977). However, assignment of the green emission to β-carotene is somehow provocative in view of the reputedly non-fluorescing property of this molecule even at low temperature (Tric and Lejeune, 1970; Song and Moore, 1974). We are left with the hypothesis that the microenvironment of this molecule in the microvillar membrane would be such as to allow some radiative deexcitation, whether the carotene remains as such or suffers a "retro" isomerism (Wallcave and Zechmeister, 1953).

The fluorescence intensity of all cell types remains stable over hours under moderate blue excitation, thus allowing scrutiny of the retinal mosaic (see section 6-8). Before we report the spectral sensitivity of these various receptor cells we first present some methods we now have on hand that allow rapid measurement of the spectral sensitivity and rapid recovery of an impaled cell.

FAST MEASUREMENT OF THE SPECTRAL SENSITIVITY OF SINGLE CELLS WITH A VOLTAGE-CLAMP METHOD

The spectral sensitivity of a receptor cell can be defined as the reciprocal of the photon flux required at each wavelength to induce a criterion response (depolarizing or hyperpolarizing receptor potential). The voltage-clamp method we have devised (Franceschini, 1979) is a straightforward application of this definition. Its principle is to have the light flux impinging upon the cell automat-ically adjusted at each wavelength in such a way that the receptor potential remains clamped at a given reference value V_{ref}. This is achieved by a neutral density wedge whose position is continuously controlled by the errorsignal between the reference voltage and the actual voltage delivered by the cell (Fig. 3).

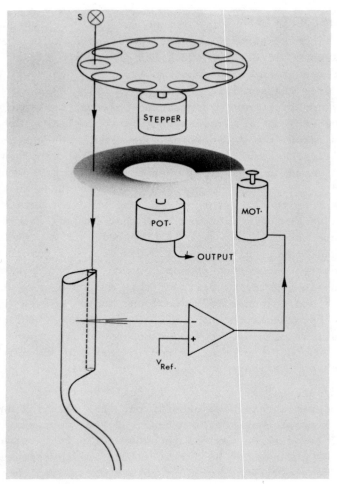

Fig. 3.   Voltage-clamp technique for fast measurement of the spectral
          sensitivity of a receptor cell (a fly photoreceptor cell of
          type Rl-6 is here schematically depicted, hit by a microe-
          lectrode). The purpose of the electromechanical feedback
          is to have the cell deliver a constant output voltage (e-
          qual to a reference voltage V_{ref}.) and to record the grey
          wedge settings (POT. = Potentiometer) which realize this
          condition for each colour. The error signal between the
          actual receptor potential and the reference voltage V_{ref}.
          is amplified by a high-gain differential amplifier whose
          output controls the rotation of a miniature DC—motor (MOT.)
          and in turn the rotation of a quartz neutral density wedge
          (optical density 0-4).

In the "open loop mode" (Fig. 4a) the grey wedge has a fixed setting
and stepping of the interference filter wheel induces a jump of receptor potential which depends upon many parameters (spectral sensitivity and characteristic curve of the cell, spectral emission of
the lamp and transmission of each filter). In the "closed loop mode"
on the other hand (Fig. 4b) any deviation of the cell's output from
the reference voltage (here V_{ref} = 8mV) is automatically nulled out.
The grey wedge (Fig. 4c) continuously searches for the setting which
yields a constant receptor potential (Fig. 4b). Under these conditions, the wedge setting D (λ), which is translated by a potentio-
meter (Fig. 3), is a useful output from which a genuine spectral
sensitivity of the cell can be determined subsequently. For this
purpose each pair λ, D is set again after the electrophysiological
experiment and a radiometer reads the corresponding light flux,
whose inverse is plotted versus wavelength as the spectral sensitivity of the cell (Fig. 4d).

The main advantage of this method lies in the rapid uptake of
the essential information required to (subsequently) determine the
spectral sensitivity. In Fig. 4, it took only 20 seconds to explore
a one-octave wavelength range in 20 discrete points. But the relatively rapid settling time ($\tau \sim 100$ ms) of the electromechanical
servo-system allows spectral sensitivity measurements to be done
within only three seconds provided the spectrum in continuously
scanned rather than discretely stepped (Franceschini, in preparation).

FAST RECOVERY OF DYE-INJECTED CELLS IN THE LIVING ANIMAL

The blindly impaled receptor cell whose spectral sensitivity
is being determined can subsequently be recovered in vivo provided
a fluorescent dye be injected into the cell at the end of the electrophysiological recording (Franceschini and Hardie, 1980).

In Fig. 2, two such cells were recovered in this way. Under
blue excitation the stained receptor cells were identified immediately after the injections by the bright (yellow) fluorescence of
their rhabdomeres (and to a lesser extent of their cell bodies)
standing out from the fainter (red or green) autofluorescence of
most rhabdomeres. The two cells were penetrated one after the other
with a micropipette filled with procion yellow. Following physiological measurements, iontophoretic injection of the dye was done in
each case by passing a negative d.c. current (2 nA for 1 min.; i.e.
$\sim 0.1 \mu$ C) across the "preparation". The two spotlighted rhabdomeres

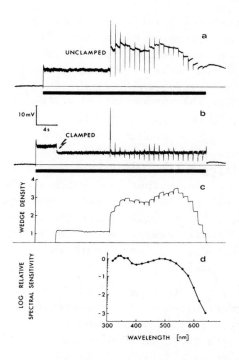

Fig. 4.   To illustrate the operation of the servo-system schematized
          in Fig. 3 (a) "open-loop mode"; the feedback is disconnected
          and the receptor potential of the cell is free to jump from
          one value to another as the interference filter wheel is
          stepped at 1 Hz. Following a steady illumination at 620 nm,
          the filter wheel successively presents its 20 interference
          filters (halfwidth <10 nm) from UV to red. At the end of
          this spectral scan, a prolonged depolarizing afterpotential
          is observed, which declines to the resting level within ∿20
          sec.

                    (b,c) "closed-loop mode". The feedback is set
          into operation after 4 sec steady red light illumination
          (620 nm, wedge maximally transparent). As the choosen ref-
          erence voltage $V_{ref.}$ (Fig. 3) is smaller than the actual
          cell output, the neutral wedge (c) immediately turns to
          the required attenuation value (D ∿ 1,2). As soon as the
          filter wheel is stepped, the wedge rapidly searches for
          the attenuations which maintain a constant receptor potential
          equal to $V_{ref.}$. Notice that the cell rapidly repolarizes
          to the dark level at the end of the scan and clamp. By
          contrast to the ill-defined light regime used in (a), the

(Fig. 2) are clearly identified as R2 and R3 (comp. Fig. 1a) and they are located in ommatidia containing a non-fluorescing and a green-fluorescing R7 rhabdomere respectively.

It takes only a few minutes after the injection to locate and identify the cell in vivo without calling upon the usual histological procedure. The lack of chemical treatment, embedding and microtomy guarantees a very high recovery rate (nearly 100%) so that routine injections into single photoreceptor cell are feasible.

Both methods described in sections 4 and 5 are characterized by their speed. In the best cases a spectral sensitivity run can be done in three seconds and, using the highly fluorescing dye lucifer yellow (Stewart, 1978), it takes only another three seconds (with 3 nA) to stain the cell sufficiently to permit a safe and rapid recovery (Franceschini and Hardie, in prep.).

---

overall light adaptation of the cell during the measurement can be here conveniently expressed by the product "receptor potential x time".

(d) dual-peak spectral sensitivity of the recorded cell (type R1-6). The ordinate represents the inverse of the relative photon flux impinging upon the cell in the voltage-clamp situation (b,c). This photon flux has been measured at each wavelength, for each corresponding value of the neutral density wedge. The dual-peak spectral sensitivity is due to the presence of two pigments housed in the same rhabdomere: a blue-green absorbing rhodopsin and an ultraviolet sensitizing pigment (see section 6).

DUAL-PEAK SPECTRAL SENSITIVITY OF CELLS 1-6

As shown in Fig. 4d, the spectral sensitivity of a cell type 1-6 curiously consists of two bands, one peaking in the blue-green ($\sim$ 490 nm) the other in the near ultraviolet ($\sim$ 350 nm). Ever since Burkhardt (1961) first obtained such spectral curves from fly receptor cells, interpretation of this odd dual-peak sensitivity has led to many conjectures.

The present interpretation is as follows. We know that the "visible" peak (490 nm) is due to the rhodopsin P490 (Hamdorf et al., 1973; Hamdorf, 1979; Stavenga et al., 1973; Kirschfeld and Franceschini, 1975). On the other hand, there is evidence that the ultraviolet peak originates from an accessory, photostable pigment housed in the same rhabdomere and playing the role of a sensitizer (Kirschfeld et al., 1977).

As discussed by Kirschfeld in this volume, energy transfer is assumed to take place from the UV-absorbing pigment (donor) to the rhodopsin (acceptor) according to the model of "inductive resonance" (Foerster, 1951). Even though this kind of transfer does not involve donor fluorescence followed by absorption of radiation by the acceptor, it nevertheless requires a spectral overlap between the emission spectrum of the donor and the absorption spectrum of the acceptor. In this context it has been interesting to observe a conspicuous, broadband fluorescence emission from rhabdomeres R 1-6 under UV-excitation (Franceschini, 1977; 1982; Franceschini et al., 1981 b; Stark et al., 1977; 1979; Stavenga et al. in prep.). This fluorescence emission has a first peak at 470 nm (Stavenga et al., in prep.) and if this were to originate from the UV-pigment it would be a sign that excitation energy can be transferred to the nearby rhodopsin by inductive resonance.

When measured with high spectroscopic resolution (which is not the case in Fig. 4d) the spectral sensitivity of receptor cells 1-6 display a conspicuous fine structure consisting of three peaks near 330, 350, 370 nm (Gemperlein et al., 1979; Kirschfeld et al., in press) which is seen also in the extinction spectrum of R 1-6 rhabdomeres determined by microspectrophotometry (Kirschfeld, this volume, Kirschfeld et al., in press).

As discussed elsewhere (Franceschini, 1982) many carotenoid-related substances could account for such a fine structure but the most interesting candidate is a retinol-protein complex. The classical, diffuse absorption spectrum of vitamin A (retinol) which peaks near 325 nm not only suffers a red shift of 25 nm upon binding to a protein but also becomes a vibrationally resolved with three peaks near, 330, 350, 370 nm. This fine structure is especially pronounced when, upon binding to the protein a "retro" retinol isomer is formed (Schreckenbach et al., 1977; Ong and Chytill, 1978; Hemley et al., 1979; Fugate and Song, 1980). An appealing hypothesis is that the retinol chromophore would be bound to the opsin itself, at a site close to the retinal chromophore. This would meet the second stringent requirement of Foerster's model which is a close proximity of donor and acceptor molecules.

From a functional standpoint the UV-sensitizing pigment extends the spectral range over which cells 1-6 are sensitive. And in making these cells 'panchromatic' it improves their quantum catch.

Thanks to the technique of optical neutralization of the cornea, the 18000 rhabdomeres R 1-6 of an eye can be screened _in vivo_ within a few hours. All of them display the same fluorescence colour (red) under blue excitation. If this red label is everywhere indicative of a dual-peak spectral sensitivity like that shown in Fig. 4d (an hypothesis of far-reaching value as shown in Section 8) it appears that the first visual subsystem, i.e. that which is driven by receptor cells 1-6 exclusively (see section 2) is spectrally homogeneous and hence cannot by itself mediate colour vision. Evidence has been produced that this visual system is implicated in movement detection (Eckert, 1971; Kirschfeld, 1972; Mc Cann and Arnett, 1972; Heidenberg and Buchner, 1977; Riehle and Franceschini, 1983).

SPECTRAL SENSITIVITY OF THE CENTRAL CELLS R7 AND R8

By contrast to the ubiquitous receptor cells R 1-6 which are spectrally homogeneous, the central cells R7 and R8 display a bewildering variety of spectral types. It is only in the last five years that we have gained a detailed knowledge about the spectral properties and mosaic organization of these cells whose tiny somata (width 3-5 μm; comp. Fig. 1a) make intracellular recordings a difficult task.

The analyses have called upon various techniques: microspectro-photometry (Langer and Thorell, 1966; Kirschfeld and Franceschini, 1977; Kirschfeld et al., 1978; Kirschfeld, 1979; Mac Intyre and Kirschfeld, 1981), fluorescence microscopy (Franceschini, 1977; Hardie et al., 1979; Franceschini and Hardie, 1980; Franceschini et al., 1981 a, b). intracellular recordings (Meffert and Smola, 1976; Hardie, 1977; 1979; Hardie et al., 1979; Smola and Meffert, 1979) and electron microscopy (Meffert and Smola, 1976; Smola and Meffert, 1979; Franceschini et al., 1981 a; Hardie et al., 1981).

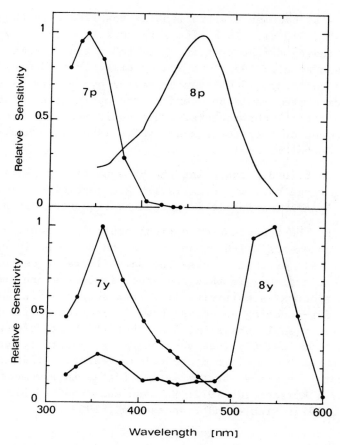

Fig. 5.   Spectral sensitivities of the central receptor cells R7
           and R8 in a fly ommatidium (see fig. 1c). From a comparison
           of the frequency of occurence of the various spectral curves
           to the frequency of occurence of the various R7 autofluor-
           escence colours (Fig. 2 and 6) and from in vivo recovery
           of intracellularly stained cells (Section 5), it is inferred
           that each ommatidium houses either a "yellow" pair (bottom
           curves) or a "pale" pair (upper curves) of R7-8 cells.
           The green fluorescence of the R7y rhabdomeres and the non-
           fluorescence of the R7p rhabdomeres allow both pairs, y and
           p to be spotted in vivo on the retinal mosaic (Fig. 2) so
           that detailed spectral maps of the retina can be drawn
           (Fig. 6). Notice that in both pairs, y and p, the spectral
           maxima are quite separate and the spectral curves sometimes
           quite sharp (e.g. 7y; 8y). Curves redrawn after Hardie et
           al., 1979, 1981; 8p from Hardie, unpublished.

The mosaic organization of the various spectral receptors (type 7 and 8) is not as crystalline as it was expected. As already shown in Fig. 2 some ommatidia house a green-fluorescing, others a non-fluorescing R7 rhabdomere. The green-fluorescing R7's are those equipped with a blue-absorbing photostable pigment (see section 3) which make them look yellow in transmitted white light (hence 7 yellow, 7y). The non-fluorescing R7's, by contrast appear pale in transmitted white light (hence 7 pale, 7p).

By taking fluorescence photographs of several adjacent retinal domains like that shown in Fig. 2, the precise mosaic organization of rhabdomere R7y and R7p could be mapped in the frontal part of both eyes (Fig. 6). These rhabdomere types appear randomly distributed and show no dorso-ventral or bilateral symmetry. Although their precise distribution is different from one fly to another the retina is systematically composed of ∿70% R7y and ∿30% R7p.

Since the voltage-clamp technique (Section 4) had not been developed yet, spectral sensitivities of cells 7 and 8 were determined by the classical method of recording the responses to isoquantal stimuli and referring them to a V/log I curve determined in the same cell (Hardie et al., 1979).

Although dye injections followed by _in vivo_ cell recovery (see section 5 and Fig. 2) allowed us to unequivocally assign some of the measured spectral sensitivities to R7 cells, distinction between 7p and 7y was not possible as the extrinsic fluorescence of the stain usually obscured the R7's natural fluorescence colour. Assignment of the measured spectral sensitivities to the various classes of cells R7 and R8 mainly relies upon a comparison between the frequency of occurrences of spectral classes and rhabdomere types. At least the counts of R7p and R7y could be made under the fluorescence microscope from the very retinal domain surrounding the impaled and recovered cells (comp. Fig. 2).

The present picture we have about these cells is the following (Hardie et al., 1979; Smola and Meffert, 1979). Cells 7 and 8 whose rhabdomeres lie in tandem (Fig. 1c) usually form two different spectral pairs 7p/8p and 7y/8y whose individual spectral properties are shown in Fig. 5. Cell 7p is a UV-sentive receptor and its underlying companion 8p is a blue-sensitive receptor. Cell 7y is again a UV-sensitive receptor but has an extended blue sensitivity. Its underlying companion 8y is a green-sensitive receptor. Even though both 7p and 7y cells are predominantly UV-sensitive, their rhodopsin/metarhodopsin system is different (Kirschfeld, 1979). As a matter

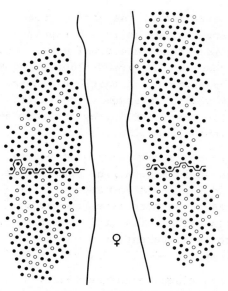

Fig. 6.   Fluorescence mapping of the distribution of the two classes
          of R7 rhabdomeres in the frontal part of both eyes in a
          <u>female</u> housefly. Each dot represents an R7 rhabdomere as
          it appears in the center of each ommatidium (see Fig. 1a
          and 2).   ●: 7y rhabdomeres, recognized from their green
          autofluorescence colour (bright central spots in Fig. 2).
          o: 7p rhabdomeres which are non-fluorescing under blue-
          excitation (dark central spots in Fig. 2). This map, which
          covers approximately 10% of the whole retinal mosaic, was
          obtained from many overlapping fluorescence photographs
          like that shown in Fig. 2, each of them beeing taken after
          a small tilt of the goniometric stage supporting the animal
          under the epi-fluorescence microscope. The female retina
          is composed of   70% R7y and   30% R7p. Notice that the
          exact distribution shows no precise symmetry between the
          two eyes or above and below the equator (represented by
          a zig-zag line). From Hardie et al., 1981

of fact the 7y spectral sensitivity seems to be mediated by the
combined efforts of three pigments, a blue-absorbing rhodopsin, a
blue-absorbing screening pigment and a UV-absorbing sensitizing pigment which all shape the spectral curve in such a way that little
remains from the original rhodopsin spectrum (Kirschfeld, 1979; Hardie et al., 1979; Hardie and Kirschfeld, in preparation).

The unusually sharp spectrum of 8y cells is accurately modelled if one assumes that they contain a rhodopsin with $\lambda_{max} \sim 520$ nm and if one takes into account the major screening action of the blue-absorbing photostable pigment contained in the overlying R7y (Hardie, 1977; Kirschfeld et al., 1978; Hardie et al., 1979). In one case the in vivo recovery technique (section 5) allowed us to correlate unequivocally the green peak of spectral sensitivity of an R8 cell with the presence of an overlying 7y cell (identified by the green autofluorescence of its rhabdomere).

To summarize these results, it appears that the second visual subsystem of the fly, which is driven by receptor cells 7 and 8, displays a great variety of spectral types that certainly provides a potential for colour vision. A remarkable fact is that the tandem-organization of rabdomeres R7 and R8 (Fig. 1C) is of no hindrance as in both pairs (p and y) the spectral maxima of cells 7 and 8 are finally quite separate. In the case of the 7y/8y pair, advantage is even taken of this tandem configuration since the blue-absorbing screening pigment incorporated in the distal cell (7y) contributes to shape the spectral sensitivity of both 7y and 8y cells.

SEX-SPECIFIC CHROMATIC ORGANIZATION OF THE RETINAL MOSAIC

The fluorescence retinal mapping shown in Fig. 6 stemmed from a female. Unexpectedly when mapping the eye of a male we observed that in a peculiar region of the retina, the green-fluorescing R7y and non-fluorescing R7p were progressively substituted for another, red-fluorescing type of R7 called R7 red or R7r (Franceschini et al., 1981 a; Hardie et al., 1981).

As shown in fig 7 (stars), these male-specific photoreceptor cells invade the frontal-dorsal part of the retina. From the red-fluorescence colour of their rhabdomeres we conjectured that these cells would have the same visual pigments and hence spectral sensitivity as their six neighbours in the ommatidium. Both microspectrophotometry and intracellular recordings confirmed this view. Cells 7r display a similar , dual-peak spectral sensitivity like that shown in Fig. 4d, and hence build a third, spectrally distinct population of receptor cells R7 which does not exist at all in the female.

Electrophysiologically the response of the male-specific 7r cells is extremely similar to that of R 1-6 cells. In particular they have the same low noise level. It proved impossible to tell them apart during recording and only subsequent recovery of blindly

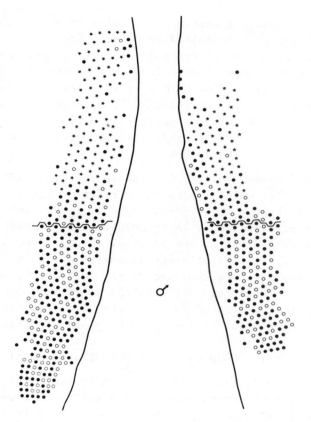

Fig. 7. Distribution of the three classes of central receptor cells
         R7 in the retina of a <u>male</u> housefly (compare to the eye of
         a female, Fig. 6). Beside the gree-fluorescing R7y (●) and
         non fluorescing R7p (o) already encountered in the female,
         a new, red-fluorescing type of R7 (★) invades the frontal-
         dorsal part of the eye, which looks upwards. Such R7r re-
         ceptor cells not only have the same, dual-peak spectral
         sensitivity as their six neighbours in the ommatidium (see
         Fig. 4d), but they project their axon to the same neuropile
         (the lamina), in contrast with the other types of R7 cells.
         From Hardie etal., (1981).

injected cells (see section 5) revealed that they had been recorded
from.

     Ultrastructural examination of such cells (first identified <u>in
vivo</u> from their red fluorescence colour) revealed that their somata
and rhabdomeres were as large and nearly as long as those of R 1-6

cells. But most surprisingly, histological recovery of Lucifer
stained 7r cells showed that their axons stopped short in the lamina
instead of running down to the medulla as do the other R7's of the
eye (section 2).

Hence 7r cells resemble R 1-6 cells not only as regards their
ultrastructure, visual pigments and electrophysiological properties
but also as regards their target neuropile. It would first look as
though all cells endowed with the same visual pigment would project
to the same neuropile. Evidence against this idea is provided however by the underlying cell 8r which again seems to house the same
visual pigments as R 1-6 cells and yet sends its axon directly to
the medulla as do the other R8's of the retina (Franceschini et al.,
1981 a; Hardie et al., 1981). R8r cells have a broadband spectral
sensitivity which can be closely modelled by the screening effect
of the rhodopsin in the 7r rhabdomere upon an R8 rhodopsin similar
to that of R 1-6 and R7r (Hardie et al., 1981).

COLOUR BLIND MALE FOVEA AND SEXUAL BEHAVIOUR

Male flies are known to chase females for mating purposes, but
they also chase other males and even unidentified flying objects,
provided they have the right dimension and speed (Land and Collet,
1974). These aerobatic chases are performed at high speed (1-4 m/sec)
and involve rapid turns of the animal (saccades) at up to 4000°/sec
as well as smooth pursuits.

The intriguing photoreceptor dimorphism described in the preceding section could well serve this exquisite piece of behaviour. A
striking feature of the male chases, as revealed by high-speed cine-
matography, is that the pursuing fly always remain below the pursued
fly (Wehrhahn, 1979). In so doing, the chasing fly probably keeps
the target in the frontal-dorsal part of its retina, that dedicated
part in which the atypical receptor cells 7r are found. The relative
position of both flies is clearly seen in Fig. 8b which shows the
frame-by-frame reconstruction of a chase filmed from the side.

This kind of behavioural act is highly demanding from the standpoint of neuro-optical signal processing. In the first place it
requires the dynamic detection of the small contrast provided by
a black spot (the leading fly) against a continuously changing background (fly chases are not only observed under the blue sky). Hence
the success of the maneuver will depend upon the contrast detectivity
of the visual system. Bearing in mind the principle of "neural superposition" of the fly's eye (section 2) the connectivity of a cell 7r

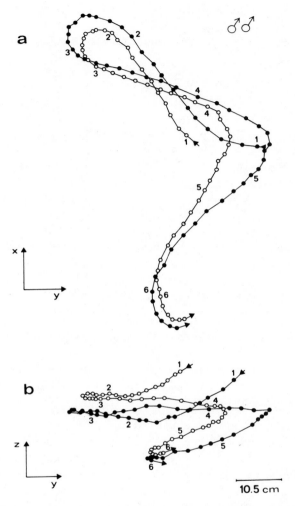

Fig. 8. Example of a chase between two male houseflies (o leading
         fly; ● chasing fly. This high speed chase (whose total du-
         ration was less than 1 sec) was filmed simultaneously from
         above (a) and from the side (b). Film speed: 80 frames
         per sec. Points at 12,5 ms intervals. Corresponding times
         are indicated by the same numbers on both flight paths.
         Notice in (b) that the chasing male remains behind and
         below the leading fly, suggesting that the target's image
         probably falls upon the frontal-dorsal retinal mosaic, in
         which the male-specific R7r receptor cells are found.
         From Wehrhahn, 1979.

is apparently such that a seventh input could now participate in the averaging process which takes place in each cartridge of the lamina. The beneficial consequence would be an improved smoothing of the photon noise at the level of the second order neurons and hence a better capability to detect small contrasts.

Several other features indeed make the frontal-dorsal part of the male retina a rather strategic region of the visual system. It is distinguished by a high acuity like the fovea of the vertebrate eye (Franceschini, 1975; Beersma et al., 1975; Collett and Land, 1975). It also distinguishes itself by an exceptionally large binocular visual field (Franceschini, 1975; Beersma et al., 1975; Franceschini et al., 1979) which is illustrated by the simultaneous microscopical observation of both deep pseudopupils (Fig. 9b). Most importantly, this eye region is known to drive a small set of higher order neurons found in the third neuropile (the lobula), which are characteristic of the male visual system (Hausen and Strausfeld, 1980). One of these neurons, whose receptive field includes the frontal-dorsal part of the retina, is the Male Lobula Giant Neuron N° 1 (MLG1), only one of which exists in each lobula (Fig. 9c).

CONCLUSION

The housefly retinal mosaic displays a rich variety of spectral receptor types (at least 6) and hence rivals the wealth of some reptilian and avian retinae (Liebman and Granda, 1971; Bowmaker and Knowles, 1977; Bowmaker, 1979).

The non-invasive technique of "ommatidial funds fluoroscopy" we have introduced allows us to discriminate individual receptor cells in vivo by their intrinsic fluorescence label (green, red or black) observed under blue excitation. As revealed by transmission microspectrophotometry, these various labels are tightly linked to the specific absorbance of the visual pigments (photosensitive or photostable) and hence constitute a reliable colour code for identifying the various spectral types of receptors. Intracellular injection of a fluorescent dye provides the recorded cell with an additional marker whose in vivo recovery (Fig. 2) facilitates the assignment of a measured spectral sensitivity to a given cell type.

Autofluorescence of vertebrate receptor cells would probably yield a similarly interesting colour code were it not dramatically fading within a few seconds (Liebman and Leigh, 1969). On the other hand, the variously coloured, photostable oil droplets of the turtle

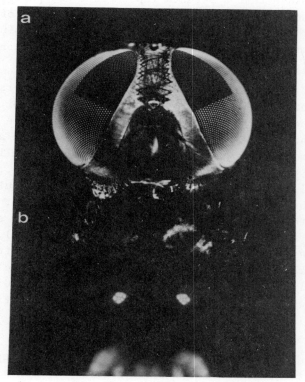

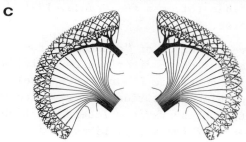

Fig. 9.   (a) Head of a male housefly photographed with a home-made
          Lieberkühn-microscope. The shaded area delineates approx-
          imately the region of the eye in which the male specific
          R7r receptor cells are frequently encountered (stars of
          Fig. 7).
          (b) The two "deep pseudopupils" (Franceschini and Kirsch-
          feld, 1971b) of another male Musca photographed in incident
          light at ∿ 30° above the equator, i.e. in the R7r region.

retina (Brown, 1969, Granda and Haden, 1970) are each associated
with a given visual pigment (Liebman and Granda, 1971) and constitute
another, transmission based colour-code (Baylor and Hodgkin, 1973;
Ohtsuka, 1978).

Several aspects in the chromatic organization of the fly retinal
mosaic deserve special attention.

Light-harvesting pigment in receptor cells R 1-6

The largely represented cells R 1-6 make up a spectrally homogeneous population. It looks as though these cells had been refined
to absorb as many quanta as possible. An ingenious solution is the
incorporation into the microvillar membrane of a slave pigment, absorbing in the UV and transferring its excitation energy to the mas-
ter, rhodopsin. It is thanks to this sensitizing pigment (which is
reminiscent of the light-harvesting pigments in photosynthesis) that
the spectral sensitivity of the cell is extended beyond the constraints set by the intrinsic absorption properties of the blue-absorbing rhodopsin.

From a functional standpoint the existence of a sensitizing
pigment in cells R 1-6 goes along the same line as the neural pooling
of several receptor signals within each cartridge of the lamina.
Both features unite to confer upon the visual system driven by these
cells a high quantum catch. Hence if a comparison were allowed with
the vertebrate retina, R 1-6 cells could be compared to rods (as did
Hanström in 1928) and not to cones (as did Sanchez in 1923).

Vertebrate visual systems too have managed to increase their
quantum catch via neural pooling. However in a camera eye, this

---

The simultaneous observation of both DPP's illustrates the
binocular overlap which is particularly large in the male.
Center-to-center distance between the two DPP's is 800 μm,
giving the scale of both figures (a) and (b). From Franceschini, (1975).
(c) Third optic ganglion (lobula plate) of each eye showing
the unique Male Lobula Giant Neuron No 1 (MLG1) whose dendritic arborization (black profile) is superimposed upon
the numerous Col A neurons. Cobalt staining. The two MLG1
neurons are encountered only in the male and their receptive
field comprises the R7r region seen in Fig. 7 and 9a. Not
to scale with (a) and (b). After Hausen and Strausfeld,
1980.

latter process is done only at the expense of acuity. The principle
of neutral superposition makes the fly retina unique in the sense that
the second order neurons of a cartridge pool signals from carefully
selected receptor cells which not only have the same spectral sensitivity but also aligned visual axes.

Variety of colour receptors among R7 and R8

The two central cells R7 and R8 (Fig. 1) constitute an obvious
deviation to the crystallinity of the compound eye. Pale (p) and
yellow (y) R7 cells can be discriminated in vivo by their different
absorption (Kirschfeld et al., 1978) or fluorescence (Franceschini
et al., 1981 b) properties. It is still questionable whether they
correspond to the two ultrastructurally distinguished types described
by Smola and Meffert (1979).

The axonal projections of the central cells R7 and R8 down to
the medulla has long suggested that these cells build a parallel
visual pathway serving a function different from that of R 1-6 cells.
The richness of their spectral types obviously suggests that they
could play a role in colour vision like the cones of the vertebrate
retina. However, the largest population of R7 cells (7 yellow) could
be involved in polarized vision too. They are equipped with a blue-
absorbing screening pigment similar to the yellow oil droplet found
in many vertebrate cones. But the molecular orientation of this
pigment in the microvillar membrane confers upon this photoreceptor
cell a remarkably high polarization sensitivity (PS~5) in the blue
range of the spectrum (Hardie et al., 1979).

The precise connectivity pattern of pale and yellow R7's and
R8's onto the ganglion cells of the medulla remains to be carefully
studied. It is noteworthy that in the primate retina some ganglion
cells are contacted by the photoreceptors themselves so that here
too a direct visual pathway exists, in parallel with the well-known
bipolar pathway (Mariani, 1982).

Ethoneurological Aspect

Obsessed as it is in the task of detecting a flying black spot,
the male housefly seems to own a retinal domain specially devoted
to this great cause. This northern retinal domain houses in nearly
every ommatidium an eccentric member of the R7 community which is
never encountered in the female. This cell distinguishes itself
by having not only the same, broadband spectral sensitivity as R 1-6
receptor cells but also the same target neuropile.

It looks as though the frontal-dorsal part of the male eye had nearly sacrificed colour vision for another, more vital kind of information processing.

Photons are at a premium not only in dim light vision but also in any rapid visual task involving detection of small contrast (Kirschfeld and Wenk, 1976; Snyder, 1977). In this context the participation of a seventh, spatially and spectrally matched input to the averaging process which takes place in a lamina cartridge would be a further improvement in the striving for quanta and hence contrast detectivity, a further weapon in the struggle for life. The argument that the improvement in signal-to-noise ratio (by factor $\sqrt{7/6}$) achieved ed in this way would be too small to be worth the trouble of a special neural circuit is probably fallacious in view of the challenge, which is to see or not to see. After all, it seems that many visual systems throughout the animal kingdom would have --by human standards-- paid a high price in terms of optical and neuronal gadgetry to finally gain a trifle of improvement, for example in quantum catch.

It is refreshing to see that sexual dimorphism can hide itself even in the retina, and even down to the level of single photoreceptor cells. This may open a promising line of study in the vertebrate retina, even if the test turns out to be positive in the human eye.

The sex-specificity encountered in the spectral organization of the fly retina illustrates how structure, mechanism and biological function of a neural circuit appear harmoniously linked when studied at the level of single cells in the context of animal behaviour. This points to the interesting possibility that studing the behavioural acts of an animal could be of considerable value for figuring out the beneficial consequences and operation of peripheral neural circuits. Thus "Ethoneurology" could be to the physiologist what Neuroethology is to the ethologist. This very "ethoneurological" approach –which is not commonly used in the laboratory studies of the vertebrate retina- could possibly shed a new light upon some enigmatic features like the electrical coupling between photoreceptor cells in the turtle and toad retina. Though the idea in mind is quite different from that of the male housefly, the turtle in ambush lies in wait for a similar flying black spot. Possibly, the strange properties of the network of electrical connections (Detwiler et al., 1978) assist in the detection of this prey and contribute to drive the ultimate tongue snap which will be little respectful of the fly's own retinal beauty.

Acknowledgement

I thank M. Wilcox for critically reading the manuscript.
Special thanks are due to C. Wehrhahn and K. Hausen for the permis-
sion to reproduce Fig. 8 and Fig. 9c, respectively. The technical
assistance of Mrs. A. Totin-Yvard and M. André and of Mr. J. Creuzet
and G. Jacquet is gratefully acknowledged.

REFERENCES

Basinger, S.F., Gordon, W.C. and Lam, D.M.K. (1979). Differential
    labelling of retinal neurones by ^{3}H-2-deoxyglucose, Nature,
    280, 682 - 684.
Baylor, D.A. and Hodgkin, A.L. (1973). Detection and resolution of
    visual stimuli by turtle photoreceptors, J. Physiol., 234,
    163 - 198.
Beersma, D.G.M., Stavenga, D. and Kuiper, J.W. (1975). Organization
    of visual axes in the compound eye of the fly Musca Domestica
    L. and behavioural consequence, J. comp. Physiol., 102, 305-329.
Boschek, B. (1971). On the fine structure of the peripheral retina
    and lamina ganglionaris of the fly Musca Domestica. Z. Zell-
    forsch. Abt. Histochem., 118, 369 - 409.
Bowmaker, J.K. (1979). Visual pigments and oil droplets in the pi-
    geon retina, as measured by microspctrophotometry, and their
    relationship to spectral sensitivity, in "Neural mechanisms
    of behavior in the pigeon", A.M. Granda and J.H. Maxwell, eds.,
    pp. 287 - 305, Plenum Publishing Corporation, New York.
Bowmaker, J.K. and Knowles, A. (1977). The visual pigments and oil
    droplets of the chicken retina, Vision Res., 17, 755 - 764.
Braitenberg, V. (1967). Patterns of projection in the visual system
    of the fly. I. Retina-lamina projections, Exp. Brain Res.,
    3, 271 - 298.
Braitenberg, V. and Strausfeld, N. (1973). Principle of the mosaic
    organization in the visual system's neuropile of Musca Dome-
    stica, in "Handbook of sensory physiology", Vol. VII/3: Central
    visual information, R. Jung ed., pp. 631 - 659, Springer,
    Berlin-Heidelberg.
Brown, K.T. (1969). A linear area centralis extending across the
    turtle retina and stabilized to the horizon by non-visual
    cues, Vision Res., 9, 1053 - 1062.
Burkhardt, D. (1962). Spectral sensitivity and other response char-
    acteristics of single visual cells in the arthropod eye, Symp.
    Soc. Expl. Biol., 16, 86 - 109.

Butler, R. (1971). The identification and mapping of spectral cell types in the retina of Periplaneta americana, Z. vergl. Physiol., 72, 67 - 80.

Cajal, S.R. and Sanchez, D. (1915). Contribucion al conocimiento de los centros nerviosos de los insectos. Parte I. Retina y centros opticos, Trab. Lab. Invest. Biol. Univ. Madrid, 13, 1 - 64.

Campos-Ortega, J.A. and Strausfeld N.J. (1972). The columnar organization of the second synaptic region of the visual system of Musca Domestica. I/ Receptor terminals in the medulla, Z. für Zellforsch, 124, 561 - 585.

Collet, T.S. and Land, M.F. (1975). Visual control of flight behaviour in the hover-fly Syritta pipiens L., J. comp. Physiol., 99, 1 - 66.

Denton, E.J. and Wyllie, J.H. (1955). Study of the photosensitive pigments in the pink and green rods of the frog, J. Physiol., 127, 81 - 89.

Detwiler, P.B., Hodgkin, A.L. and Mc Naughton, P.A. (1978). A surprising property of electrical spread in the network of rods in the turtle retina, Nature, 274, 562 - 565.

Eckert, H. (1971) Spektrale Empfindlichkeit des Komplexauges von Musca, Kubernetik, 9, 145 - 156.

Eckert, H., Bishop, L.G. and Dvorak, D.R. (1970). Spectral sensitivities of identified receptor cells in the blowfly Calliphora, Naturwiss., 63, 47 - 48.

Fernald, R.D. (1981). Chromatic organization of a cichild fish retina, Vision Res., 21, 1749 - 1753.

Foerster, T. (1951). "Fluoreszenz organischen Verbindungen", Vandenhoeck and Ruprecht, Göttingen.

Franceschini, N. (1975). Sampling of the visual environment by the compound eye of the fly: Fundamentals and applications, in "Photoreceptors optics", A.W. Snyder and R. Menzel, eds. Springer, Berlin, Heidelberg.

Franceschini, N. (1977). In vivo fluorescence of rhabdomeres in an insect eye, Proc. Int. Union Physiol. Sc. XIII. XXVIIth Int. Congr. Paris, 237.

Franceschini, N. (1979). Voltage clamp by light, Invest. Ophthalm., Suppl. May. p. 5.

Franceschini, N. (1982). In vivo microcpectrofluorometry of visual pigments, in: "Biology of photoreceptors", D. Cosens ed., Cambridge University press, Cambridge (in press).

Franceschini, N. and Hardie, R. (1980). In vivo recovery of intracellularly stained cells, J. Physiol. (Lond.), 301, 59p.

Franceschini, N. and Kirschfeld, K. (1971a). Etude optique in vivo
    des éléments photorécepteurs dans l'oeil composé de Drosophila,
    Kybernetik, 8, 1 - 13.

Franceschini, N. and Kirschfeld, K. (1971 b). Les phénomènes de
    pseudopupille dans l'oeil composé de Drosophila Kybernetik,
    9, 159 - 182.

Franceschini, N. Kirschfeld, K. and Minke, B. (1981 b). Fluorescence
    of photoreceptor cells observed in vivo, Science, 213, 1264 -
    1267.

Franceschini, N. Münster, A. and Heurkens, G. (1979). Equatorial and,
    binocular vision in the fly Calliphora Erythrocephala, Verh.
    Dtsch. Zool. Ges. Gustav Fischer, Stuttgart, p. 209.

Franceschini, N. Hardie, R., Ribi, W. and Kirschfeld, K. (1981).
    Sexual dimorphism in a photoreceptor, Nature, 291, 241 - 244.

Fugate, R. D. and Song, P.S. (1980). Spectroscopic characterization
    of -lactoglobulin-retinol complex, Biochem. Biophys. Acta, 625,
    28 - 42.

Gemperlein, R. Paul, R. Lindauer E. and Steiner A. (1980). UV-fine
    structure of the spectral sensitivity of flies visual cells
    revealed by FIS (Fourier Interferometric stimulation), Natur-
    wiss., 67, 565 - 566.

Granda, A. M. and Haden, K. W. (1970). Retinal oil globiles counts
    and distributions in two species of turtles: Pseudemys Scripta
    Elegans (Wied) and Chelonia Mydas Mydas (Linnaeus), Vis. Res.
    10, 79 - 84.

Gribakin, F. G. (1969). Cellular basis of colour vision in the Honey
    Bee, Nature 223, 639 - 641.

Hamdorf, K. (1979). The physiology of invertebrate visual pigments,
    in: "Handbook of sensory physiology", Vol. VII/6A. H. Autrum
    ed., pp 145 - 224, Springer, Berlin-Heidelberg.

Hamdorf, K., Paulsen, R. and Schwemer, J. (1973). Photoregeneration
    and sensitivity control of photoreceptors of invertebrates, in:
    "Biochemistry and physiology of visual pigments". H. Langer
    ed., p. 155, Springer, Berlin-Heidelberg.

Hanström, B. (1928). "Vergleichende Anatomie des Nervensystems der
    Wirbellosen Tieren", Springer, Berlin-Heidelberg.

Hardie, R. C. (1977). Electrophysiological properties of R7 and R8
    in Dipteran retina, Z. Naturforsch., 32C, 887 - 889.

Hardie, R. C. (1979). Electrophysiological analysis of fly retina.
    I. Comparative properties of R1-6 and R7 and R8, J. comp.
    Physiol., 129, 19 - 33.

Hardie, R. C., Franceschini, N. and Mac Intyre, P. (1979). Electro-
    physiological analysis of fly retina. II. Spectral and polar-
    ization sensitivity in R7 and R8, J. comp. Physiol. 133, 23-39.

Hardie, R.C., Franceschini, N., Ribi, W. and Kirschfeld, K. (1981).
    Distribution and properties of sex-specific photoreceptors in
    the fly Musca Domestica, J. comp. Physiol., 145, 139 - 152.

Hausen, K. and Strausfeld, N. (1980). Sexually dimorphic interneuron
    arrangements in the fly visual system, Proc. R. Soc. Lond.
    (Biol.), 208, 57 - 71.

Heisenberg, M. and Buchner, E. (1977). The rôle of retinula cell
    types in visual behavior of Drosophila melanogaster, J. comp.
    Physiol., 117, 127 - 162.

Hemley, R., Kohler, B.E. and Siviski, P. (1979). Absorption spectra
    for the complexes formed from vitamin-A and β-lactoglobulin,
    Biophys. J., 28, 447-455.

Horridge, G.A. and Meinertzhagen, I.A. (1970). The accuracy of the
    patterns of connections of the first- and second-order neurons
    of the visual system of Calliphora, Proc. Roy. Soc. Lond. B,
    175, 69 - 82.

Järvilehto, M. (1971). "Lokalisierte Intrazelluläre Ableitungen aus
    den Axonen der 8-ten Sehzelle der Fliege Calliphora Erythroce-
    phala", Dissertation, Universität München.

Kirschfeld, K. (1967). Die Beziehung zwischen dem Raster der Omma-
    tidien und dem Raster der Rhabdomere im Komplexauge von Musca,
    Exp. Brain Res., 3, 248 - 270.

Kirschfeld, K. (1972). The visual system of Musca: studies on optics,
    structur and function. in: "Information processing in the
    visual systems of Arthropods" R. Wehner ed., pp 61 - 74,
    Springer, Berlin, Heidelberg.

Kirschfeld, K. (1979). The function of photostable pigments in fly
    photoreceptors, Biophs. Struct. Mechanism, 5, 117 - 128.

Kirschfeld, K. and Franceschini, N. (1968). Optische Eigenschaften
    der Ommatidien im Komplexauge von Musca, Kybernetik, 5, 47-52.

Kirschfeld, K. and Franceschini, N. (1975). Microspectrophotometry
    of fly rhabdomeres, Conf. on visual Physiology, Günzburg
    (Germany).

Kirschfeld, K and Franceschini, N. (1977). Photostable pigments
    within the membrane of photoreceptors and their possible role,
    Biophys. Struc. Mechanism, 3, 191 - 194.

Kirschfeld, K. and Wenk, P. (1976). The dorsal compound eye of
    Simuliid flies: An eye specialized for the detection of small,
    rapidly moving objects, Z. Naturforsch., 31c, 764 - 765.

Kirschfeld, K. Feiler, R. and Franceschini, N. (1978). A photostable
    pigment within the rhabdomere of fly photoreceptor N° 7, J.
    comp. Physiol., 125, 275 - 284.

Kirschfeld, K. Franceschini, N. and Minke, B. (1977). Evidence for
    a sensitizing pigment in fly photoreceptors, Nature, 269, 386 -
    390.

Kirschfeld, K., Feiler, R., Hardie, R., Vogt, K., and Franceschini,
    N. (1982). The sensitizing pigment of fly photoreceptors:
    properties and candidates, Biophys. Struct. Mechanism, (in
    press).

Kolb, M. and Jones, J. (1982). Light and electron microscopy of the
    photoreceptors in the retina of the red-eared slider, Pseudemys
    Scripta Elegans, J. comp. Neurol., 209, 331 - 338.

Land, M. F., Collett, T. S. (1974). Chasing behaviour of house flies
    (Fannia canicularis): a description and analysis, J. comp.
    Physiol., 89, 331 - 357.

Langer, H. and Thorell, B. (1966). Microspectrophotometry of single
    rhabdomeres in the insect eye, Exp. cell Res., 41, 673 - 677.

Levine, J. S., MacNichol, E. F. Jr., Kraft, T. and Collins, B. A.
    (1979). Intraretinal distribution of cone pigments in certain
    teleost fishes, Science, 204, 523 - 526.

Liebman, P. A. and Granda, A. M. (1972). Microspectrophotometric
    measurements of visual pigments in two species of turtle
    Pseudemys scripta and chelonia Mydas, Vis. Res., 11, 105 - 114.

Liebman, P. A. and Leigh, R. A. (1969). Autofluorescence of visual
    receptors, Nature, 221, 1249 - 1251.

Marc, R. E. and Sperling, H. G. (1976). Color receptor identities
    goldfish cones, Science, 191, 487 - 489.

Mariani, A. P. (1982). Biplexiform cells: ganglion cells of the
    primate retina that contact photoreceptors, Science, 216,
    1134 - 1136.

Mariani, A. P. and Leure-Du Pree, A. E. (1978). Photoreceptors and
    oil droplet colors in the red area of the pigeon retina, J.
    comp. Neur., 182, 821 - 838.

Mc Cann, G. D. and Arnett, D. W. (1972). Spectral and polarization
    sensitivity of the dipteran visual system, J. Gen. Physiol.,
    59, 534 - 558.

McIntyre, P. and Kirschfeld, K. (1981). Absorption of a photostable
    pigment (P456) in rhabdomere 7 of the fly, J. comp. Physiol.,
    143, 3 - 15.

Meffert, P. and Smola, U. (1976). Electrophysiological measurements
    of spectral sensitivity of central visual cells in eye of
    blowfly, Nature, 260, 342 - 344.

Menzel, R. (1972). The fine structure of the compound eye of Formica
    Polyctena: Functional morphology of a hymenopteran eye, in:
    "Information processing in the visual system of Arthropods",
    R. Wehner ed. p. 37 - 49, Springer, Berlin-Heidelberg.

Meyer, D. B. and May, H. C. (1973). The topographical distribution
    of rods and cones in the adult chicken retina, Exp. eye Res.,
    17, 347 - 355.
Monasterio, F. M. de, Schein, S. J. and McCrane, E. P. (1981).
    Staining of blue-sensitive cones of the macaque retina by a
    fluorescent dye, Science, 213, 1278 - 1279.
Ohtsuka, T. (1978). Combination of oil droplets with different types
    of photoreceptor in a freshwater turtle, Geoclemys reevesii,
    Sens. Process., 2, 321 - 325.
Ong, D. E. and Chytil, F. (1978). Cellular retinol-binding protein
    from rat liver, J. Biol. Chem., 253, 828 - 832.
Riehle, A. and Franceschini N. (1983). Response of a movement sensi-
    tive neuron to microstimulation of two photoreceptor cells
    (in preparation).
Sanchez y Sanchez, D. (1923). Action spécifique des Bâtonnets réti-
    niens des insectes, Trav. Labor. Rech. Biol. Univ. Madrid, 21,
    143 - 167.
Scholes, J. (1969). The electrical responses of the retinal recep-
    tors and the lamina in the visual system of the fly Musca,
    Kybernetik, 6, 149 - 162.
Scholes, J. (1975). Colour receptors and their synaptic connexions
    in the retina of a cyprinid fish, Phil. Trans. R. Soc. Lond.
    B, 270, 61 - 118.
Schreckenbach, T., Walckhoff, B. and Oesterhelt, D. (1977). Studies
    on the retinal-protein interaction in bacterio-rhodopsin, Eur.
    J. Biochem., 76, 499 - 511.
Shaw, S. R. (1981). Anatomy and physiology of identified non-spiking
    cells in the photoreceptor-lamina complex of the compound eye
    of insects, especially Diptera, in: "Neurones without impul-
    ses", A. Roberts and B. M. Bush eds., Cambridge Univ. Press,
    Cambridge, New-York.
Smola, U. and Meffert, P. (1975). A single-peak UV-receptor in the
    eye of Calliphora erythrocephala, J. comp. Physiol., 103, 353 -
    357.
Smola, U. and Meffert, P. (1979). The spectral sensitivity of the
    visual cells R7 and R8 in the eye of the blowfly Calliphora
    erythrocephala, J. comp. Physiol., 133, 41 - 52.
Snyder, A. (1977). Acuity compound eyes: physical limitations and
    design, J. comp. Physiol., 116, 161 - 182.
Song, P. S. and Moore, T. A. (1974). On the photoreceptor pigment
    for phototropism and phototaxis: is a carotenoid the most
    likely candidate ?, Photochem. Photobiol., 19, 435 - 441.

Sperling, H. G., Johnson, C. and Harwerth, R. S. (1980). Differential spectral photic damage to primate cones, Vision Res., 20, 1117 - 1125.

Stark, W. S. Ivanyshyn, A. M. and Greenberg, R. M. (1977). Sensitivity and photopigments of R1-6, a two-peaked photoreceptor, in Drosophila, Calliphora and Musca, J. comp. Physiol., 121, 289 - 305.

Stark, W. S., Stavenga, D. G. and Kruizinga, B. (1979). Fly photoreceptor fluorescence is related to UV sensitivity, Nature, 280, 581 - 583.

Stavenga, D., Franceschini, N. and Kirschfeld, K. (1982). Fluorescence of visual pigments studied in the eye of intact flies, (in preparation).

Stavenga, D. G., Zantema, A. and Kuiper, J. (1973). Rhodopsin processes and the function of the pupil mechanism in flies, in: "Biochemistry and physiology of visual pigments", H. Langer ed., pp. 175 - 180, Springer, Berlin-Heidelberg.

Stewart, W. W. (1978). Functional connections between cells as revealed by dye-coupling with a highly fluorescent naphthalimide tracer, Cell 14, 741 - 759.

Tric, C. and Lejeune, V. (1970). Les carotènes fluorescent-ils?, Photochem. Photobiol., 12, 339 - 343.

Trujillo-Cenoz, O. and Melamed, J. (1966). Electron microscope observations on the peripheral and intermediate retinas of Dipterans. in: "The functional organization of the compound eye. Part. IV: Integration of visual input", G. G. Bernhard ed., pp. 338 - 361, Pergamon Press, London.

Vigier, P. (1909). Mécanisme de la synthèse des impressions lumineuses recueillies par les yeux composés des Diptères, C. R. Acad. Sci. Paris, 148, 1221 - 1223.

Wallcave, L. and Zechmeister, L. (1953). Coversion of dehydrocarotene, via boron trifluoride complex, into an isomer of cryptoxanthin, J. Amer. Chem. Soc., 75, 4495 - 4498.

Wehrhahn, C. (1979). Sex-specific differences in the chasing behaviour of free flying houseflies (Musca), Biol. Cybern., 32, 239 - 241.

Zeil, J. (1979). A new kind of neural superposition eye: the compound eye of male Bibionidae, Nature, 278, 249 - 250.

VISUAL CONTROL OF FLIGHT IN THE FLY

Werner Reichardt

Max-Plank-Institut für biologische Kybernetik

Spemannstrasse 36, 7400 Tubigen, FRG

The nervous system of the fly is estimated to consist of about 10^6 neurons. It is a complex system that can be studied at several different levels. The first level may be characterized as that at which the nature of the overall computation is expressed in the behavior of the organism. At the second level are the algoritms that implement a computation, whereas the third level deals with the realization of the algorithms at the cellular level.

It is clear that the nature of the overall computation is determined and confined by the problem the organism solves, whereas the particular algorithms involved depend on the problem and the available neural mechanisms.

The part of the nervous system underlying visually guided movements is especially attractive for a quantitative analysis at the three levels mentioned above, because it represents a complete information-processing system, from visual input to motor output. The analysis of visually guided movements in insects offers a good example of the understanding one can achieve at the different levels of behavioral organization.

Level I. Overall Computations

Flies fixate small, contrasted patterns and track moving ob- jects. The theoretical analysis of this control system relied almost completely on experiments performed in the laboratory with a flight-simulator, shown in Fig. 1. The setup allows one to sim-

351

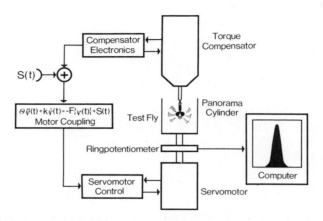

FIg. 1. Simplified scheme of the basic closed-loop flight simulator
        setup. A fly, suspended from the torque compensator,
        controls the velocity of a cylindrical panorama by its own
        torque signal. The transfer properties of the compensator,
        the motor coupling block and the servomotor approximate
        free flight dynamics. The instantaneous position of the
        panorama is signalled by a ring potentiometer for further
        data processing.

ulate free-flight conditions in one degree of freedom, namely,
rotation around the vertical axis. Results obtained with this device, in which the fly is fixed with the head glued to the thorax
can be extended to free-flight conditions, under the assumptions
that nonvisual input play a negligible role, that body control does
not depend on the head-movement system, and that there are no other
effective degrees of freedom, because these are mechanically blocked
(Reichardt, 1973).

     The flight dynamic is well approximated by the following equa-
tion

$$\Theta \, \ddot{\alpha}_f(t) + K \, \dot{\alpha}_f(t) = F(t) \tag{1}$$

where Θ and K are the moment of inertia and an aerodynamic friction
constant of the fly, respectively, and $F(t)$ is the instantaneous
torque produced by the fly's wings. The angular velocity of the fly
α_f is essentially instantaneously proportional to the torque since
$\Theta/K = 8 \cdot 10^{-3}$ sec. α_f designates the instantaneous direction of
flight with respect to an arbitrary zero direction in the horizontal

plane. If we designate with α_p the istantaneous angular position
of an object, then $\psi = \alpha_f - \alpha_p$ is referred to as the error angle (in
the horizontal plane). ψ represents the angular position of the
object with respect to the coordinate system of the fly. If the
head is fixed relative to the thorax, $\psi(t)$ is the location of the
image of the object on the retina of the fly at instant t. Trans-
lation effects are neglected, that is to say the object is far away
from the fly. Equation (1) can now be rewritten as

$$\Theta \ddot{\psi}(t) + K \dot{\psi}(t) = - F(t) + S(t) \text{ with } S(t) = \Theta \ddot{\alpha}_\phi(t) + K \dot{\alpha}_\phi(t) \qquad (2)$$

$S(t)$ reflects the trajectory of the object p. Thus the fly controls
its angular velocity through its torque F. The central problem
here is to determine how F depends on the visual input, that is,
which control system is used by the fly (Reichardt and Poggio, 1976).

A series of experiments has led to the following conclusions:
A. The underlying torque process is stationary under normal experimental conditions, implying that there is no switching between
different control systems. B. $F(t)$ can be approximated as a sum
of two terms: a strictly visually evoked response $R_t \{\psi(s)\}$, that
is, a function of the error angle history, and a component that can
be characterized stochastically as a Gaussian process. Thus

$$F(t) = R_t \{\psi(s)\} + N(t) \qquad (3)$$

C. The visually-induced response depends in a smooth way on the
error angle history $\psi(s)$. Under this condition R_t can be approximated by a function of $\psi(t)$ and its derivatives. The first order approximation is

$$R_t \{\psi(s)\} = D(\psi) + r(\psi) \dot{\psi}. \qquad (4)$$

It has been verified experimentally that Equation (4) is a satisfactory approximation under a wide range of conditions. The terms
$D(\psi)$ and $r(\psi)$ are shown in Fig. 2. The reaction shows a very small
delay of $\epsilon = 20$ msec. Thus Equation (2) becomes

$$\Theta \ddot{\psi}(t) + K \dot{\psi}(t) = - D[\psi(t-\epsilon)] - r(\psi)\dot{\psi}(t-\epsilon) + N(t) + S(t) \qquad (5)$$

where $r(\psi) \dot{\psi}$ is the result of a velocity computation: $D(\psi)$ carries
the position information and represents an actractiveness profile
associated with the specific pattern. All these terms have been

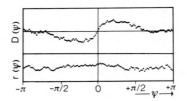

Fig. 2.   The terms $D(\psi)$ and $r(\psi)$ characterizing the position and
         the velocity computation elicited by a narrow vertical
         black stripe segment in <u>Musca</u> females.

characterized quantitatively through independent experiments.
Equation (5) is a stochastic nonlinear equation. Its solution has
several interesting aspects. Through Equation (5) the theory can
predict nontrivial behavior in quantitative detail. An example of
the predictive power of Equation (5) is shown in Fig. 3. The theory
predicts, in a stochastic sense, the angular trajectory of a fly
fixating or tracking patterns. The experimental data agree with
the theoretical predictions.

      Perhaps the most significant aspect of the phenomenological
theory presented here is the fact that (closed-loop) orientation
behavior can be quantitatively predicted from knowledge of the
open-loop response (the terms $D(\psi)$ and $r(\psi)$ of the fly which means
that the Reafferenz-Prinzip (Mittelstaedt, 1971) seems not to be
necessarily required at the level of the behavior described here.
One may argue that the fly may therefore not to be able to distinguish between self movement and object movement. That this is not
so will be discussed later in connection with the phenomenon of
figure-ground discrimination.

      Many more experimental data can be accounted for by the validity
of Equation (5). For instance, the gaze of the fly toward rather
complex patterns in quantitatively predictable in connection with
a superposition rule. The justification for this rule and its range
of validity depend on the algorithms for computing $D(\psi)$ and $r(\psi)$.
The most dramatic validation of the theory, however, comes from
free-flight experiments.

      Land and Collett (1974) have filmed chases of male flies
(<u>Fannia cancularis</u>) pursuing other flies. These data led to the
conclusion that the control system used by the chasing fly is a
continuously operating device that can be described essentially by

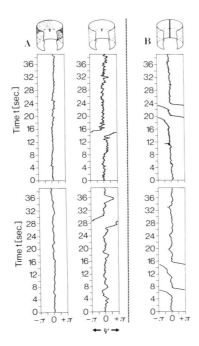

Fig. 3.A. Dynamics of fixation of two different patterns by Musca
females as measured (upper part) and as predicted (lower
part) by Equation (5) with standard values for the parameters. B. The trajectory Ψ (t) for tracking of a black
stripe rotating at constant angular velocity as measured
(upper part) and predicted (lower part) in a stochastic
sense by the same equation.

Equation (5) by neglecting N(t) and setting $D(\psi) = \beta \, \psi$. They have
also been able to show that Equation (5) can correctly simulate the
trajectory of the chasing fly, given that of the leading fly. A
later analysis of the flight behavior in the hoverfly (Collett and
Land, 1975 a, 1975 b) uncovered different control systems used by
the fly in various circumstances. One of them is again a smooth
system, phenomenologically identical to the control system in Fannia
and Musca, that relies on angular position and movement information
to control flight torque continuously. Thus the control system
described by the Reichardt-Poggio theory is equivalent to the control system used in free flight by male Fannia and, often by Syritta.
This does not mean that the male tracking system is identical to
the female smooth tracking and fixation system at the level of the
neural circuitry. The problem of functional equivalence is logical-

ly separate from the problem of identity at the circuitry level.

The difference between chasing in males and females does not necessarily imply a unique male-specific neural circuit specifically designed for chasing in males. Collett and Land's conjecture that there should be male-specific visual interneurons in the optic lobe has now been supported by Hausen and Strausfeld (see Hausen, 1977). Wehrhahn's (1979) recent demonstration that during chasing male flies keep the target in the superior frontal part of the visual field, while female flies chase with the inferior frontal part of the eye, is consistent with the anatomical evidence of Hausen and for females with measurements of $D(\psi)$ and the correspondent term $L(\theta)$ for the lift component by Wehrhahn and Reichardt (1975). The fact that males and females use different parts of the eye strongly suggests that the neural circuitry of the male chasing system is distinct from the neural circuitry underlying normal fixation and chasing in females and males.

The phenomenological theory (Reichardt and Poggio, 1976) outlined before is restricted to one degree of dynamic freedom, namely, rotation around the vertical axis. It has been shown that the vertical degree of freedom, involving the fly's lift, can be described by an equation similar to Equation (5) (Wehrhahn and Reichardt, 1975). The results allow a quantitative decription of fixation and tracking behavior in two degrees of freedom. In addition, taking into account the observation that in chasing the velocity of the chasing fly is about proportional to the distance between the leading and the chasing fly, one can make computer reconstructions of flight trajectories, given the trajectories of the leading flies. An example of this is shown in Fig. 4.

The analysis sketched here of a part of the fly's orientation behavior is independent of lower levels of understanding. Physiological information is not needed to arrive at an understanding of the principles of basic information processing. This analysis, however, is quite important for, and in a sense preliminary to, a study at the algorithmic and cellular or circuitry level.

Level II. The Algorithms

The phenomenological theory outlined so far deals with the basic logical organization of the visual control system of the fly. It requires the neural network between the receptors and the flight muscles to perform two main computations on the visual input. One

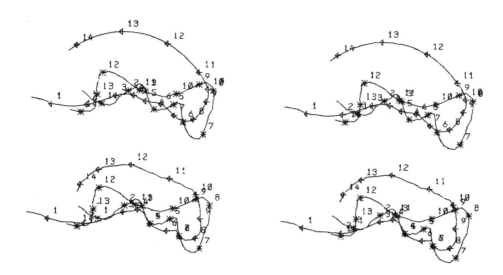

Fig. 4. A 1440 msec chase of flies (<u>Musca domestica</u>) flying freely. The bottom stereo plot shows the 3-dimensional trajectories of the two flies (* leading fly, Δ chasing fly). The top stereo pair shows a computer simulation of the flight of the chasing fly, according to the theory sketched here (film by H. Wagner).

computation extracts movement information (the term $r(\psi)\dot{\psi}$), the other provides position information (the term $D(\psi)$). The question at level II is how these computations are performed in the neural network of the visual system of the fly (Poggio and Reichardt, 1976).

It is obvious that for the computation of directional movement, signals from at least two photoreceptors must be compared. More- over, since it is required that the time-averaged response is direc-

tion selective, the interaction between the two inputs must be nonlinear, because the time-averaged response of a linear system is a
linear combination of the input's averages. The simplest operation
that can perform movement detection is thus a multiplication-like
interaction between the two inputs from two photoreceptors or two
groups of photoreceptors. The interaction must be asymmetric, in
the sense that the two channels are not equivalent, since otherwise
the output would not be different for different directions of motion.
The simplest model of this type is in fact a pure multiplication
of the two signals, as shown in Fig. 5a, after delaying or low-pass
filtering one of the two. In the meantime it is now well established that the computation of directional movement is carried out in
the visual systems of the fly and other insects through such an
algorithm, proposed first by Hassenstein and Reichardt (1956). If
the output of a movement detector is completely antisymmetric, the
overall corresponding interaction is also antisymmetric. It is
always possible to synthetize an antisymmetric interaction from an
asymmetric one, as shown in Fig. 5b, which represents a version of
the original model proposed by Reichardt and Hassenstein (see also
Götz, 1972).

The task of the position computation is the detection and the
localization of a small contrasted object. The output of the
computation is required to drive an eye-centering servomechanism.
Thus the sign of the output must depend on whether the image of the
target is in the right or left eye. An array of modules distributed
in the eye, each receiving input from an individual photoreceptor,
can perform this computation. Each module has a weight or an
amplification factor parametrized by its position in the eye (see
Fig. 2). The modules could operate in a linear fashion. In order,
however, that stabilized retinal images give a zero average output
such one-input modules must be nonlinear, for instance of degree
two (see Fig. 5c). This simple one-input algorithm seems to underly
position computation in the fly. Experimental evidence has been
provided by Pick (1974), who showed that more complex interactions
are not necessary.

More recently (Reichardt and Poggio, 1979) it has been shown
(see data plotted in Fig. 6) that a fly can not only detect motion
and position but also relative motion, as, for instance, the motion
of an object in front of a textured background. Clearly, one-input
modules can not consistently detect a small object moving in front
of a moving texture. However, 2- and 4-input, 4th-order inhibitory

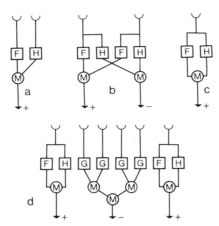

Fig. 5a. A part of the algorithm for movement detection of Hassans-
tein and Reichardt. The two inputs are multiplied after
low-pass filtering with different time constants. If an
average operation is made on the output, the overall operation is equivalent to a weighted cross-correlation of the
two inputs. b. The output of this and its complementary
scheme represents the behavioral optomotor response of the
whole insect. While the interaction between input 1 and
2 is asymmetric in a, the scheme shown in b is antisymmetric: reversal of the direction of motion simply reverses
the sign of the output. c. The algorithm for position
detection. Each of these modules has a weight or amplification factor parametrized by its position in the eye. d.
The algorithm for relative movement or figure-ground discrimination consisting of position detectors and symmetric
movement detectors. The coherence of the two movement
fields is measured by a symmetric detector.

modules together with the position detectors, can detect relative
object or figure-ground motion. The argument is easy to understand
intuitively. If relative motion is perceived, all position detectors
in the eye of the fly must be inhibited, except for those near the
discontinuities in the velocity field. Thus, besides the position
detectors, this computation needs a center-surround organization
of directionally-selective movement detectors to inhibit the position detectors where there is the same movement in the center as in
the periphery. A rigorous analysis shows that the interaction of
direction-insensitive movement detectors or even flicker detectors
can play a similar role. Considering the behavioral experiment in

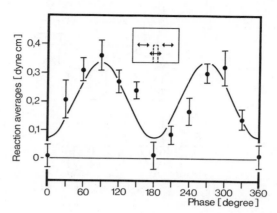

Fig. 6.   Phase dependence of the figure-ground discrimination effect.
Average torque response of ten flies to sinusoidally oscillating figure and ground patterns. The figure consists
of a black, vertically oriented stripe, 3° wide, positioned
in the lower part of the panorama, oscillated around the
mean position ψ = +30°. The ground pattern consists of a
random-dot texture which can be moved independently of the
stripe. The oscillation amplitude of stripe and ground
amounted to ±1° at 2,5 Hz frequency. The continuous line
is the component K_{FG} cos 2 $\emptyset$ derived from a Fourier analysis
of the data plotted in the figure, with $\emptyset$ the relative
phase between the figure and ground oscillations.

Fig. 6, the time-averaged response of the fly is well approximated
by

$$\overline{R} = K_G + K_F - K_{FG} \cos 2 \emptyset \qquad\qquad (6)$$

a result consistent with the algorithm drawn in Fig. 5d.

The algorithmic principle used by the fly to discriminate
figure from ground motion makes it understandable why the "Reafferenz
-Prinzip" is not needed for a discrimination between self- and non-
self motion in a natural environment.

The three algorithms discussed here provide the necessary
movement, position and relative movement information to the flight-
control system of the fly. It is important to mention that the
visual control of flight certainly relies on other algorithms as
well, like the algorithms underlying landing or distance evaluation.

Several of these new algorithms may be based on computations carried out on the movement field, as measured by the movement detectors, briefly described here.

Level III. Neuronal Circuitry

In recent years, Poggio and Torre (1978) have developed a theory of synaptic interactions in so-called local circuits consisting of neurons whose activity is entirely expressed in graded potentials but not in action potentials. In this connection they have proposed a specific synaptic interaction mechanisms which could be responsible for movement and position computation (Torre and Poggio, 1978). The mechanisms proposed rest on a physiological process known as shunting inhibition.

More recently Poggio, Reichardt and Hausen (1981) have proposed a neuronal circuitry for the operation of relative movement or figure-ground discrimination by the visual system of the fly. The circuitry may be located in the third optical ganglion; it is shown in Fig. 7. The proposed circuitry has a retinotopic array of elementary movement detectors as its input-channels. The usual assumption was made that all cells carry only positive signals: in particular, detectors for progressive movement are separate from detectors for regressive movement. Large-field cells (S_L and S_R) summate the outputs of the elementary movement detectors over a large part of the visual field and receive a similar contralateral input. They inhibit, by shunting inhibition, the single elementary detector signals, irrespective of their preferred direction. After shunting inhibition the signals are then summated by another large field cell (X_L and X_R). Before summation, each input undergoes a nonlinear transformation like a squaring operation, representing either the nonlinear presynaptic-postsynaptic characteristic at the synapse or local active properties of the postsynaptic membrane. The last cells would then directly drive the behavioral response.

Extensive computer simulations suggest that the basic features of the proposed circuitry are so far sufficient to account well for all the main properties of the figure-ground effect. Fig. 8, for instance, shows the computer response for two characteristic phase situations ($0°$ and $90°$). The comparison with the behavioral torque response is indeed satisfactory in all experimental situations, including the relevant time-averaged responses.

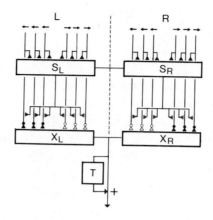

Fig. 7.   The outline of a neuronal circuitry for the right (R) and
          for the left (L) eye. A retinotopic array of elementary
          movement and position detectors serves as input channels
          to the neural circuitry. In the right eye a pool neuron
          (S_R) summates the detector output responding to progressive
          (regressive) motion, as well as the input from its
          contralateral homologue (S_L). Its output is assumed to
          undergo a saturation effect and to shunt each elementary
          detector output via presynaptic inhibition. The synapses
          involved (▷─) should therefore inhibit (opening ionic
          channels with an equilibrium potential close to the resting
          potential) the output terminal of each elementary detector
          channel. The output cell X summates the progressive
          (excitatory ▲) and the regressive (inhibitory, ☖)
          detectors. Progressive channels have a higher amplification
          than regressive ones, possibly because of the different
          ionic batteries involved. The synapses on the X cell are
          assumed to operate with a nonlinear input-output
          characteristic, leading to postsynaptic signals that are
          about the square of the inputs. The motor ourput is
          controlled by the X cell via a direct channel and a channel
          T computing the running average of the X cell's output lead-
          ing to the DC shift of responses to relative movement.

Great effort is now being made to find parts, or the entire
network, in the fly's visual system, especially in the lobular
complex. Recently Hausen has shown that the equatorial horizontal
cell in the HS-cell system of <u>Calliphora</u> responds to relative motion
of figure and ground in such a way that the shunting inhibition
process must have taken place prior to the cell tested. Other experimental tests on different cells are presently being undertaken
by M. Egelhaaf.

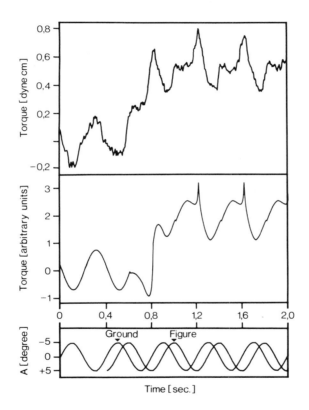

Fig. 8.a. A typical response of a fly in a figure-ground experiment.
A textured stripe of 12° angular width is sinusoidally
oscillated in front of 360° textured ground, which oscillates with the same amplitude and the same frequency
(2,5 Hz). The stripe oscillates around the mean position
ψ = 30° that is in front of the right eye. Oscillation
amplitudes amount to +5°. The time courses of the figure
and the ground oscillations (their positions) are plotted
in the lower part of the figure. At time 0,4 sec the
(continued)

Fig. 8.a. cont.

relative phase between figure and ground switches from
0° to 90°. The response of the fly increases after the
phase has shifted, and oscillates around a positive average
response level with 2,5 Hz. The increase of the response
means that the fly is attracted by the oscillating figure.
b. Computer simulation of the figure-ground experiment
reported in Fig. 8.a. The running average time is one
period of response or 360 relative time units. The figure-
ground phase amounts to $\emptyset = 0°$ and $\emptyset = 90°$. The phase
changes from 0° to 90° at 360 time units. The transition
phase is completed at 720 time units.

REFERENCES

Collett, T.S., and Land, M. (1975 a). Visual control of flight
     behaviour in the hoverfly, Syritta pipiens, J. Comp. Physiol.,
     99, 1-66.

Collett, T.S. and Land M. (1975 b). Visual spatial memory in a hover
     hoverfly, J. Comp. Physiol.,100, 59-84.

Götz, K.G.. Principles of optomotor reactions in insects, Biblthca
     ophthal., 82, (1972), 251-259.

Hassenstein, B. and Reichardt, W. (1956). Systemtheoretische Analyse
     der Zeit-Reihenforlgen- und Vorzeichenauswertung bei der
     Bewegungsperzeption des Rüsselkafers Chlorophanus, Z. Natur-
     forschg., 11b, 513-524.

Hausen, K.. Signal processing in the insect eye (1977). in:
     "Function and Formation of Neural Systems", Life Sciences
     Research Report. Vol. b. Stent, G.S., ed. Berlin: Dahlem
     Konferenzen, 81-110.

Land, M.F., and Collett, T.S.. Chasing behaviour of houseflies
     (Fannia canicularis): A description and analysis, J. Comp.
     Physiol. 89, (1974), 331-357.

Mittelstaedt, H.. Reafferenzprinzip-Analogie un Kritik. In: Vorträge
     der Erlanger Physiologentagung, Keidel, W.D., and K.H. Plattig,
     eds. Berlin: Springer-Verlag (1971).

Pick, B. (1974). Visual flicker induces orientation behaviour in
     the fly Musca, Z. Naturforschg., 29c, 310-312.

Poggio, T., and Reichardt, W. (1976). Visual control of orientation
     behaviour in the fly. Part II. Towards the underlying neural
     interactions, Quart. Rev. Biophysics,9, 3, 311-375.

Poggio, T., and Torre, V. (1978). A new approach to synaptic inter-
    action. in: Lecture Notes in Biomathematics, Vol. 21. Theo-
    retical Approaches to Complex Systems. R. Heim and G. Paim,
    eds. Berlin: Springer-Verlag, 89-115.
Reichardt, W. (1973). Musterinduzierte Flugorientierung.
    Verhaltensversuche an der Fliege Musca domestica, Naturwissen-
    schaften 60, 122-138.
Reichardt, W., and Poggio, T. (1976). Visual control of orientation
    behaviour in the fly. Part I. A quantitative analysis, Quart.
    Rev. Biophysics, 9, 3, 311-375.
Reichardt, W., and Poggio, T. (1979). Figure-ground discrimination
    by relative movement in the visual system of the fly. Part I,
    Experimental results, Biol. Cybern. 35, 81-100.
Torre, V., and Poggio, T. (1978). A synaptic mechanism possibly
    underlying directional selectivity to motion, Proc. Roy.
    Soc. B 202, 409-416.
Wehrhahn, C., and Reichardt, W. (1975). Visually induced height
    orientation of the fly Musca domestical, Biol. Cybern., 20,
    37-50.
Wehrhahn, C. t1979). Sex specific differences in the orientation
    behaviour of houseflies, Biol. Cybern., 32, 239-241.

CONTRIBUTORS